ACCESS YOUR ONLINE RESOURCES

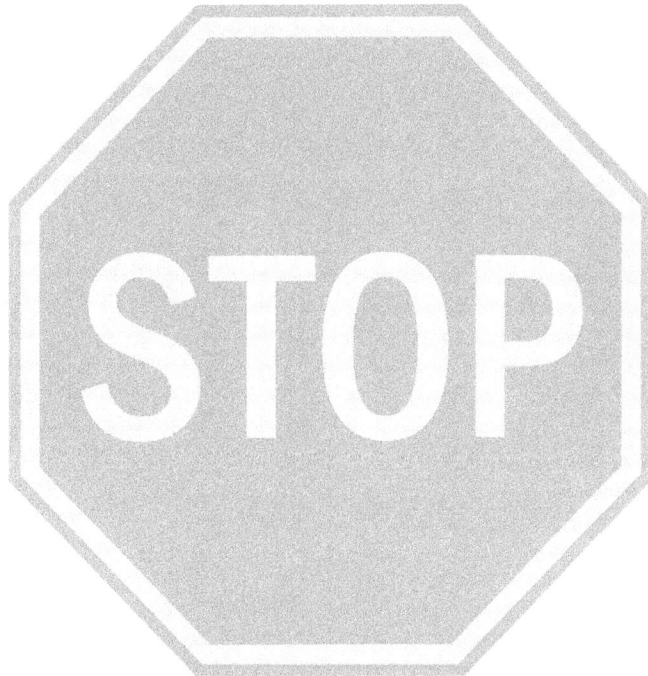

DON'T MISS OUT ON THE ONLINE RESOURCES INCLUDED WITH YOUR PURCHASE!

Your purchase of this product unlocks access to our Online Resources page. Elevate your study experience with our **interactive practice test interface**, along with all of the additional resources that we couldn't include in this book.

Flip to the Online Resources section at the end of this book to find the link and a QR code to get started!

Mometrix
TEST PREPARATION

Sonography
Exam Review
Secrets

Study Guide
Your Key to Exam Success

**Sonography Review Book for the
ARRT® Sonography Exam**

Practice Test Questions

Detailed Answer Explanations

M⊘metrix
T E S T   P R E P A R A T I O N

Written and edited by the Mometrix Sonography Registration Test Team

Mometrix offers volume discount pricing to institutions. For more information or a price quote, please contact our sales department at sales@mometrix.com or 888-248-1219.

Paperback
ISBN 13: 978-1-5167-1008-9
ISBN 10: 1-5167-1008-8

Hardback
ISBN 13: 978-1-5167-1904-4
ISBN 10: 1-5167-1904-2

DEAR FUTURE EXAM SUCCESS STORY

First of all, **THANK YOU** for purchasing Mometrix study materials!

Second, congratulations! You are one of the few determined test-takers who are committed to doing whatever it takes to excel on your exam. **You have come to the right place.** We developed these study materials with one goal in mind: to deliver you the information you need in a format that's concise and easy to use.

In addition to optimizing your guide for the content of the test, we've outlined our recommended steps for breaking down the preparation process into small, attainable goals so you can make sure you stay on track.

We've also analyzed the entire test-taking process, identifying the most common pitfalls and showing how you can overcome them and be ready for any curveball the test throws you.

Standardized testing is one of the biggest obstacles on your road to success, which only increases the importance of doing well in the high-pressure, high-stakes environment of test day. Your results on this test could have a significant impact on your future, and this guide provides the information and practical advice to help you achieve your full potential on test day.

Your success is our success

We would love to hear from you! If you would like to share the story of your exam success or if you have any questions or comments in regard to our products, please contact us at **800-673-8175** or **support@mometrix.com**.

Thanks again for your business and we wish you continued success!

Sincerely,
The Mometrix Test Preparation Team

Need more help? Check out our flashcards at:
http://mometrixflashcards.com/Sonography

TABLE OF CONTENTS

Introduction

Thank you for purchasing this resource! You have made the choice to prepare yourself for a test that could have a huge impact on your future, and this guide is designed to help you be fully ready for test day. Obviously, it's important to have a solid understanding of the test material, but you also need to be prepared for the unique environment and stressors of the test, so that you can perform to the best of your abilities.

For this purpose, the first section that appears in this guide is the **Secret Keys**. We've devoted countless hours to meticulously researching what works and what doesn't, and we've boiled down our findings to the five most impactful steps you can take to improve your performance on the test. We start at the beginning with study planning and move through the preparation process, all the way to the testing strategies that will help you get the most out of what you know when you're finally sitting in front of the test.

We recommend that you start preparing for your test as far in advance as possible. However, if you've bought this guide as a last-minute study resource and only have a few days before your test, we recommend that you skip over the first two Secret Keys since they address a long-term study plan.

If you struggle with **test anxiety**, we strongly encourage you to check out our recommendations for how you can overcome it. Test anxiety is a formidable foe, but it can be beaten, and we want to make sure you have the tools you need to defeat it.

1

Secret Key #1 – Plan Big, Study Small

There's a lot riding on your performance. If you want to ace this test, you're going to need to keep your skills sharp and the material fresh in your mind. You need a plan that lets you review everything you need to know while still fitting in your schedule. We'll break this strategy down into three categories.

Information Organization

Start with the information you already have: the official test outline. From this, you can make a complete list of all the concepts you need to cover before the test. Organize these concepts into groups that can be studied together, and create a list of any related vocabulary you need to learn so you can brush up on any difficult terms. You'll want to keep this vocabulary list handy once you actually start studying since you may need to add to it along the way.

Time Management

Once you have your set of study concepts, decide how to spread them out over the time you have left before the test. Break your study plan into small, clear goals so you have a manageable task for each day and know exactly what you're doing. Then just focus on one small step at a time. When you manage your time this way, you don't need to spend hours at a time studying. Studying a small block of content for a short period each day helps you retain information better and avoid stressing over how much you have left to do. You can relax knowing that you have a plan to cover everything in time. In order for this strategy to be effective though, you have to start studying early and stick to your schedule. Avoid the exhaustion and futility that comes from last-minute cramming!

Study Environment

The environment you study in has a big impact on your learning. Studying in a coffee shop, while probably more enjoyable, is not likely to be as fruitful as studying in a quiet room. It's important to keep distractions to a minimum. You're only planning to study for a short block of time, so make the most of it. Don't pause to check your phone or get up to find a snack. It's also important to **avoid multitasking**. Research has consistently shown that multitasking will make your studying dramatically less effective. Your study area should also be comfortable and well-lit so you don't have the distraction of straining your eyes or sitting on an uncomfortable chair.

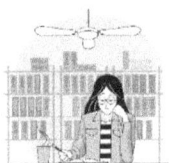

The time of day you study is also important. You want to be rested and alert. Don't wait until just before bedtime. Study when you'll be most likely to comprehend and remember. Even better, if you know what time of day your test will be, set that time aside for study. That way your brain will be used to working on that subject at that specific time and you'll have a better chance of recalling information.

Finally, it can be helpful to team up with others who are studying for the same test. Your actual studying should be done in as isolated an environment as possible, but the work of organizing the information and setting up the study plan can be divided up. In between study sessions, you can discuss with your teammates the concepts that you're all studying and quiz each other on the details. Just be sure that your teammates are as serious about the test as you are. If you find that your study time is being replaced with social time, you might need to find a new team.

Secret Key #2 – Make Your Studying Count

You're devoting a lot of time and effort to preparing for this test, so you want to be absolutely certain it will pay off. This means doing more than just reading the content and hoping you can remember it on test day. It's important to make every minute of study count. There are two main areas you can focus on to make your studying count.

Retention

It doesn't matter how much time you study if you can't remember the material. You need to make sure you are retaining the concepts. To check your retention of the information you're learning, try recalling it at later times with minimal prompting. Try carrying around flashcards and glance at one or two from time to time or ask a friend who's also studying for the test to quiz you.

To enhance your retention, look for ways to put the information into practice so that you can apply it rather than simply recalling it. If you're using the information in practical ways, it will be much easier to remember. Similarly, it helps to solidify a concept in your mind if you're not only reading it to yourself but also explaining it to someone else. Ask a friend to let you teach them about a concept you're a little shaky on (or speak aloud to an imaginary audience if necessary). As you try to summarize, define, give examples, and answer your friend's questions, you'll understand the concepts better and they will stay with you longer. Finally, step back for a big picture view and ask yourself how each piece of information fits with the whole subject. When you link the different concepts together and see them working together as a whole, it's easier to remember the individual components.

Finally, practice showing your work on any multi-step problems, even if you're just studying. Writing out each step you take to solve a problem will help solidify the process in your mind, and you'll be more likely to remember it during the test.

Modality

Modality simply refers to the means or method by which you study. Choosing a study modality that fits your own individual learning style is crucial. No two people learn best in exactly the same way, so it's important to know your strengths and use them to your advantage.

For example, if you learn best by visualization, focus on visualizing a concept in your mind and draw an image or a diagram. Try color-coding your notes, illustrating them, or creating symbols that will trigger your mind to recall a learned concept. If you learn best by hearing or discussing information, find a study partner who learns the same way or read aloud to yourself. Think about how to put the information in your own words. Imagine that you are giving a lecture on the topic and record yourself so you can listen to it later.

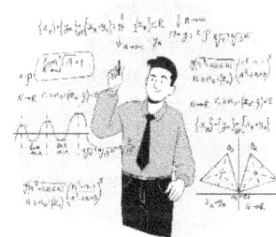

For any learning style, flashcards can be helpful. Organize the information so you can take advantage of spare moments to review. Underline key words or phrases. Use different colors for different categories. Mnemonic devices (such as creating a short list in which every item starts with the same letter) can also help with retention. Find what works best for you and use it to store the information in your mind most effectively and easily.

3

Secret Key #3 – Practice the Right Way

Your success on test day depends not only on how many hours you put into preparing, but also on whether you prepared the right way. It's good to check along the way to see if your studying is paying off. One of the most effective ways to do this is by taking practice tests to evaluate your progress. Practice tests are useful because they show exactly where you need to improve. Every time you take a practice test, pay special attention to these three groups of questions:

- The questions you got wrong
- The questions you had to guess on, even if you guessed right
- The questions you found difficult or slow to work through

This will show you exactly what your weak areas are, and where you need to devote more study time. Ask yourself why each of these questions gave you trouble. Was it because you didn't understand the material? Was it because you didn't remember the vocabulary? Do you need more repetitions on this type of question to build speed and confidence? Dig into those questions and figure out how you can strengthen your weak areas as you go back to review the material.

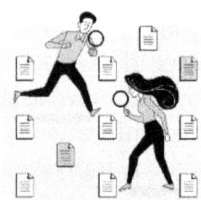

Additionally, many practice tests have a section explaining the answer choices. It can be tempting to read the explanation and think that you now have a good understanding of the concept. However, an explanation likely only covers part of the question's broader context. Even if the explanation makes perfect sense, **go back and investigate** every concept related to the question until you're positive you have a thorough understanding.

As you go along, keep in mind that the practice test is just that: practice. Memorizing these questions and answers will not be very helpful on the actual test because it is unlikely to have any of the same exact questions. If you only know the right answers to the sample questions, you won't be prepared for the real thing. **Study the concepts** until you understand them fully, and then you'll be able to answer any question that shows up on the test.

It's important to wait on the practice tests until you're ready. If you take a test on your first day of study, you may be overwhelmed by the amount of material covered and how much you need to learn. Work up to it gradually.

On test day, you'll need to be prepared for answering questions, managing your time, and using the test-taking strategies you've learned. It's a lot to balance, like a mental marathon that will have a big impact on your future. Like training for a marathon, you'll need to start slowly and work your way up. When test day arrives, you'll be ready.

Start with the strategies you've read in the first two Secret Keys—plan your course and study in the way that works best for you. If you have time, consider using multiple study resources to get different approaches to the same concepts. It can be helpful to see difficult concepts from more than one angle. Then find a good source for practice tests. Many times, the test website will suggest potential study resources or provide sample tests.

Practice Test Strategy

If you're able to find at least three practice tests, we recommend this strategy:

UNTIMED AND OPEN-BOOK PRACTICE

Take the first test with no time constraints and with your notes and study guide handy. Take your time and focus on applying the strategies you've learned.

TIMED AND OPEN-BOOK PRACTICE

Take the second practice test open-book as well, but set a timer and practice pacing yourself to finish in time.

TIMED AND CLOSED-BOOK PRACTICE

Take any other practice tests as if it were test day. Set a timer and put away your study materials. Sit at a table or desk in a quiet room, imagine yourself at the testing center, and answer questions as quickly and accurately as possible.

Keep repeating timed and closed-book tests on a regular basis until you run out of practice tests or it's time for the actual test. Your mind will be ready for the schedule and stress of test day, and you'll be able to focus on recalling the material you've learned.

5

Secret Key #4 – Pace Yourself

Once you're fully prepared for the material on the test, your biggest challenge on test day will be managing your time. Just knowing that the clock is ticking can make you panic even if you have plenty of time left. Work on pacing yourself so you can build confidence against the time constraints of the exam. Pacing is a difficult skill to master, especially in a high-pressure environment, so **practice is vital**.

Set time expectations for your pace based on how much time is available. For example, if a section has 60 questions and the time limit is 30 minutes, you know you have to average 30 seconds or less per question in order to answer them all. Although 30 seconds is the hard limit, set 25 seconds per question as your goal, so you reserve extra time to spend on harder questions. When you budget extra time for the harder questions, you no longer have any reason to stress when those questions take longer to answer.

Don't let this time expectation distract you from working through the test at a calm, steady pace, but keep it in mind so you don't spend too much time on any one question. Recognize that taking extra time on one question you don't understand may keep you from answering two that you do understand later in the test. If your time limit for a question is up and you're still not sure of the answer, mark it and move on, and come back to it later if the time and the test format allow. If the testing format doesn't allow you to return to earlier questions, just make an educated guess; then put it out of your mind and move on.

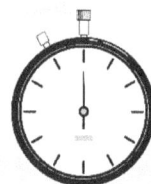

On the easier questions, be careful not to rush. It may seem wise to hurry through them so you have more time for the challenging ones, but it's not worth missing one if you know the concept and just didn't take the time to read the question fully. Work efficiently but make sure you understand the question and have looked at all of the answer choices, since more than one may seem right at first.

Even if you're paying attention to the time, you may find yourself a little behind at some point. You should speed up to get back on track, but do so wisely. Don't panic; just take a few seconds less on each question until you're caught up. Don't guess without thinking, but do look through the answer choices and eliminate any you know are wrong. If you can get down to two choices, it is often worthwhile to guess from those. Once you've chosen an answer, move on and don't dwell on any that you skipped or had to hurry through. If a question was taking too long, chances are it was one of the harder ones, so you weren't as likely to get it right anyway.

On the other hand, if you find yourself getting ahead of schedule, it may be beneficial to slow down a little. The more quickly you work, the more likely you are to make a careless mistake that will affect your score. You've budgeted time for each question, so don't be afraid to spend that time. Practice an efficient but careful pace to get the most out of the time you have.

Secret Key #5 – Have a Plan for Guessing

When you're taking the test, you may find yourself stuck on a question. Some of the answer choices seem better than others, but you don't see the one answer choice that is obviously correct. What do you do?

The scenario described above is very common, yet most test takers have not effectively prepared for it. Developing and practicing a plan for guessing may be one of the single most effective uses of your time as you get ready for the exam.

In developing your plan for guessing, there are three questions to address:

- When should you start the guessing process?
- How should you narrow down the choices?
- Which answer should you choose?

When to Start the Guessing Process

Unless your plan for guessing is to select C every time (which, despite its merits, is not what we recommend), you need to leave yourself enough time to apply your answer elimination strategies. Since you have a limited amount of time for each question, that means that if you're going to give yourself the best shot at guessing correctly, you have to decide quickly whether or not you will guess.

Of course, the best-case scenario is that you don't have to guess at all, so first, see if you can answer the question based on your knowledge of the subject and basic reasoning skills. Focus on the key words in the question and try to jog your memory of related topics. Give yourself a chance to bring the knowledge to mind, but once you realize that you don't have (or you can't access) the knowledge you need to answer the question, it's time to start the guessing process.

It's almost always better to start the guessing process too early than too late. It only takes a few seconds to remember something and answer the question from knowledge. Carefully eliminating wrong answer choices takes longer. Plus, going through the process of eliminating answer choices can actually help jog your memory.

Summary: Start the guessing process as soon as you decide that you can't answer the question based on your knowledge.

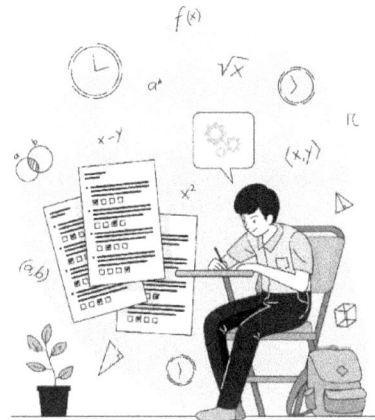

7

How to Narrow Down the Choices

The next chapter in this book (**Test-Taking Strategies**) includes a wide range of strategies for how to approach questions and how to look for answer choices to eliminate. You will definitely want to read those carefully, practice them, and figure out which ones work best for you. Here though, we're going to address a mindset rather than a particular strategy.

Your odds of guessing an answer correctly depend on how many options you are choosing from.

Number of options left	5	4	3	2	1
Odds of guessing correctly	20%	25%	33%	50%	100%

You can see from this chart just how valuable it is to be able to eliminate incorrect answers and make an educated guess, but there are two things that many test takers do that cause them to miss out on the benefits of guessing:

- Accidentally eliminating the correct answer
- Selecting an answer based on an impression

We'll look at the first one here, and the second one in the next section.

To avoid accidentally eliminating the correct answer, we recommend a thought exercise called **the $5 challenge**. In this challenge, you only eliminate an answer choice from contention if you are willing to bet $5 on it being wrong. Why $5? Five dollars is a small but not insignificant amount of money. It's an amount you could afford to lose but wouldn't want to throw away. And while losing $5 once might not hurt too much, doing it twenty times will set you back $100. In the same way, each small decision you make—eliminating a choice here, guessing on a question there—won't by itself impact your score very much, but when you put them all together, they can make a big difference. By holding each answer choice elimination decision to a higher standard, you can reduce the risk of accidentally eliminating the correct answer.

The $5 challenge can also be applied in a positive sense: If you are willing to bet $5 that an answer choice *is* correct, go ahead and mark it as correct.

Summary: Only eliminate an answer choice if you are willing to bet $5 that it is wrong.

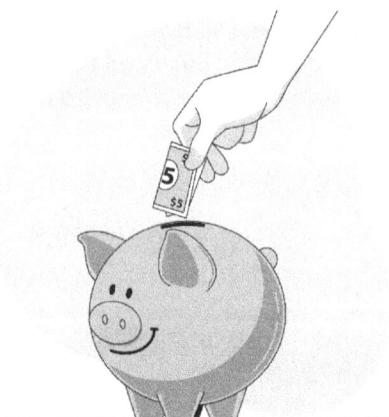

Which Answer to Choose

You're taking the test. You've run into a hard question and decided you'll have to guess. You've eliminated all the answer choices you're willing to bet $5 on. Now you have to pick an answer. Why do we even need to talk about this? Why can't you just pick whichever one you feel like when the time comes?

The answer to these questions is that if you don't come into the test with a plan, you'll rely on your impression to select an answer choice, and if you do that, you risk falling into a trap. The test writers know that everyone who takes their test will be guessing on some of the questions, so they intentionally write wrong answer choices to seem plausible. You still have to pick an answer though, and if the wrong answer choices are designed to look right, how can you ever be sure that you're not falling for their trap? The best solution we've found to this dilemma is to take the decision out of your hands entirely. Here is the process we recommend:

Once you've eliminated any choices that you are confident (willing to bet $5) are wrong, select the first remaining choice as your answer.

Whether you choose to select the first remaining choice, the second, or the last, the important thing is that you use some preselected standard. Using this approach guarantees that you will not be enticed into selecting an answer choice that looks right, because you are not basing your decision on how the answer choices look.

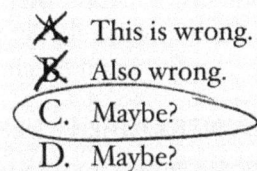

X This is wrong.
X Also wrong.
C. Maybe?
D. Maybe?

This is not meant to make you question your knowledge. Instead, it is to help you recognize the difference between your knowledge and your impressions. There's a huge difference between thinking an answer is right because of what you know, and thinking an answer is right because it looks or sounds like it should be right.

Summary: To ensure that your selection is appropriately random, make a predetermined selection from among all answer choices you have not eliminated.

Test-Taking Strategies

This section contains a list of test-taking strategies that you may find helpful as you work through the test. By taking what you know and applying logical thought, you can maximize your chances of answering any question correctly!

It is very important to realize that every question is different and every person is different: no single strategy will work on every question, and no single strategy will work for every person. That's why we've included all of them here, so you can try them out and determine which ones work best for different types of questions and which ones work best for you.

Question Strategies

⦸ READ CAREFULLY

Read the question and the answer choices carefully. Don't miss the question because you misread the terms. You have plenty of time to read each question thoroughly and make sure you understand what is being asked. Yet a happy medium must be attained, so don't waste too much time. You must read carefully and efficiently.

⦸ CONTEXTUAL CLUES

Look for contextual clues. If the question includes a word you are not familiar with, look at the immediate context for some indication of what the word might mean. Contextual clues can often give you all the information you need to decipher the meaning of an unfamiliar word. Even if you can't determine the meaning, you may be able to narrow down the possibilities enough to make a solid guess at the answer to the question.

⦸ PREFIXES

If you're having trouble with a word in the question or answer choices, try dissecting it. Take advantage of every clue that the word might include. Prefixes can be a huge help. Usually, they allow you to determine a basic meaning. *Pre-* means before, *post-* means after, *pro-* is positive, *de-* is negative. From prefixes, you can get an idea of the general meaning of the word and try to put it into context.

⦸ HEDGE WORDS

Watch out for critical hedge words, such as *likely, may, can, often, almost, mostly, usually, generally, rarely*, and *sometimes*. Question writers insert these hedge phrases to cover every possibility. Often an answer choice will be wrong simply because it leaves no room for exception. Be on guard for answer choices that have definitive words such as *exactly* and *always*.

⦸ SWITCHBACK WORDS

Stay alert for *switchbacks*. These are the words and phrases frequently used to alert you to shifts in thought. The most common switchback words are *but, although*, and *however*. Others include *nevertheless, on the other hand, even though, while, in spite of, despite*, and *regardless of*. Switchback words are important to catch because they can change the direction of the question or an answer choice.

⊘ FACE VALUE

When in doubt, use common sense. Accept the situation in the problem at face value. Don't read too much into it. These problems will not require you to make wild assumptions. If you have to go beyond creativity and warp time or space in order to have an answer choice fit the question, then you should move on and consider the other answer choices. These are normal problems rooted in reality. The applicable relationship or explanation may not be readily apparent, but it is there for you to figure out. Use your common sense to interpret anything that isn't clear.

Answer Choice Strategies

⊘ ANSWER SELECTION

The most thorough way to pick an answer choice is to identify and eliminate wrong answers until only one is left, then confirm it is the correct answer. Sometimes an answer choice may immediately seem right, but be careful. The test writers will usually put more than one reasonable answer choice on each question, so take a second to read all of them and make sure that the other choices are not equally obvious. As long as you have time left, it is better to read every answer choice than to pick the first one that looks right without checking the others.

⊘ ANSWER CHOICE FAMILIES

An answer choice family consists of two (in rare cases, three) answer choices that are very similar in construction and cannot all be true at the same time. If you see two answer choices that are direct opposites or parallels, one of them is usually the correct answer. For instance, if one answer choice says that quantity *x* increases and another either says that quantity *x* decreases (opposite) or says that quantity *y* increases (parallel), then those answer choices would fall into the same family. An answer choice that doesn't match the construction of the answer choice family is more likely to be incorrect. Most questions will not have answer choice families, but when they do appear, you should be prepared to recognize them.

⊘ ELIMINATE ANSWERS

Eliminate answer choices as soon as you realize they are wrong, but make sure you consider all possibilities. If you are eliminating answer choices and realize that the last one you are left with is also wrong, don't panic. Start over and consider each choice again. There may be something you missed the first time that you will realize on the second pass.

⊘ AVOID FACT TRAPS

Don't be distracted by an answer choice that is factually true but doesn't answer the question. You are looking for the choice that answers the question. Stay focused on what the question is asking for so you don't accidentally pick an answer that is true but incorrect. Always go back to the question and make sure the answer choice you've selected actually answers the question and is not merely a true statement.

⊘ EXTREME STATEMENTS

In general, you should avoid answers that put forth extreme actions as standard practice or proclaim controversial ideas as established fact. An answer choice that states the "process should be used in certain situations, if..." is much more likely to be correct than one that states the "process should be discontinued completely." The first is a calm rational statement and doesn't even make a definitive, uncompromising stance, using a hedge word *if* to provide wiggle room, whereas the second choice is far more extreme.

11

⊘ Benchmark

As you read through the answer choices and you come across one that seems to answer the question well, mentally select that answer choice. This is not your final answer, but it's the one that will help you evaluate the other answer choices. The one that you selected is your benchmark or standard for judging each of the other answer choices. Every other answer choice must be compared to your benchmark. That choice is correct until proven otherwise by another answer choice beating it. If you find a better answer, then that one becomes your new benchmark. Once you've decided that no other choice answers the question as well as your benchmark, you have your final answer.

⊘ Predict the Answer

Before you even start looking at the answer choices, it is often best to try to predict the answer. When you come up with the answer on your own, it is easier to avoid distractions and traps because you will know exactly what to look for. The right answer choice is unlikely to be word-for-word what you came up with, but it should be a close match. Even if you are confident that you have the right answer, you should still take the time to read each option before moving on.

General Strategies

⊘ Tough Questions

If you are stumped on a problem or it appears too hard or too difficult, don't waste time. Move on! Remember though, if you can quickly check for obviously incorrect answer choices, your chances of guessing correctly are greatly improved. Before you completely give up, at least try to knock out a couple of possible answers. Eliminate what you can and then guess at the remaining answer choices before moving on.

⊘ Check Your Work

Since you will probably not know every term listed and the answer to every question, it is important that you get credit for the ones that you do know. Don't miss any questions through careless mistakes. If at all possible, try to take a second to look back over your answer selection and make sure you've selected the correct answer choice and haven't made a costly careless mistake (such as marking an answer choice that you didn't mean to mark). This quick double check should more than pay for itself in caught mistakes for the time it costs.

⊘ Pace Yourself

It's easy to be overwhelmed when you're looking at a page full of questions; your mind is confused and full of random thoughts, and the clock is ticking down faster than you would like. Calm down and maintain the pace that you have set for yourself. Especially as you get down to the last few minutes of the test, don't let the small numbers on the clock make you panic. As long as you are on track by monitoring your pace, you are guaranteed to have time for each question.

⊘ Don't Rush

It is very easy to make errors when you are in a hurry. Maintaining a fast pace in answering questions is pointless if it makes you miss questions that you would have gotten right otherwise. Test writers like to include distracting information and wrong answers that seem right. Taking a little extra time to avoid careless mistakes can make all the difference in your test score. Find a pace that allows you to be confident in the answers that you select.

⊘ Keep Moving

Panicking will not help you pass the test, so do your best to stay calm and keep moving. Taking deep breaths and going through the answer elimination steps you practiced can help to break through a stress barrier and keep your pace.

Final Notes

The combination of a solid foundation of content knowledge and the confidence that comes from practicing your plan for applying that knowledge is the key to maximizing your performance on test day. As your foundation of content knowledge is built up and strengthened, you'll find that the strategies included in this chapter become more and more effective in helping you quickly sift through the distractions and traps of the test to isolate the correct answer.

Now that you're preparing to move forward into the test content chapters of this book, be sure to keep your goal in mind. As you read, think about how you will be able to apply this information on the test. If you've already seen sample questions for the test and you have an idea of the question format and style, try to come up with questions of your own that you can answer based on what you're reading. This will give you valuable practice applying your knowledge in the same ways you can expect to on test day.

Good luck and good studying!

Patient Care

PROPER PATIENT IDENTIFICATION

Proper patient identification is important because it can prevent a critical error like misidentifying a patient specimen which could result in harm or death to a patient. Patient identification includes asking a patient to state their name and date of birth, and then you check the identification band and the requisition to see if they match. Verbal identification should never be relied on alone although it is important since patients can be hard of hearing, ill, or mentally incompetent and may give incorrect information. Also, check the identification band since it is possible for a patient to be wearing the wrong ID band. If there is no ID band, notify the nurse and have her confirm the patient's identity and attach an ID band before the blood is drawn. If there is any discrepancy on the ID band, information given by the patient or on the requisition, a reconciliation of the discrepancy must be made before a collection is taken. More than one patient may have the same name. Usually a name alert is placed on the chart but not in all cases.

ADVANCE DIRECTIVES

In accordance to Federal and state laws, individuals have the right to self-determination in health care, including decisions about end of life care through **advance directives** such as living wills and the right to assign a surrogate person to make decisions through a durable power of attorney. Patients should routinely be questioned about an advanced directive as they may present at a healthcare provider without the document. Patients who have indicated they desire a do-not-resuscitate (DNR) order should not receive resuscitative treatments for terminal illness or conditions in which meaningful recovery cannot occur. Patients and families of those with terminal illnesses should be questioned as to whether the patients are Hospice patients. For those with DNR requests or those withdrawing life support, staff should provide the patient palliative rather than curative measures, such as pain control and/or oxygen, and emotional support to the patient and family. Religious traditions and beliefs about death should be treated with respect.

BENEFICENCE AND NONMALEFICENCE

Beneficence is an ethical principle that involves performing actions that are for the purpose of benefitting another person. In the care of a patient, any procedure or treatment should be done with the ultimate goal of benefitting the patient, and any actions that are not beneficial should be reconsidered. As conditions change, procedures need to be continually reevaluated to determine if they are still of benefit.

Nonmaleficence is an ethical principle that means healthcare workers should provide care in a manner that does not cause direct intentional harm to the patient:

- The actual act must be good or morally neutral.
- The intent must be only for a good effect.
- A bad effect cannot serve as the means to get to a good effect.
- A good effect must have more benefit than a bad effect has harm.

SUBPOENA DUCES TECUM

Subpoena duces tecum literally means bring [it] with you under penalty of punishment. It is a court order for a witness to produce documents. The judge must carefully consider if *subpoena duces tecum* transgresses the patient's HIPAA rights.

15

HANDLING WOUNDS OF VIOLENCE AND CHILD ABUSE

The physician and other health professionals must report to authorities:

- Gunshot wounds
- Possible terrorist incidents, especially if they involve the spread of disease
- Known or suspected abuse of a child, senior, or disabled person
- Sexual assault of a juvenile or disabled person
- Poisoning
- Wounds intentionally caused by knives and sharp objects
- Criminal violence, including domestic violence
- Client-specific information for the central cancer registry
- Specific contagious diseases determined by each state

The facility must keep a written record of the patient's information that was disclosed to authorities.

GOOD SAMARITAN ACT AND DUTY OF CARE

Good Samaritan Act: There are two kinds of Good Samaritan Acts:

I. A first aider who provides unpaid assistance to the injured in an emergency and acts as "a reasonable man" up to his/her level of training is protected by state law from unfair prosecution for death, disability, or disfigurement. A judge would dismiss assault and battery charges. A *Good Samaritan Act* is not a duty to assist law, except in Vermont and Minnesota. Nevada and California may adopt a duty to assist clause.

II. A living donor who offers a non-directed donation of an organ to the transplant center is a Good Samaritan. The following organs can be donated by a living donor: kidneys; liver lobes; lung lobes; pancreas segments; and small bowel segments. Non-direct donors do not have anyone particular in mind whom they would like to receive their donated organ. The donation is usually anonymous and the Good Samaritan is blameless for complications the recipient suffers.

Duty of care: One must act as "a reasonable man" and meet the standard of care to avoid negligence charges. This means being watchful, attentive, cautious, and prudent at work.

MEDICOLEGAL TERMS/DOCTRINES

Medicolegal terms/doctrines include:

- Subpoena: A legal writ (order) requiring a person to come to court, to testify in court, and/or to produce documents or evidence. Failure to do so may result in fine or jailing.
- *Res ipsa loquitur* ("the thing speaks for itself"): The principle of law that allows the use of circumstantial evidence as proof.
- *Locum tenens* ("to substitute for"): Allows one medical professional to serve temporarily in place of another. For example, a physician's practice may be covered by another physician usually for a few days up to 6 months when the first goes on vacation or takes leave. Companies specialize in providing *locums* physicians to work on a contract basis.
- Deposition: This is a sworn out-of-court witness statement taken under oath, usually in an attorney's office prior to a court case to document what the witness knows and to preserve the statements for use in court.

16

RESPONDEAT SUPERIOR

Respondeat Superior is Latin for "let the master answer". The *Doctrine of Respondeat Superior* means if a technician is involved in a legal action resulting from work, then the doctor is ultimately responsible for the technician's actions or losses incurred. However, the technician employer is also held accountable for due diligence.

EXCEPTIONS TO INFORMED CONSENT

There are some exceptions to the rule of informed consent. They are as follows:

- Emergencies: If the patient's life is at stake, they are unconscious, and the procedure is widely accepted a necessary for treatment, there is no need to get informed consent.
- Emotional Distress/not able to process information: Informed consent is not necessary if a patient is unable to understand the information given to him by the doctor, whether it is because of a mental handicap or the patient has become emotionally distraught.
- Legal Incompetence: Informed consent is waived if a judge rules a patient incompetent.
- Minor Age Status: Informed consent may be waived if the patient is a minor and getting parental consent is not a possibility. If the procedure is not a matter of life or death, it may be postponed until a legal guardian can consent to it.

INFORMED CONSENT REQUIREMENTS

In order for a procedure to be performed, the ordering doctor must provide the patient with all necessary information and get their consent to have it done. The following are the requirements for getting informed consent for a procedure:

- The physician ordering the procedure got consent to do so from the patient.
- Risk/Benefit information was provided to the patient.
- Other treatment possibilities were discussed with patient.
- Patient informed of possible outcome if the procedure is not done.
- Patient was informed using understandable language.
- The place that provided the service also provided patient with information about risks.
- State-mandated rules regarding time between signing consent and performing procedure were followed.
- The patient was not scared or forced into having the procedure performed.

HIPAA

HIPAA is the Health Insurance Portability and Accountability Act approved by congress and signed into law in 1996. HIPAA was enacted to protect the privacy of personal health information by setting limits on the use and disclosure of such information without patient authorization. The Act also gives patients rights over their health information, including the right to examine and obtain copies of their health records and the right to request corrections.

PATIENT PRIVACY

Every patient has a right to privacy during a procedure. The basics of patient privacy for any procedure are as follows:

- Provide a private area for changing or dressing.
- Provide a dressing gown that has closures (use two gowns if the patient is large).
- Cover the patients' exposed legs and feet. Provide slippers if necessary.
- Only expose parts of the body that are necessary for the procedure.

- Allow only necessary personnel in the room during the procedure.
- Do not have personal conversations with other personnel in front of the patient.
- Show the patient's chart to only necessary personnel and do not discuss the patient with others.
- Respect patient confidentiality.

PATIENT'S RIGHTS

Even if a physician writes an order to perform a procedure, it is ultimately up to the patient to decide if the procedure will be performed. Every patient has the right to refuse any medical procedure. This patient's right, among others, stems from the Patient's Bill of Rights. In 1973, the American Hospital Association developed the first Patient's Bill of Rights. It was a document that outlined a patient's rights when it comes to choices in healthcare. This Bill of rights has been updated and adopted, in some form, by most states, and it is the responsibility of the technician to become familiar with their local version. It covers topics such as informed consent, advanced directives, living wills, appointment of surrogates, confidentiality, privacy, access to medical records, and access to healthcare.

REQUIREMENTS FOR RESEARCH PARTICIPATION

Research participation requires precise documentation for every step, not only for the subject's safety and rights but also to protect the validity of the study being conducted. The pretrial documentation should include the brochures for the trial and how they recruited subjects, compensation, certificates that outline how products will be shipped along with their purity, and signed consent forms. During the trial, standard operation procedure (SOP) and specific protocols should be in place along with the confidential list of participants and any records pertaining to the patient's care (e.g., prescriptions, labs, radiology exams, and notes kept by the subject). After the trial, a case study is produced explaining the results of the trial. It is communicated if subjects will need follow-up care, and all supplies are accounted for and returned to the vendor. All of the documentation should be the original paperwork that was filed during the trial. If the original files cannot be provided, a certified copy should be used. The paperwork should also have signatures to identify who filed the paperwork along with the dates.

ARRT STANDARDS OF ETHICS, RULES OF ETHICS, AND ADMINISTRATIVE PROCEDURES

ARRT STANDARDS OF ETHICS

The American Registry of Radiological Technologists has developed a code of ethics that acts as a guideline for performing in the best possible manner. The eleven principles of this code of ethics are as follows:

1. Act in a professional manner.
2. Respect the dignity of everyone.
3. Deliver healthcare without discrimination.
4. Be a competent technician.
5. Make decisions that take into consideration the needs of your patients.
6. Diagnosis and interpretation are not your job or responsibility.
7. Be aware of and practice current technical and safety procedures.
8. Practice ethical behavior that provides quality care.
9. Respect patient privacy and confidentiality.
10. Be involved in continuing education.
11. Refrain from drug abuse

RULES OF ETHICS

The Rules of Ethics is a further detailing and defining of the professional conduct expectations consisting of the following 8 subjects:

- Fraud or Deceptive Practices
- Subversion
- Unprofessional Conduct
- Scope of Practice
- Fitness to Practice
- Improper Management of Patient Records
- Violation of State or Federal Law or Regulatory Rule
- Duty to Report

ADMINISTRATIVE PROCEDURES

The Administrative Procedures cover the definitions processes surrounding infractions of the Standard of Practice. The following are the 7 areas the procedures cover:

- Ethics Committee
- Hearings
- Appeals
- Adverse Decisions
- Publication of Adverse Decisions
- Procedure to Request Removal of a Sanction
- Amendments to the Standards of Ethics

VERBAL AND NONVERBAL MODES OF COMMUNICATING WITH PATIENTS

Because the technician is usually the only person to have contact with a patient during a procedure, it is important that they effectively communicate all important information, collect the necessary patient history, as well as make the patient feel as comfortable as possible. This is all done using various verbal and nonverbal modes of communication. The verbal ways that we communicate with others are obvious-we ask questions, provide information, clarify misunderstandings. Some of the ways that we communicate nonverbally are less obvious, yet equally as important. Nonverbal communication ranges from the organization and cleanliness of the technician and the room, to the ways in which the patient is touched or transferred for the procedure. It is important to convey to the patient an attitude of understanding, caring, and competency.

CULTURAL CONSIDERATIONS

HISPANIC PATIENTS

Many areas of the country have large populations of **Hispanic** and Hispanic-Americans. As always, it's important to recognize that cultural generalizations don't always apply to individuals. Recent immigrants, especially, have cultural needs that the nurse must understand:

- Many Hispanics are Catholic and may like the nurse to make arrangements for a priest to visit.
- Large extended families may come to visit to support the patient and family, so patients should receive clear explanations about how many visitors are allowed, but some flexibility may be required.
- Language barriers may exist as some may have limited or no English skills so translation services should be available around the clock.

- Hispanic culture encourages outward expressions of emotions, so family may react strongly to news about a patient's condition, and people who are ill may expect some degree of pampering, so extra attention to the patient/family members may alleviate some of their anxiety.

MIDDLE EASTERN PATIENTS

Caring for **Middle Eastern** patients requires understanding of cultural differences:

- Families may practice strict dietary restrictions, such as avoiding pork and requiring that animals be killed in a ritual manner, so vegetarian or kosher meals may be required.
- People may have language difficulties requiring a translator, and same-sex translators should be used if at all possible.
- Families may be accompanied by large extended families that want to be kept informed and whom patients consult before decisions are made.
- Most medical care is provided by female relatives, so educating the family about patient care should be directed at females (with female translators if necessary).
- Outward expressions of grief are considered as showing respect for the dead.
- Middle Eastern families often offer gifts to caregivers. Small gifts (candy) that can be shared should be accepted graciously, but for other gifts, the families should be advised graciously that accepting gifts is against hospital policy.
- Middle Easterners often require less personal space and may stand very close.

ASIAN PATIENTS

Caring for **Asian** patients requires understanding of cultural differences:

- Patients/families may not show outward expressions of feelings/grief, sometimes appearing passive. They also avoid public displays of affection. This does not mean that they don't feel, just that they don't show their feelings.
- Families often hide illness and disabilities from others and may feel ashamed about illness.
- Terminal illness is often hidden from the patient, so families may not want patients to know they are dying or seriously ill.
- Families may use cupping, pinching, or applying pressure to injured areas, and this can leave bruises that may appear as abuse, so when bruises are found, the family should be questioned about alternative therapy before assumptions are made.
- Patients may be treated with traditional herbs.
- Families may need translators because of poor or no English skills.
- In traditional Asian families, males are authoritative and make the decisions.

CULTURAL COMPETENCE

Different cultures view health and illness from very different perspectives, and patients often come from a mix of many cultures, so the acute care nurse must be not only accepting of cultural differences but must be sensitive and aware. There are a number of characteristics that are important for a nurse to have **cultural competence:**

- **Appreciating diversity:** This must be grounded in information about other cultures and understanding of their value system.
- **Assessing own cultural perspectives:** Self-awareness is essential to understanding potential biases.
- **Understanding intercultural dynamics:** This must include understanding ways in which cultures cooperate, differ, communicate, and reach understanding.

- **Recognizing institutional culture:** Each institutional unit (hospital, clinic, office) has an inherent set of values that may be unwritten but is accepted by the staff.
- **Adapting patient service to diversity:** This is the culmination of cultural competence as it is the point of contact between cultures.

MIDDLE EASTERN PATIENTS

There are considerable cultural differences among **Middle Easterners,** but religious beliefs about the segregation of males and females are common. It's important to remember that segregating the female is meant to protect her virtue. Female nurses have low status in many countries because they violate this segregation by touching male bodies, so parents may not trust or show respect for the nurse who is caring for their family member. Additionally, male patients may not want to be cared for by female nurses or doctors, and families may be very upset at a female being cared for by a male nurse or physician. When possible, these cultural traditions should be accommodated:

- In Middle Eastern countries, males make decisions, so issues for discussion or decision should be directed to males, such as the father or spouse, and males may be direct in stating what they want, sometimes appearing demanding.
- If a male nurse must care for a female patient, then the family should be advised that *personal care* (such as bathing) will be done by a female while the medical treatments will be done by the male nurse.

ASIAN PATIENTS

There are considerable differences among different **Asian** populations, so cultural generalizations may not apply to all, but nurses caring for Asian patients should be aware of common cultural attitudes and behaviors:

- Nurses and doctors are viewed with respect, so traditional Asian families may expect the nurse to remain authoritative and to give directions and may not question, so the nurse should ensure that they understand by having them review material or give demonstrations and should provide explanations clearly, anticipating questions that the family might have but may not articulate.
- Disagreeing is considered impolite. "Yes" may only mean that the person is heard, not that they agree with the person. When asked if they understand, they may indicate that they do even when they clearly do not so as not to offend the nurse.
- Asians may avoid eye contact as an indication of respect. This is especially true of children in relation to adults and younger adults in relation to elders.

THERAPEUTIC COMMUNICATION TECHNIQUES
USE WITH THE HEARING IMPAIRED

Hearing impaired patients may have some hearing and may use hearing aids while **deaf** patients typically have little or no hearing. Some patients are able to use lip reading to various degrees, so the technician should always face the patient (at 3-6 feet) and speak slowly and clearly, using gestures (not excessively) to augment speech:

- Hearing impaired: Assistive devices (hearing aids, writing material) should be available and used during communication. Use a normal tone of voice and speak in short sentences. Minimize environmental noises.

Mometrix

- <u>Deaf:</u> If patients are deaf, sign language interpreters should be used for important communication (face the patient, not the interpreter). Assistive devices, such as writing materials, TDD phone/relay service, should be available for use. Always announce presence on entering a room by waving, clapping, tapping the foot (whatever works best for the patient). Ensure alarms have visual feedback (lights). Do not chew, smoke, or eat while speaking to the patient.

USE WITH THE VISION IMPAIRED

Visual impairment is unrelated to intelligence or hearing, so the technician should speak with age-appropriate vocabulary in a normal tone of voice, facing the patient so the technician can observe facial expression. Depending on the degree of visual impairment the patient may not be able to see gestures or materials, so alternate forms of materials (braille handouts or enlarged text) or manipulatives must be considered. The field of vision may be impaired so that the patient sees shapes or has better vision in some areas than others, and the technician should try to position herself/himself for the patient's advantage. The technician should also announce his/her presence, explain actions and movement ("I'm putting your dressing supplies on the counter."), announce position ("I'm at your right side.") and always tell the patient if intending to touch the patient ("I'm going to take your blood pressure on your right arm").

USE WITH THE INTELLECTUALLY DISABLED AND ILLITERATE

Communicating with patients who are **intellectually disabled** can be challenging, and patients may have very different and individual responses, so observation of the patient must serve as a guide. Patients may be apprehensive and frightened, so the technician should maintain a friendly normal tone of voice and should speak with the patient often to establish rapport, even if the response is not clear. The technician should always ask the patient before touching his/her things. Initiating communication by talking about familiar things (family, pictures, the past) may be comforting for the patient. If responses are unclear or inappropriate, the technician can say, "I didn't understand that" but should not laugh or indicate frustration. Communicating with patients who are **illiterate** is not different than with most patients because the patients may be quite intelligent, but the technician should take care to explain procedures and provide verbal rather than written instructions.

PROPER THERAPEUTIC RESPONSES TO PEDIATRIC/ADOLESCENT, GERIATRIC, AND TERMINALLY ILL PATIENTS

Therapeutic responses include:

- <u>Pediatric/Adolescent</u>: Use vocabulary appropriate to age and encourage adolescents to make decisions whenever possible ("Which arm should I use?"). Avoid approaching young children too abruptly but chat with the child and caregiver to ease the child's fear. Explain in advance any actions to be taken, such as temperature or BP, and allow the child to see and hold the equipment when possible.
- <u>Geriatric</u>: Treat patients with respect, address them by their names ("Mrs. Jones") and avoid terms like "honey," and "dear." Be alert for barriers, such as hearing deficit, to communication, and encourage patients to ask questions and discuss concerns. Avoid rushing and interrupting and utilize active listening skills.
- <u>Terminally ill</u>: Avoid being excessively sympathetic ("You poor thing"), but remain patient and empathetic. Utilize active listening and allow patient time to express feelings or concerns. Understand that patients may be in pain, weak, frightened, nauseated, and/or depressed and may over-react or under-react.

COMMUNICATION TECHNIQUES WHEN ASSESSING UNDERSTANDING

Communication techniques used when assessing patient's understanding and communication include:

- Reflection: Refers to both the meaning of the patient's words and the emotions. If a patient states, "I understand how to monitor my blood pressure," a reflecting question might be: "You feel confident that you know how to take your blood pressure and when to notify the physician?"
- Restatement: Restates or paraphrases something a patient said, "I've been having dizzy spells for two weeks?" Restatement might be: "You've been having dizzy spells for 2 weeks."
- Clarification: Asks for more information. If a patient states, "I haven't been feeling well," a clarifying question might be: "What exactly do you mean when you say you haven't been feeling well?"
- Feedback: Responds to something a patient has said or done, letting them know that the message/information was received: "You have kept very accurate records of your blood pressure and pulse."

DISTRACTIONS THAT DISRUPT THE COMMUNICATION CYCLE

Distractions (interference) that disrupt the communication cycle include:

- Internal: The communicator's or recipient's emotional status, such as increased anxiety or anger, can negatively impact communication. Biases, prejudices, and belief systems may also interfere with a person's ability to attend to the ideas of another person. Pain and hunger can be so distracting that the person is unable to focus on communication. When under stress, the brain may process information differently, interfering with comprehension.
- External: Noise in the environment (conversation, traffic, alarms, air conditioning) can make it hard for some people to hear clearly, especially those with hearing impairment, and may make concentration difficult. Additionally, people may find noise very stressful to the point that they have difficulty thinking. Other environmental factors, such as extremes of heat or cold, may cause physical discomfort that interferes with the ability to communicate.

COMMUNICATION TECHNIQUES IN THERAPEUTIC RELATIONSHIPS

The following are four appropriate communication techniques to encourage in therapeutic relationships:

1. **Use active listening** – Paraphrase and repeat back information transmitted by your patient. Ask for clarification when the message is confusing. Summarize what you agreed to at the end of your conversation.
2. **Watch for nonverbal cues** – Nonverbal cues are gestures, grimaces, posturing, appearance, and eye movements that comprise 85% of all communication. Nonverbal cues denote pain, fear, lying, depression, or subterfuge by a caregiver. Gently ask your patient to clarify when verbal and nonverbal cues do not match. Children and psychiatric patients may develop tic disorders (involuntary gestures and movements). If you cannot decipher which movements are truly cues and which are tics, ask the doctor.
3. **Ask open-ended questions** – Get your patient to 'open up', rather than ask questions that require only a yes or no answer.
4. **Consider influences** – Put communication in the context of your patient's: Developmental age; emotions; values; ethics; health; education; culture; environment; social and family status; and drug levels.

23

COMMUNICATION TECHNIQUES TO AVOID

The following are ten *inappropriate* communications techniques to avoid in therapeutic relationships:

1. **Ask leading questions** – Never shape the patient's answers to questions, or try to change the patient's interpretation of the situation by "putting words into the patient's mouth"
2. **Demand an explanation** – Do not ask "why" questions in an accusing tone
3. **Give advice** – The physician advises and the technician supports
4. **Demand an immediate response** – Allow the patient sufficient time for silent reflection before responding
5. **Disinterested body language** – Do not appear distracted or make the patient feel inconsequential by impatient motions, bored posture, or rolling your eyes
6. **Minimize the patient's feelings** – Do not compare feelings and experiences
7. **Negatively empower** – Do not help your patient to manipulate another person
8. **Make false promises** – Never promise the patient that the doctor will definitely cure the condition, or make promises that cannot be kept
9. **Play into stereotypes** – Racist, sexist, and religious prejudice must not influence your treatment of the patient
10. **Deliberately mislead** – Always disclose upcoming treatments, tests, or procedures

EXPLAINING PROCEDURES TO PATIENTS

It is very important that the patient fully understands the procedure that is to be done. A patient cannot be expected to consent to a procedure that they do not understand. There are different ways that a technician can communicate the information to the patient. Because everyone has a different level of education and understanding of medical procedures, a technician must tailor their explanation to the patient's needs. The following steps should be taken to assure that the patient is adequately informed:

- Ask is the patient is familiar with the procedure.
- Find out if the procedure has already been explained to them.
- Provide a simple and concise explanation using language they will understand.
- Explain if the patient is to do anything during the procedure (not move, hold breath).
- Have the patient explain any important instructions back to you.
- Allow the patient to ask questions.

MRI

MRI stands for magnetic resonance imaging and is a procedure that does not use ionizing radiation. Instead, it uses magnetic fields and computer software to produce an image. The dye gadolinium is used as a contrast medium for the procedure. MRI is particularly useful in imaging soft tissue. Because it does not used ionizing radiation, there are, in general, fewer risks associated with MRIs. However, because it uses magnetism, any metal objects in the room or on/in the patient can become sources of injury. Also, because an MRI must be conducted within a close distance to the patient, many people experience claustrophobia. It is sometimes necessary to medicate the patient so that they remain still long enough to get a quality image.

CT

CT stands for computed tomography and is a highly specific application of radiation and computer analysis that is used to get a detailed, three-dimensional image. Because the primary beam of radiation is highly collimated (restricted) and delivered in a helical (spiral) fashion using slip ring technology, it can be precisely targeted to the area of interest to provide a multi-layered image. An iodinated contrast medium allows for the visual differentiation of different tissues. In order to get the quality image necessary for diagnosis, it is very important that a patient remain still for a CT procedure. It is sometimes necessary to medicate the patient so that they remain still long enough to get a quality image.

ULTRASOUND PROCEDURES

Ultrasound (or medical sonography) creates an image by recording the echo of sound waves as they bounce off the anatomy to which they are applied. It is primarily a non-invasive procedure that does not carry with it the risk of exposure to ionizing radiation. For this reason, it is the primary means of visualizing the fetus during pregnancy. It can, however, be used in invasive procedures such as biopsy, intravaginal imaging, transesophageal echocardiography. To improve imaging, water is sometimes consumed so that the full bladder acts to magnify the anatomy being imaged. This is particularly helpful in fetal imaging.

NUCLEAR MEDICINE PROCEDURES

In nuclear medicine, instead of the patient being exposed to radiation externally, they are injected with a radioactive isotope. Once the body begins to emit gamma radiation, the image is captured by a scintillation camera and analyzed by a computer. Because of the potential danger in working with radioactive materials, only nuclear medicine technologists are authorized to inject the radioisotope. It is a procedure that is extensively regulated by the NRC (nuclear regulatory committee). A department must keep very accurate records and properly dispose of nuclear waste in order to maintain a license to practice nuclear medicine.

MAMMOGRAPHY

Used to detect breast cancer, mammography uses tissue compression and low doses of radiation to image breast tissue. It has become a highly regulated area of radiography that requires additional training and continuing education. The Mammography Quality Control Standards Act (MQSA) of 1994 and American College of Radiology (ACR) regulations provide the guidelines for mammography use and interpretation. Because breast tissue can be difficult to image using mammography alone, ultrasound, nuclear medicine, and MRI combined with the use of a breast coil can help give more accurate results. A biopsy (surgical or needle) is used to confirm the presence of cancer. Appropriate film-screen combinations are necessary to get the best image. A computer image does not provide enough detail for an accurate diagnosis.

STEPS TO MAKE PATIENTS FEEL LESS ANXIOUS ABOUT ULTRASOUND EXAMS

It is important to show empathy during an ultrasound exam. Often, the patient is nervous about the procedure, so it is up to the sonographer to help the patient feel more comfortable. Upon having correctly identified the patient, the sonographer should introduce themselves to the patient, explain the exam that will be performed, and answer any questions that may arise. An important step prior to the exam is to get a thorough history from the patient and find out if any prior exams have been done for comparison. Make sure the patient is as comfortable as possible, and during the exam check in and ask him/her how they are doing. Once the exam is over, make sure that all of the gel is wiped off. It is also important to discuss how the patient will receive their results and when to expect them. A sonographer should not relay any of the associated findings with the patient because they must come from the ordering physician or radiologist. Patients often appreciate being shown back to the waiting room after the exam is finished.

ASKING PATIENTS ABOUT PRIOR IMAGING STUDIES

Often, an ultrasound exam may be performed as a follow-up to a disorder that has already been diagnosed with another imaging modality or prior ultrasound. If a patient has already had prior imaging (magnetic resonance imaging [MRI], computed tomography [CT], ultrasound, etc.), it is important to look at the images and read the report so that the sonographer knows exactly what is to be interrogated. It is also important that the radiologist has this information because ordering physicians appreciate and expect comparative reports. Ultrasound is useful as a follow-up modality because it does not subject the patient to ionizing radiation like CT and X-ray do. The facility may use a technique called fusion imaging, which allows side-by-side ultrasound imaging with comparative CT or MRI studies that have already been performed. This technique allows more confidence that the lesion visualized on ultrasound is the exact same lesion found on a previous study.

PATIENT SAFETY

It is important that all medical procedures are safe for the patient. The basics of patient safety for medical procedures are as follows:

- Be sure to properly identify the patient.
- Conduct patient needs assessment.
- Use proper body mechanics so as not to injure yourself or the patient.
- Use safety straps, side rails, and immobilization devices properly and when necessary.
- Be aware of the location of the patient when moving equipment.
- Properly label and store patient personal belongings.
- Document any patient injury or property loss/damage immediately.

RISK OF INJURY TO PATIENT DURING ULTRASOUND

Ultrasound labs must perform routine preventative maintenance on their equipment to make sure that all parameters are within the acceptable standards for ultrasound equipment. It is up to the sonographer to make sure that all parts of the equipment are inspected on a regular basis. Sonographers should make sure that the machine is plugged into the correct electrical outlets and the cords do not present a trip hazard. There are many fundamental pieces of the machine that may be connected to the patient at the same time. The transducer is an integral part of the ultrasound machine and is the component that is always directly on or within the patient. This contact would account for the greatest risk of injury to the patient during an exam. Not only could a damaged transducer degrade the quality of an image, but a cracked transducer could also impart an electrical shock to the patient.

IMPORTANCE OF MONITORING TI DURING SONOGRAM

Patient safety is a primary concern during an ultrasound. Bioeffects can occur if an increase in tissue temperature occurs as a result of the interactions of tissue with the ultrasound beam. The thermal index (TI) is displayed on the screen for users as an indicator of a possible increase in tissue temperature. Research has shown that an increase in temperature of some tissues by as little as 2 to 4 degrees can cause bioeffects. This, of course, depends on the tissue type as well as the amount of time the tissue is exposed. The TI is directly related to the acoustic output of the machine. There are three types of thermal indices that serve as the best in vivo indicators of a rise in temperature: the soft-tissue thermal index (TIS), bone thermal index (TIB), and cranial bone thermal index (TIC). Obstetrical exams are of great concern because adverse effects have been identified with an elevated TI value.

DECREASING MI

The mechanical index (MI) reading on an ultrasound machine determines the probability of bioeffects when gas bubbles in the tissue interact with the ultrasound beam. This is a phenomenon known as cavitation. The significance of a system displaying a high MI is that there is a better chance that bioeffects will occur. If a sonographer notices that the MI is too high, it is helpful to decrease the output power on the machine in order to reduce the amount of voltage sent to the transducer. The operator should also increase the frequency of the transducer because the frequency and MI have an inverse relationship. These adjustments are effective in reducing the display because lower frequency and pressure are two properties of the beam that tend to raise the MI.

SPTA

The term in vivo involves observing possible bioeffects that take place inside a living body. The spatial peak temporal average (SPTA) is the intensity that is referred to in the Statement on Mammalian Biological Effects of Ultrasound In Vivo of the American Institute of Ultrasound in Medicine. Unfavorable outcomes have been observed in exploratory conditions. Many experiments have been carried out in the lab setting pertaining to the possible bioeffects that ultrasound has on the body. Lab mammals are used to help experts better comprehend the associated risks that ultrasound has on the body. Lower ultrasound frequencies pose no threat to human tissue during in vivo trials. During controlled trials, it has been confirmed that as long as a focused beam's SPTA intensity does not exceed 1 W/cm^2 and an unfocused beam's SPTA intensity stays less than 100 mW/cm^2, then bioeffects should not occur.

PROPER DOCUMENTATION OF ROUTINE MONITORING

Proper documentation must be performed to provide the best patient care possible during the exam. Documentation also provides pertinent information that may be reviewed by clinicians and staff when follow-up studies are to be performed. When injecting a patient with contrast during exams, it is important to document the contrast media, dose, and any reactions the patient experienced. Routine monitoring requires the technologist to check for any change in the patient's mental status or other important vitals. Many symptoms can be monitored just by looking at or speaking with the patient. If the patient is suddenly having difficulty breathing, sweating profusely, bleeding, developing hives, or having a hard time speaking because of laryngeal edema, these are all signs that he or she is having a reaction to the contrast.

CREATING A SAFE WORKPLACE ENVIRONMENT

The technician should take an active role in creating a **safe workplace environment** and preventing accidents:

- Slips: Most slips occur when the floor is wet or lacks adequate traction. Common causes include spills (water, urine, soap), oily substances (leaking oil), loose rugs and mats, and excessive floor waxing. Slips are especially a risk during wet weather as people may track water or snow in from outside. Floors should be checked and kept clean and dry,
- Trips: Most trips occur when the foot encounters obstacles (wrinkled rugs, cables, cords, clutter), view/walkway is obstructed, or lighting is poor. Traffic areas should be kept clear of clutter and lighting checked. Uneven steps should have warning signs.
- Falls: Many falls result from slipping or tripping, but some occur from a height, such as from a ladder or stairs. Patients who are unstable should always be assisted when walking and assisted at an appropriate pace.

IMPORTANCE OF FALL PREVENTION

Patient falls are a considerable problem in the health care setting. Injuries resulting from a fall are considered to be a primary cause of morbidity in older adults. The loss of coordination and bone density as people age puts them at an increased risk for breaking bones after a fall; the resultant loss of independence may lead to a decline in health and eventual death. Yet falling is not a normal part of aging. Proper prevention can greatly decrease a patient's risk of falling. As a nurse aide, it is important to follow fall precautions to prevent patient falls within the hospital setting.

Review Video: <u>Fall Prevention</u>
Visit mometrix.com/academy and enter code: 972452

NECESSARY SAFETY PRECAUTIONS FOR BED-BOUND PATIENTS

Patients who are bedridden have a particularly high risk of falling.

- While the patient is in bed, make sure the side rails are up to prevent the patient from climbing out of bed.
- If necessary, a bed alarm may be placed in the bed to alert the nurse aide that the patient is attempting to get out of bed without assistance.
- The patient's call light should be placed within reach, as well as the patient's tray table and any other items the patient might need.
- Toileting should be offered at least every two hours, and the patient should be turned every two hours to prevent bedsores.

PRECAUTIONS TO PREVENT FALLS

There are a number of precautions that can be taken to prevent patient falls.

- The first step of prevention is identifying the needs of the patient.
- If the patient has been determined to be a fall risk, a sign should be placed on the door so the staff knows the patient has special mobility needs.
- While the patient is in bed, at least two side rails should be kept in the raised position to prevent the patient from falling out of bed.
- Prior to standing with assistance, patients should be allowed to sit or dangle at the side of the bed to prevent dizziness that may result from the change in position.
- The patient should also wear rubber-soled shoes or socks.
- The floor should be kept free of all hazards, including puddles of water and small rugs that can cause slipping.
- While the patient sits in or stands up from the chair or wheelchair, the brakes should be kept locked.

PHYSICAL SIGNS AND SYMPTOMS TO MONITOR

Technologists should always monitor patients for any sign of reaction to contrast or any decline of health during a procedure. Specifically, has there been a change in the patient's level of consciousness? Is the patient alert enough to comprehend and answer questions asked? Are there any indications of hives or cyanosis when looking at the patient's skin? Is the patient's breathing of normal rate and rhythm? A patient's pulse ox can easily be monitored should the technologist find it necessary to check. Technologists should be aware of any seizures that the patient may experience. Blood pressure is yet another important vital sign to monitor along with heart rate to determine the severity of a reaction to contrast, when caring for trauma patients, or during routine monitoring of a patient during an exam. If intravenous contrast was used, check for any signs of extravasation.

MEDICATION RECONCILIATION

Medication reconciliation is an important step while obtaining a patient's history. It provides important data to clinicians about the current medications (prescription and over the counter), reasons for taking the drugs, dosage, and how often the medication is taken. Medication reconciliation is a safety measure to prevent any harm to patients but can be a difficult task as, often, patients are not able to give a complete history (unless they bring in the packages for all of their medications) and may see more than one provider. Technologists should ask patients about any medications that they are taking to make sure that there aren't any contraindications when injections or oral contrast media is to be used. Often, patients may be confused as to why they take a certain medication, so technologists should become familiar with medications to provide additional insight regarding diseases or disorders the patient may have.

IMPLEMENTATION OF PROPER ERGONOMIC TECHNIQUES FOR ULTRASOUND LAB

Ultrasound managers are aware of the astronomical costs associated with new employee hiring, training, and workers' compensation claims. Ergonomics awareness is a must in the ultrasound lab in order to maintain a sonographer's health and avoid work-related musculoskeletal injuries. Often, these injuries are career ending (20%), and almost 75% of sonographers tend to have symptoms of pain, numbness, tingling, swelling. These symptoms do not occur only while scanning; they may also be felt throughout the day and while away from the lab. These injuries are difficult to treat especially if sonographers continue to scan the same way. Employers must make sure that their staff has the equipment necessary to prevent these injuries from occurring along with continuing education concerning these risk factors. An imaging manager should allow for breaks between ultrasound exams to give each employee time to stretch. The number of exams should be closely monitored so that injuries do not occur as a result of inadequate rest time. The ultrasound lab should also be equipped with ergonomic tables and chairs, and the machine itself should be adjusted so the staff can safely and comfortably perform exams.

PROPER BODY MECHANICS TO PREVENT PERSONNEL AND/OR PATIENT INJURY

Because patients are often ill or physically impaired and equipment can be heavy or bulky, it is important that a technician understands the basics of proper body mechanics so as not to injure themselves or the patient when moving a load. The basics of body mechanics are the same whether the load is a person or piece of equipment. Personnel must assess if the load can be lifted alone, with mechanical help, or with the help of another person. When moving anything, it is important to maintain a wide stance with a straight back and lift with the knees. Keeping the load close to your body and being sure that there is nothing that will impede movement will assure proper transfer of the load. When transferring a patient to or from a wheelchair or bed, always check to see if the wheel locks are set. Finally, make sure you clearly explain to the patient what you are going to do so that they do not hinder the move.

PROPER TECHNIQUE FOR FALLING WITH A PATIENT

Even with all necessary precautions properly observed while ambulating, the patient is still at risk for falling. A fall may result if the patient's legs give out from under him or if he were to lose consciousness while ambulating. If a sudden fall were to occur, it is important to protect the patient and yourself from harm.

- Support the patient using the gait belt and your free arm, and gently lower the patient to the floor or to a nearby chair, taking care to protect the patient's head.
- If the fall is uncontrolled as a result of loss of balance, focus on supporting the patient as much as possible while keeping yourself safe.
- Try to avoid tensing up prior to impact as this may cause additional injury.

DEVICES TO PROMOTE PATIENT SAFETY

Common devices to promote patient safety include:

- **Lifts**: Utilizing lifts, such as the Hoyer lift, to assist in moving and lifting patients reduces the risk of falls and injuries.
- **Assistive devices**: Various assistive devices, such as canes, walkers, wheelchairs, grabbers, reaching devices, and medication dispensers, help to prevent falls, facilitate mobility, and promote safety.
- **Alarms**: Many types of sensors with alarms are available, including floor mat sensors, chair sensors, seatbelt sensors, and movement sensors. Door alarms may sound when doors are opened to alert staff.
- **Wander management systems**: Systems such as *Wanderguard®* and *RoamAlert®* require the patient to wear a device (such as a bracelet) that contains a locator and may also have a door controller to automatically lock doors as the patient approaches them or to sound alarm if the patient passes through an open door.

PATIENT COMFORT

Many procedures can be uncomfortable due to equipment and positioning. This can be made worse by the illness or injury of the patient. It is the responsibility of personnel to ease discomfort as much as possible. This includes the use of cushions, pillows, and sponges, as well as positioning considerations. A technician should also attend to basic patient needs such as allowing them going to the bathroom (and assisting when necessary), providing drinking water, warm blankets, a damp cloth, lip balm, and necessary personal cleanliness. If the patient is uncomfortable in any way, they are more likely to move and movement can compromise the quality of the image making a repeat procedure necessary. Thus, by making a patient as comfortable as possible, you enhance both the patient's experience and the quality of the image.

MEDICAL EMERGENCIES ASSOCIATED WITH PATIENT SAFETY AND INFECTION CONTROL

Patients who are hospitalized, seen in the emergency room, or treated on an outpatient basis should be monitored in case a medical emergency arises. All technicians and hospital personnel caring for patients should be trained in basic cardiac life support. In addition, the hospital should have an emergency response system and protocol in place that any technician and/or health care practitioner can initiate, which may involve a hospital emergency response team or protocol. Health care practitioners and technicians should be trained in the protocol and system to be put into effect if a medical emergency occurs when caring for or performing a diagnostic approach on a patient.

LATEX ALLERGY

Latex products can cause mild to sever allergic reactions in patients. The reaction can be to the proteins in the latex itself, or to the other chemicals added to latex in processing. There are three types of reactions that can occur when a person is sensitive to latex products:

- Irritant Contact Dermatitis – Mild skin irritation that is characterized by dry, itch areas. This is not considered a true allergic reaction.
- Allergic Contact Dermatitis – Also called delayed hypersensitivity. Usually occurs 24-48 hours after exposure. Causes a rash to oozing blisters.
- Latex Allergy – Also called immediate hypersensitivity. Occurs within minutes to hours after exposure. Reaction can be mild to serious.

Common medical equipment that could contain latex are disposable gloves, tourniquets, blood pressure cuffs, stethoscopes, IV tubing, oral and nasal airway tubing, enema tips, endotracheal tubes, syringes, electrode pads, catheters, wound drains, and injection ports.

SURGICAL ASEPSIS

There are basic principles that govern surgical asepsis. They are in place to help keep an environment sterile, thus preventing and controlling the spread of infection. The most important (and basic) principle is that sterile objects remain sterile only when they come into contact with other sterile objects. No matter how clean the object it comes into contact with is, if it is not sterile, it should be considered a contaminant. If you are not sure if an object is sterile, or if the object is out of your field of view, it should be treated as contaminated.

ASEPTIC AND STERILE TECHNIQUES OF VENIPUNCTURE

During the physical act of administering medication, the practitioner should be aware of the basic tenets of sterilization. The medication or contrast agent must be injected with consideration for power injectors, other comparable methods, extravasation and treatment, and use of an IV pump. Any adverse reactions to contrast dyes, latex, or sedation and the treatment required for such reactions should be analyzed and included in the patient's documentation. The practitioner should always adhere to aseptic techniques and should verify that the area is free of pathogenic microorganisms so that infection can be prevented, according to the standards and guidelines set forth by the medical facility in which the venipuncture is being performed. All medical facilities must meet certain health codes regarding asepsis.

COMMUNICABLE INFECTIONS AND NOSOCOMIAL INFECTIONS

Communicable Infection - An illness caused by the direct or indirect transmission of a specific infectious agent or the toxins it produces from an infected person, animal, or inanimate host to a susceptible body; indirect transmission can be via a vector, intermediate plant or animal host, or the inanimate environment.

Nosocomial Infection - Hospital-acquired illness not resulting from the original reason for the patient to be admitted.

CYCLE OF INFECTION

The cycle of infection starts with the presence of a pathogen (a disease-causing organism) and an environment that allows it to grow and multiply. Aside from being able to grow and multiply, the conditions must allow it to be passed on (transmission) from one organism (host) to another. Transmission can be either direct or indirect. Direct transmission occurs when the infection is passed from one infected host to another. There are several different possible modes of indirect transmission. An object can become contaminated and a person becomes infected when they touch the contaminated object (called a fomite). A vector can be employed by the pathogen, infecting an intermediate host where it can multiply and develop before being passed on to a new host. The pathogen can become airborne before finding a new host to infect. In any mode of transmission, there must be a way for the pathogen to enter the new host and the host must be susceptible to the infection.

RESERVOIR

Medical professionals must understand all components of the cycle of infection to prevent the spread of disease. All of these factors must be present for an infection to transpire: an **infectious agent**, a **reservoir host**, **portal of exit**, **method of transmission**, **route of entrance**, and a **susceptible host**. The first aspect takes place when a microorganism (pathogen) latches onto a living host. This living host is referred to as a reservoir host and may be a human, an insect, or even an animal. A reservoir's body will offer the proper nourishment for the pathogen for it to live and/or proliferate. When humans serve as the reservoir hosts, they become carriers of the disease but are often oblivious that they have been infected and can easily transmit the disease to other people. When there is evidence of a disease in a reservoir host, one may be more aware of hand washing and other methods to prevent the spread of disease.

PORTAL OF ENTRY

A portal of entrance is the fourth step that must take place for an infection to occur known as the cycle of infection. As the microorganism exits the reservoir host, it must have an entrance portal to infect the susceptible host. Examples of entrance portals are similar to exit routes and include any mucous membrane such as the nose, mouth, rectum, or vagina. These pathogens can also enter via the integumentary system when the skin is no longer intact. The eyes are yet another entrance portal, and conjunctivitis is a very contagious disease that is spread via this entrance method. Urinary tract infections are another common infection seen, especially in females. This occurs as bacteria from the rectum are transferred to the urethra because of the close proximity of these structures. It is important to practice proper hygiene whether it is wiping after using the toilet or hand washing to prevent the transfer of bacteria and other pathogens.

PORTAL OF EXIT

The second step that must take place for an infection to occur is that the reservoir host provides a portal of exit. This describes the method in which the microorganism leaves the reservoir host to continue on to infect another organism, known as the susceptible host. The most prevalent avenues for exiting the body are via the mouth, nose, blood, urine, vaginal or seminal fluid, feces, and even the eyes. Often the portal of exit is the exact same as the entrance portals, which is the fourth step in the cycle of infection.

SUSCEPTIBLE HOST

A susceptible host is the fifth and final component in the cycle of infection. A susceptible host is an individual that is unable to fight off an infection and will enable the cycle to continue when this individual passes the pathogen onto another person. There are many factors that determine whether the susceptible host will become infected. These may include the strength of the immune system, overall health, and level of nourishment. Age is another important factor as infants and the elderly are more susceptible to certain diseases. Hygiene practices as well as living conditions are yet another determining factor that may induce an infection. For example, perhaps the host employs great hand-washing techniques but is forced to wash with water that is contaminated while living in a house with rodents and insects. Sometimes the susceptible host, regardless of how healthy he or she is, may be infected with a microorganism so potent that the host is unable to fight it off even with a strong immune system.

MODES OF TRANSMISSION

DROPLET

Droplet (mucous) particles may be transmitted when the reservoir host sneezes or coughs. It is known that the reservoir host does not need to be in close proximity to the susceptible host as droplet particles can travel several feet in the air. Respiratory diseases such as influenza and tuberculosis may be transmitted via a direct airborne method when the susceptible host inhales the droplets of the infected person. These types of infections may sweep through a population rapidly, so it is important to practice proper techniques to prevent airborne transmission. This includes coughing or sneezing into a tissue when possible. If a tissue is not available, one should sneeze or cough into the crook of the elbow and then perform proper hand washing. Often, patients who have a respiratory infection are asked to wear a mask to prevent the spread of infected droplets.

DIRECT CONTACT

Bloodborne transmission may occur by direct mode if blood from the infected reservoir host comes into contact with the susceptible host's mucous membranes or when the integrity of the skin is compromised. Healthcare workers must always practice universal precautions and utilize personal protective equipment (PPE) such as gloves, gowns, masks, eye protection, and face shields to prevent blood from reaching these mucous membranes or from getting into any cut in the skin. The most common bloodborne pathogens that may be transmitted in a healthcare setting are hepatitis B (HBV), hepatitis C (HCV), and the human immunodeficiency virus (HIV). Healthcare professionals should assume and treat all bodily fluids as if they are contaminated, and any PPE should be managed and disposed of properly. Another example of direct transmission is when a pregnant female passes on a sexually transmitted infection (STI) onto her baby via the placenta or during a vaginal delivery, such as gonorrhea, herpes, or syphilis.

AIRBORNE MODE

The spread of microorganisms can take place when particles are dispersed from the respiratory system of the reservoir host and inhaled by another individual. This is known as airborne transmission. An example of airborne transmission is inhaling droplets when an infected individual coughs or sneezes. It is known that people do not need to be located right next to each other as these droplets are capable of traveling several feet following a cough or sneeze. This is a common method in which influenza, tuberculosis, or even chickenpox is spread. People may also become ill after the inhalation of bacteria or fungi within water that is contaminated. One example of this type of airborne infection is Legionnaires' disease. This is not spread from person to person but rather when somebody inhales water droplets that contain the bacteria. This is often heard of in contaminated water supplies such as in hotels, resorts, or air-conditioning systems of apartment complexes.

VEHICLE-BORNE FOMITE

A fomite is referred to any inanimate object that can spread a pathogen from one person to the next. Common examples of fomites that aid in the transmission of disease are doorknobs, drinking fountains, water glasses, pens, toys, books, and shopping carts. With these examples, it is easy to see why schools or child-care centers can readily spread germs among individuals. Note that this transmission is carried out in an indirect fashion as body membranes do not need to touch each other. Examples of vehicle-borne fomites in the medical industry could be instruments used in clinical care settings such as tools used for surgical procedures or patient care. Other examples of a vehicle-borne fomite in the medical field could be blood, biopsy specimens, or organs and tissues used for transplants or grafting material.

VECTOR-BORNE MECHANICAL OR BIOLOGICAL MODE

A vector-borne method of transmission occurs when pathogens are spread from one living organism to another. Vectors are commonly insects that act as couriers that transport bacteria and other common pathogens from one individual to the next. Examples of vectors are mosquitoes, flies, ticks, and fleas. Mosquitoes are known for spreading West Nile virus. Flies can mechanically transmit disease as they continuously land on food and people. Infected ticks are widely known for spreading Lyme disease when they bite a person. Another disease that ticks may spread is Rocky Mountain spotted fever, which may be deadly if not diagnosed correctly. Fleas are the culprits in transferring pathogens that allow people and animals to contract the plague. Mosquitoes, ticks, and fleas tend to fall under the biological mode of transmission as they tend to become infected because they feed on the blood of their hosts.

INFECTION PREVENTION AND CONTROL

UNIVERSAL/STANDARD PRECAUTIONS

Universal (also called standard) precautions were developed in 1991 when, to help prevent and control the spread of infection, OSHA (Occupational Health Administration) and the CDC (Centers for Disease Control) mandated that every patient and specimen be treated as if it is contaminated. These precautions apply to all blood and bodily fluids (including peritoneal, amniotic, vaginal, seminal, cerebrospinal, synovial and saliva, pleural and pericardial fluids). Care should be taken when handling any of these fluids, or items contaminated with these fluids. Personal protective equipment (PPE), hand washing, and preventative measures should be employed.

MEDICAL ASEPSIS

In order to prevent or control the spread of infection, the cycle of infection must be broken. The cycle of infection refers to the conditions that allow infection to spread. These conditions (presence of pathogen, growth and reproduction, transmission to host, susceptibility of host) must all be present in order for an infection to exist. Medical asepsis (also called clean or aseptic technique) refers to cleanliness practices in a non-sterile environment. The point is to remove as many pathogens as possible from the environment and prevent the spread of those that do exist. The biggest thing that can be done in medical asepsis is the washing of hands. The basic technique of hand washing is the use of warm water, antiseptic cleaner, the removal of jewelry, and specific cleaning of fingernails. Hands should be washed before and after contact with a patient, after contact with organic materials or contaminated equipment, after removing sterile or non-sterile gloves.

CONTACT ISOLATION PRECAUTIONS

Standard/Universal precaution measures should always be used when coming into contact with patients and bodily fluids. Certain diseases, however, require more stringent isolation precautions because of their highly contagious nature. Infections of MRSA, Salomonella, E. coli, hepatitis A, severe herpes simplex, lice, and scabies all require contact isolation precautions. These precautions require that gloves and gown always be used when entering the patient's room. Gloves must be changed when they come into contact with infectious material. Essentially, there should always be a barrier (gloves, mask, gown) between you and the patient, and the barrier material must be disposed of properly

DROPLET, AIRBORNE, AND REVERSE ISOLATION PRECAUTIONS

Droplet isolation precautions should be used when coming into contact with diseases that are spread by droplets (includes meningitis, Mycoplasma pneumonia, rubella, group A strep). Patients should be placed in private rooms. Masks and gloves must be worn when treating the infected patient, and gloves worn when coming into contact with every patient. Airborne isolation precautions should be used for tuberculosis, measles, and varicella. These are diseases that are spread by microscopic particles that must be filtered out of the air with special equipment. Patients must be completely isolated in negative pressure rooms. Contact precautions (gloves, gowns) must be employed and respiratory masks worn when in the infected patient's room. Reverse isolation precautions are designed to protect a patient from the healthcare worker. They are employed in cases when a patient is immunocompromised (leukemia patient, organ transplant patient). These patients should be isolated in positive pressure rooms that keep outside air and contaminants away from them.

BLOODBORNE PATHOGENS

Bloodborne pathogens are microorganisms in the blood or other body fluids that can cause illness and disease in people. These microorganisms can be transmitted through contact with contaminated blood and body fluids. The majority of the population immediately refers to the HIV virus or AIDS when defining bloodborne pathogens. However, hepatitis B and C are much more common in the medical setting.

EXPOSURE IN MEDICAL PROFESSIONALS

A medical professional can be exposed to bloodborne pathogens by accidental puncture wounds from needles, scalpels, broken glass or razor blades. An individual can also be exposed if contaminated body fluids come into contact with an open wound on the skin. The hepatitis B virus can actually be transmitted indirectly when a medical professional touches dried or caked-on blood and then touches the eyes, nose, or mouth.

DISPOSAL OF BIOHAZARDOUS MATERIALS

Biohazardous materials include anything that has been soiled with blood or other bodily fluids. They must be placed in special biohazard waste receptacles so that they can then be disposed of properly. Sharps must be placed in the designated sharps container. Radioactive material must be allowed to decay before being disposed of. None of these items are a part of the normal trash pick-up. In fact, facilities spend large sums of money on biohazardous waste disposal. Heavy fines are the result if not disposed of properly. Biohazardous waste disposal is regulated by the EPA (Environmental Protection Agency), OSHA (Occupational Health Administration), and NRC (Nuclear Regulatory Committee).

SAFE HANDLING OF CONTAMINATED EQUIPMENT AND SURFACES

There are levels of disinfection for contaminated medical equipment and surfaces. These factors largely depend on equipment manufacturer guidelines and whether the supplies can be heat sterilized. High-level disinfection is one method that can be used for equipment that cannot be sterilized with heat, but it is not appropriate for surface disinfection. Regardless of which level necessary, all items are to be rinsed, sanitized, and then per the vendor's suggestions utilize only the disinfecting agents mentioned. Products used for high-level disinfection are considered to be sporicidal agents, are extremely virulent, and should also be rinsed with water and dried after the chemicals are used. Intermediate-level disinfection will kill tuberculosis but will not be effective at eliminating the bacterial spores. Low-level disinfection is used for surface areas and instruments such as stethoscopes, blood pressure cuffs, electrocardiogram (EKG) leads and wires, and so on that do not touch the mucous membranes of the patient.

DISINFECTANTS AND ANTISEPTICS

Disinfectants are used to kill possible pathogens. They are bactericidal corrosive compounds composed of chemicals. Some disinfectants are capable of killing viruses such as HIV and HBV. These are not used on humans to disinfect skin. A common disinfectant is bleach in a 1:10 dilution. Antiseptics are chemical compounds that inhibit or prevent the growth of microorganism microbes usually applied externally. Antiseptics attempt to prevent sepsis but do not necessarily kill bacteria and viruses. Antiseptics are used on human skin. Common antiseptics include 70% isopropyl alcohol, betadine, and benzalkonium chloride with isopropyl alcohol being the most commonly used. Betadine is used when a sterile draw is needed.

EQUIPMENT STERILIZATION

Equipment must be sterilized if it will be used during any procedure that requires a sterile field. Instruments that can be sterilized are typically stainless steel and hold up well to sterilization techniques to be used again. The most common method of sterilization for tools used in the medical industry is an autoclave. This method utilizes steam and pressure to rid the tools of any microorganisms that are present. Once a procedure has ended the tools must first be rinsed, sanitized, and dried per the department's protocols. Some tools must then be wrapped in a special paper that is porous enough for the moisture to reach the tools or placed in special pouches that may be placed in the autoclave. The autoclave typically has presets that can be chosen pertaining to the materials used. Once the cycle is finished, be sure to place the tools in a cool, dry place, and be cognizant of the expiration date as many will expire after 30 days.

DISINFECTION OF ENDOCAVITY PROBES

Sonographers can prevent nosocomial (hospital-acquired) infections by using probe covers when using an endocavity transducer. Once the protective covering is applied, the user should look for any tears or cracks. Upon removal from the body, the probe cover is removed, excess gel is wiped off, and the transducer is disinfected with a germicide. This process is considered to be high-level disinfection. CIDEX OPA is a common disinfectant agent used in ultrasound labs for endocavity transducers (see the solution information regarding the amount of time necessary for disinfecting). Regardless of the type of transducer used, it is important to properly disinfect between patients. For those transducers that are not inserted into a patient, a low-level disinfection will suffice. The ultrasound manufacturer will recommend certain solutions to prevent damage to transducers.

EQUIPMENT DISINFECTION

The majority of supplies utilized in clinical settings tend to be disposable, but for those that can be reused, they must be properly disinfected or sterilized prior to another procedure. There are different levels of disinfection, but high-level disinfection is used when the equipment used has possibly been exposed to human immunodeficiency virus (HIV), hepatitis B virus (HBV), or hepatitis C virus (HCV). The steps for proper disinfection are as follows: remove equipment from the patient, remove any protective cover from the equipment, wipe off any excess fluid, rinse under water while using a soap containing a germicidal solution, immerse (when allowed) equipment into disinfecting agent for the suggested time (check equipment manufacturer for suggested disinfection solutions), rinse with water, and dry. Caution must be taken to allow enough time between patients for the equipment to be properly disinfected.

STANDARD PRECAUTIONS, TRANSMISSION-BASED PRECAUTIONS, AIRBORNE PRECAUTIONS, DROPLET PRECAUTIONS, AND CONTACT PRECAUTIONS

Standard precautions are guidelines that should be followed to prevent exposure to blood or body fluids from all patients. These provide standards for protective gear to be worn, disposable of sharps, cleaning body fluid spills, and isolation room guidelines.

Transmission-based precautions are used when a specific disease state is known. They are guidelines followed to prevent transmission of this disease. An example of this would be the isolation room requirements and protective gear used when caring for patients with tuberculosis.

Airborne precautions outline the procedures to prevent transmission of diseases which are transmitted through the air. This includes any special masks that should be worn. An example of this is chicken pox (Varicella virus).

<u>Droplet precautions</u> outline what guidelines should be followed to prevent transmission of diseases which are transmitted by exposure to respiratory droplets. An example of this is tuberculosis.

<u>Contact precautions</u> are followed when caring for patients who have diseases that are transmitted through contact with the individual. An example of this is a MRSA skin infection.

INFECTION-CONTROL PROCEDURES FOR PATIENT AND TECHNICIAN

The technician must practice good hand-washing techniques from patient to patient. Masks may be worn for suspected fluid splatter as well as gowns or goggles. Disposal of fluid soaked linen, garbage, or specimens must be handled carefully and following the institution's policies. The sonographer may need to follow specific isolation precautions depending on the patient and the diagnosis. The scanning probe and transducers must be cleansed with appropriate cleaners; taking care to clean the cords, cable, and head of the transducer. It is usually advised to use a partial bleach solution to clean equipment and carts, counters, and sinks after completion of the examination and when the patient has left. The technician is responsible for knowing how to provide sterile techniques when appropriate.

IMPORTANT TERMS

Statute of Limitations—A law defining the maximum period the complainant or appellant can wait before filing a lawsuit. The limitation date varies according to the type of case and if it falls within state or federal jurisdiction. Usually, the limitation is 1 to 6 years. Homicide has no limitation. If the complainant misses the deadline, then the right to sue is "stats barred" (dead). Rarely, a judge will "toll" (extend) the deadline if the injury was discovered late or a trusted person hid misuse of funds or failure to pay. Minors' rights to bring negligence charges are tolled until the age of 18.

Assumption of Risk—(A.) A defense against an accusation of negligence. The defendant states the situation was obviously hazardous, so the complainant should have realized injury could result. (B.) An insurance company takes the risk of extending coverage, realizing the policyholder might make a claim, but it is statistically more likely to make a profit from the premiums.

Arbitration Agreement—The patient agrees to give up the right to sue the doctor. An arbiter (arbitrator) awards damages if injury results. Settlement is faster for the patient, and the doctor gets a malpractice insurance discount. Both parties save on legal fees.

Negligence—Taking an unreasonable, careless action that could foreseeably cause harm. Failing to exercise due care for others that a prudent, reasonable person would do. Negligence is *accidental*. Negligence is not an intentional tort, such as trespass or assault. Business errors, miscalculations, and failure to act can be negligent.

Contributory Negligence—If a person is injured partially because of his/her own negligence—even if it is slight—then the person who caused the accident does not pay *any* damages (money) to the injured person. Forty-four states recognize that applying the rule of contributory negligence could lead to unfair acquittal of genuinely negligent defendants, so they now use a comparative negligence test as a more balanced approach. In the 6 states that still have contributory negligence rules, juries tend to ignore it as unfair.

Comparative Negligence—A rule used in accident cases to calculate the *percentage* of responsibility of each person (joint tortfeasors) directly involved in the accident. Damages (money compensation) are awarded based on a complex formula.

Defamation—Defaming a person exposes him or her to public ridicule or tarnishes his or her memory through untrue and malicious statements. The defamed person can lose business due to loss of his or her good name.

Slander—*Oral* statements that damage someone's reputation. It is a form of defamation.

Libel—A *written* statement that harms an individual's character, name, or reputation. A defamatory libel statement may be true, but is published maliciously (without just cause).

Invasion of Privacy—Unsolicited or unauthorized exposure of patient information.

Malpractice—Professional misconduct, resulting in failure to provide due care. Most malpractice lawsuits are related to professional negligence, the failure to perform what is considered standard care.

Fraud—Intentional dishonesty for unfair or illegal gain.

Assault and Battery—Assault is declaring or threatening your intent to touch a patient inappropriately or to cause physical harm. Battery is the actual act of inappropriate touching.

Physical Principles of Ultrasound

TRANSDUCER DESIGN IN IMAGING AND NONIMAGING TRANSDUCERS

One of the main differences in transducer design for imaging and nonimaging transducers is that imaging transducers contain a layer called backing material. This is used to create short pulses by inhibiting the amount of time that the PZT crystals are vibrating. Short pulses create diagnostic quality images, but the layer of backing material tends to lessen the sensitivity. Nonimaging transducers do not contain this backing material; therefore, they either produce a wave that is continuous, or they tend to have very long pulses. Neither of these two types will be effective in producing an ultrasound image. Probes that are capable of producing diagnostic-quality exams are referred to as low Q (quality factor), and they have a wide bandwidth.

MATCHING LAYER

A transducer is shaped similar to a cylinder and changes one form of energy into a different form. The matching layer is located in front of the transducer's active element (PZT). Gel along with the matching layer serves to improve the propagation of sound into the body as well as add extra protection to the PZT crystals. Because PZT has an impedance of nearly 20 times more than the impedance found in skin, there must be a matching layer for sound transmission. If there was no matching layer, the sound would be reflected back to the PZT and prevent an image from ever being created. To overcome this mismatch of impedances and allow for sound transmission to occur, the thickness of the matching layer is one-fourth of the wavelength of sound within the matching layer.

TRANSDUCER PARTS

The transducer has five parts, a crystal, the matching layers, damping material, the transducer case, and the electric cable. The crystal converts the electrical voltage into sound energy to transmit and then reverses the sound energy into electrical energy when the sound beam returns or echoes back to the transducer. The matching layers lie before the transducer element and make the acoustic connection between the skin and the transducer. The damping material, such as rubber, acts as insulation and decreases extra vibrations. The transducer case houses the entire crystal, damping material, and insulation from interference with the electrical noise. The electrical cable contains the wires to conduct and transmit the electrical impulses from circuit source.

INVERSE RELATIONSHIP OF WAVELENGTH AND FREQUENCY

The definition of wavelength is the length of one cycle. Wavelength will be displayed in any unit of distance, but the usual range in diagnostic ultrasound imaging is 0.1 to 0.8 mm. Sonographers should know that the medium and the sound source are factors that determine the wavelength. Wavelength is not a control on the ultrasound system that a sonographer can change. Rather, wavelength changes when changing transducers that have a different frequency. As the frequency increases, the wavelength will become shorter. Wavelength and frequency are inversely related as long as the biologic tissue stays the same. In order to calculate the wavelength of a sound beam in soft tissue, the following formula can be used:

$$\text{wavelength in soft tissue} = \frac{1.54}{\text{frequency}}$$

Using this formula, users can also visualize the inverse relationship between the wavelength and frequency.

MAIN FREQUENCY

If a 10 MHz transducer can be bumped up to 12 MHz and lowered to 8 MHz, what will the main frequency be?

The main frequency of a transducer is the frequency that is being emitted from the probe into the body of the patient. Modern technology enables users to easily change the frequency without switching probes. In the above example, the main frequency (also known as the resonant frequency) is 10 MHz; however, the range of frequencies transmitted is 8 to 12 MHz. The bandwidth can also be determined from this example. Bandwidth refers to the frequency range within a sound beam. This can be calculated by subtracting the lowest possible frequency from the highest available frequency. In this case, the bandwidth would be $12 - 8 = 4\ MHz$. Because imaging transducers can produce many frequencies, they tend to have a wide bandwidth.

BACKING MATERIAL

Ultrasound labs use transducers that contain backing material. The backing material (also referred to as the damping element) is used to optimize the axial resolution. This is accomplished by attaching a mix of epoxy resin and tungsten particles to the back of the active element or piezoelectric lead zirconate titanate (PZT) crystal. This will decrease the length of the pulse duration because it inhibits the amount of time that the crystal will vibrate. Short pulses increase the axial resolution and create higher quality images. Nonimaging probes do not contain backing material. Using backing material will decrease the sensitivity of the transducer and create a wide bandwidth, and the result will be referred to as having a low quality factor. Continuous-wave Doppler and therapeutic ultrasound transducers are known as high-Q because they have a narrow bandwidth.

STEERING LINEAR SEQUENTIAL TRANSDUCERS

The image that is created with a linear sequential-array transducer is in the shape of a rectangle because the pulses are sent straight out from the transducer in groups. Due to the beam formers of modern phased-array technology, these transducers can be steered. These transducers are electronically steered and produce an image that is in the shape of a parallelogram when steering is implemented. Sound beams are sent out from a small arrangement of active elements on the transducer face. These transducers will never create images that are wider than the footprint.

THICKNESS OF THE MATCHING LAYER

The matching layer should be one-fourth of the wavelength of sound. This layer offers protection for the crystals because the matching layer is located in front of the active element. The matching layer is also used (along with ultrasound gel) to increase the transmission capabilities of vibrations from the PZT crystals and the tissue being interrogated. Impedance (a number that is calculated by multiplying the speed of sound by the density of the medium) influences the reflections produced as sound travels from one medium to another. The matching layer enables the ultrasound energy to make a smooth transition from the probe into the patient's body.

FOCUSING LINEAR SEQUENTIAL-ARRAY TRANSDUCERS

Earlier versions of the linear sequential-array transducers used fixed-focus techniques. This meant that either a lens was placed in front of the crystals or the active element was molded into an arc shape. In these examples, the user could not adjust them. Today's linear sequential (switched)-array transducers are electronically focused using phased technology. This technology allows the PZT crystal to send out pulses at different times. Certain returning reflections are postponed so that they don't all return to the probe at the same time. This phasing allows for signals to be returned constantly, which allows focusing at all depths.

FOCUSING TECHNIQUES FOR ULTRASOUND TRANSDUCERS

There are various techniques that are used in order to focus an ultrasound beam. Focusing is a method used to improve resolution of an ultrasound image by creating a sound beam that is narrow. External focusing using a lens is one way to improve lateral resolution. This is an example of fixed focusing or the conventional method in which a lens is embedded in front of the active element that will provide a narrow beam in the region of the focus. A more common method of fixed focusing that does not need a lens is internal focusing. This form includes a crystal that has a curved shape, but it also results in an ultrasound beam that is tapered. Electronic focusing by using phased-array technology allows the sonographer to adjust the focus. This is only available on probes that have many PZT crystals.

EFFECTS OF FOCUSING ON ULTRASOUND BEAM

When a sonographer applies focusing during an exam, many changes take place within the ultrasound beam. Focusing is used to optimize the lateral resolution of the exam. When focusing is used, the energy of the beam is concentrated into one small area (focus), thus improving the lateral resolution. An ultrasound beam that is focused will create a focal zone that is more compact than a beam that is not focused. A focused beam also tends to move the focal point closer to the face of the probe being used. This will result in a near zone that is shorter when compared to an unfocused beam. Although the ultrasound beam's shape changes, the width is also changed. The beam's diameter will diverge in the far field, but it tends to be smaller in the near zone with the smallest possible component at the focus.

PZT

The piezoelectric effect is the creation of voltage as the result of applied pressure to these piezoelectric substances. Some piezoelectric materials can be found naturally; however, lead zirconate titanate (PZT) is man-made and is the most commonly used material in transducers because it can readily be manufactured. PZT is often referred to as the active element or the crystal in an ultrasound transducer. PZT is created when a strong electrical current and heat are administered to the active element. This process creates an active element that is polarized. Depolarization can occur if the transducers are exposed to high temperatures, so sonographers should be aware that they cannot be sterilized because the crystals will lose their piezoelectric properties. The thickness of the active element should be half of the wavelength found in the active element.

IDENTICAL LINE DENSITY IN THE NEAR AND FAR FIELDS WITH LINEAR SEQUENTIAL PROBES

Curvilinear array transducers tend to create an image that appears to be sector or fan shaped. As the ultrasound beam diverges further into the body, the line density increases because there is a larger gap between every scan line. As a result of these gaps, the far field demonstrates lower lateral resolution. Linear sequential (switched) probes have a large footprint, and the shape of the image is a rectangle. The crystals in linear sequential transducers are arranged beside each other, and the pulses sent into the body will move straight ahead. Because the scan lines are evenly spaced and parallel to each other, the line density in the near and far fields will be identical.

OBTAINING LARGEST POSSIBLE FIELD OF VIEW IN NEAR AND FAR FIELDS

In order to obtain the largest possible field of view in both the near and far fields, a sonographer would want to choose a convex-array transducer. These probes are also known as curvilinear or curved-array transducers. The image display from a linear sequential probe is one that is in the shape of a rectangle because of the arrangement of the active elements. They form a straight line that directs the pulses in front, but the curved array is a sector shape that is blunted at the top. The bowed shape at the top of the image directly correlates with the curved shape of the transducer. Because these images do not form a sharp peak at the top, they tend to allow for a wider field of view in the near field as well as the far field.

ADVANTAGES OF LINEAR PHASED-ARRAY TRANSDUCERS

There are many advantages of using any transducer with phased-array technology. For example, the sonographer can electronically focus the ultrasound beam at all depths during an exam. This allows the operator to customize the ultrasound system's settings based on what is required of them. Focusing can be optimized regardless of the depth of the anatomical structure being interrogated. Steering is also controlled electronically. With linear sequential-array transducers, the part that touches the patient is flat, but the beam is sent into the body in a nonlinear fashion. In other words, the pulses can also reach structures in the body that are not directly in front of them. Linear sequential phased-array probes have very small footprints. This is great for cardiac or pediatric scanning when the user is attempting to image via the intercostal spaces.

FIRING OF PZT CRYSTALS IN A PHASED ARRAY

Transducers that offer phased-array technology are considered to be very advanced technology because they offer focusing in all planes and at all depths. Phase delays are implemented with phased-array technology. Every active element is connected to the ultrasound machine's electronic circuit component. The PZT crystals can be activated in groups to produce signals that have to be returned to the receiver. These groups of elements are excited at time intervals that are very close to the next group thus creating very small time delays.

IMAGE SHAPE WHEN USING A LINEAR PHASED-ARRAY PROBE

When a sonographer selects a linear phased-array transducer, the shape will be a sector shape that narrows to a sharp point at the top (fan shaped) although the face of the probe is flat. The footprint of a linear phased-array transducer is quite small, which enables the user to scan between the ribs; however, numerous elements are squeezed together within its compact size. The number of active elements ranges from 100 to 300. The shape of the linear phased array differs from that of a convex phased array because the curvilinear probe produces an image that is sector shaped but at the top it has a curved portion that matches the arc of the transducer face.

TRANSDUCER FORMATS USED IN REAL-TIME IMAGING

Linear array is a format offering a rectangular image of an area. It is most useful in small parts of the anatomy and in vascular imaging. It may offer additional formatting in beam steering and in virtual format, offering the ability to look at a trapezoid image shape which will give a wider view of the area. The Vector format offers a trapezoid image shape as well and is often used in abdominal, gynecological, and obstetric exams. The sector image is pie shaped and can be used in cardiac or abdominal imaging. The curved array provides a large field of view helpful in abdominal or obstetrical imaging. Modern advances to equipment and the development of specific transducers and formats help imaging to be specific and accurate.

LINEAR ARRAY TRANSDUCER AND VECTOR TRANSDUCER

The linear array transducer provides the image in a rectangle. It is used when ultrasounding small parts and for vascular imaging. Some linear array transducers can be used for beam steering, giving the ability to guide the gray scale picture more accurately. A trapezoid image shape can be displayed as well from a linear array, making the visual format wider and better for attaining measurements. A vector transducer also gives a trapezoid image and is useful in gynecological, obstetrical, and abdominal examinations. The sector picture is pie shaped, lending itself to cardiac, transcranial, and obstetrical examinations. The curved array allows for a large field of vision and is more commonly used in obstetrics.

BEAM DIAMETER AT THE PROXIMAL PORTION OF THE FAR FIELD

The far field (Fraunhofer zone) is the region that is beyond the focus. The proximal portion of the far field is the area that is located closest to the focus. In fact, half of the focal zone includes this proximal portion of the far field, and it is the narrowest portion of the ultrasound beam. This is the region that offers the best image detail, and the images that result at this depth are more accurately portrayed than those at other imaging depths. The beam tends to taper at the focus and, therefore, the proximal portion of the far field. In this area, the beam is half as wide as the diameter of the transducer and offers the greatest amount of detail.

NEAR FIELD

The shape and width of the ultrasound beam changes shape as it moves. The near zone is also known as the Fresnel zone, and it is the area located between the transducer and the focus. The diameter of the beam is the narrowest at the focus, which is at the distal portion of the near field; therefore, the beam gradually tapers as it gets closer to the focus. The width of the ultrasound beam near the transducer will be equal to the transducer diameter. At the focus, the width of the ultrasound beam is equal to half of the beam diameter. The length of the near zone is also known as the focal depth and is the region from the transducer to the focus.

SOUND BEAM'S FOCAL ZONE

The focal zone of an ultrasound beam is the section of the ultrasound beam that is surrounding the focus (focal point). Because the focal zone is a more generalized area than the actual focal point, it is located in the near and far zones of the ultrasound beam. In fact, the focal zone is divided equally so that half is within the near zone and half is located in the far zone. It is recognized that the diameter of the ultrasound wave is fairly narrow in the focal zone, so objects that are imaged are considered to be more reliable than objects visualized at other scanning depths. This is turn results in better resolution; however, keep in mind that the focal point is where the beam diameter is tapered the most, so the best resolution is located here.

PRF

Pulse repetition frequency (PRF) is the number of ultrasonic pulses occurring in one second. This value is usually expressed in kilohertz (kHz). Doppler ultrasound scanners use pulsed wave systems. The major advantages of using a pulsed wave system is that it allows measurement of depth and that the sample volume can be adjusted by the operator. For these reasons, pulsed wave ultrasound is used to provide data for color flow images. A limitation of pulsed wave ultrasound is that the maximum Doppler frequency that can be accurately measured (without aliasing) is only one half of the pulse repetition frequency.

EFFECTS ON PRP WHEN THE OPERATOR CHANGES THE DEPTH

The pulse repetition period (PRP) consists of the time the pulse is on (send) and the off time (listening) as pulses are sent out of the transducer. There is a direct relationship between the scanning depth and the PRP. If a sonographer is attempting to scan an object located deep in the body, there will be more listening (receive) time and a lower pulse repetition frequency (PRF). If the reflector being examined happens to be shallower, the PRP is shorter because the listening time is decreased. Sonographers, of course, can change the imaging depth with a control on the ultrasound system. The PRP and PRF are reciprocals of each other and have an inverse relationship.

Spatial Pulse Length

Spatial pulse length has units of distance and describes how long a pulse is from its beginning to the end. The normal value of the spatial pulse length in diagnostic ultrasound ranges from 0.1 to 1.0 mm. The pulse length depends on the sound source and the medium, but it cannot be adjusted by the ultrasound user. The scanning depth has no effect on the spatial pulse length. Operators should be aware that shorter pulse lengths produce images that are more truthful. Short pulse lengths are created when a decrease in the number of cycles is contained within the pulse. The wavelength is also determined by the sound source and the medium; therefore, if shorter wavelengths are present, then shorter pulses are created.

Duty Factor

Duty factor is the percentage or amount of time that a system is transmitting sound. The duty factor is calculated by the following equation:

$$\text{duty factor} = \frac{\text{pulse duration}}{\text{pulse repetition period}} \times 100$$

Duty factor is a calculation that has no units; rather, it will be expressed as a percentage. The ranges of duty factor for clinical imaging are from 0.002 to 0.005 or from 0.2% to 0.5%. These ranges of diagnostic ultrasound indicate that a small percentage of time is spent transmitting a pulse and a large percentage is used for listening. For continuous-wave systems, the duty factor is 1% or 100% because a signal is always being sent, but of course it cannot create an image because there are not any signals received. A system with a duty factor of 0% means that a transducer is not being used.

Increase of PRF

The duty factor is the percentage of time that a transducer is actively transmitting a signal. The pulse repetition frequency (PRF) is defined as the number of pulses sent into the body in one second. Duty factor and PRF are both affected by the imaging depth and will have a direct relationship with each other. The PRF is inversely related to the depth of the object being studied as is the duty factor. As the depth decreases, the PRF increases because new pulses are constantly being sent because the listening time is less. If the depth increases, the PRF decreases (as will the duty factor) because there is more listening time, so the return time has to be greater. If the PRF increases, the duty factor also increases because the amount of time that the system is "on" or transmitting a pulse increases.

Relationship Between Penetration Depth and Frequency

Two main items influence the amount of attenuation that a sound wave will sustain. The depth or distance that sound travels in the body is the first component. If a sound beams travel a greater distance, this will result in greater attenuation. More attenuation equates to a decrease in intensity of the sound beam. The frequency of the wave is the second item that determines the amount of soft-tissue attenuation. There is more attenuation in sound beams that have a higher frequency; therefore, lower frequency sound will provide less attenuation. Attenuation is directly related to distance and frequency. In order to provide optimal diagnostic images, one should use the highest frequency waves possible and still be able to visualize them at the depth where they are located.

Axial Resolution

Resolution refers to how precisely an object is being portrayed during a scan. Axial resolution allows the ultrasound system to distinguish between two structures that are parallel to the ultrasound beam (located in front of each other). Axial resolution will determine how close two structures can be yet correctly be portrayed as two separate reflectors on the ultrasound display.

44

Axial resolution is measured in distance, and the units are typically in millimeters. Image quality and factuality are represented with axial distances that are lower numbers. In diagnostic ultrasound, the measurements of axial resolution typically lie in the 0.1 to 1 mm range. Shorter pulses and brief pulse durations will enhance the axial resolution. Axial resolution is considered to be superior to lateral resolution because pulse lengths are shorter than the width of the beam. Axial resolution is also known as longitudinal, range, radial, and depth resolution.

Axial resolution identifies reflectors that are parallel to the ultrasound wave, and it is determined by the pulse length and duration of the pulse. If more focal zones are added, the pulse length will become longer, which can degrade the axial resolution. Shorter pulses demonstrate better axial resolution as does less ringing in the pulse. If the sonographer increases the number of focal zones, there will be better lateral resolution, however, because the width of the beam is narrow. It is important to note that if a sonographer wishes to maximize spatial resolution, this will incorporate axial and lateral resolution.

Pulses that are short will generate images with improved axial (longitudinal, range, radial, depth) resolution. Shorter pulses are established by using a transducer that offers a higher frequency, which will automatically result in shorter wavelengths. Diagnostic imaging transducers contain backing material that will limit the amount of ringing in a pulse. This is also a way to create a short pulse and improve axial resolution. Although images cannot be produced from therapeutic ultrasound or continuous wave Doppler for many reasons, one reason is that they do not incorporate backing material. As opposed to imaging transducers, they are considered to have a high quality (Q)-factor and narrow bandwidth.

CALCULATING AXIAL RESOLUTION
EXAMPLE

Calculate the axial resolution while examining structures in the body using a 3.5 MHz transducer with a pulse length of 6 mm.

The axial resolution will be equal to half of the spatial pulse length, and the following formula can be used to calculate it:

$$\text{axial resolution} = \frac{\text{spatial pulse length}}{2}$$

In this example, the pulse length is 6 mm:

$$\text{axial resolution} = \frac{6}{2} = 3 \text{ mm}$$

Depending on the available information, the axial resolution may also be calculated by the following formula:

$$\text{axial resolution} = \frac{\text{wavelength} \times \text{number of cycles in the pulse}}{2}$$

To determine the axial resolution in soft tissue:

$$\text{axial resolution} = \frac{0.77 \times \text{number of cycles in the pulse}}{\text{frequency}}$$

Remember: When the axial resolution is calculated to be a lower number, better image quality will be demonstrated because the pulses are short.

LATERAL RESOLUTION

Resolution refers to how precise an object is being portrayed during a scan. Lateral resolution allows a user to visualize two distinct reflectors when they are perpendicular to the sound beam and lying beside each other. This type of resolution will determine how close two structures can be to each other and still be visualized as two separate objects on the ultrasound display. The units of lateral resolution will be any form of a distance measurement. Values that are smaller will represent echoes that are more precise. The narrowest part of the beam (focus) is where the lateral resolution will be optimal. Lateral resolution is also known as angular, azimuthal, and transverse resolution.

The lateral resolution tends to change with the depth of the ultrasound beam. However, the region of the sound beam in which the lateral resolution is the best is at the focus. At the focus, the beam is, of course, the narrowest. Lateral resolution refers to just how close two objects can be to each other while lying perpendicular to the sound beam where the system can determine that they are separate reflectors instead of one. At the focal point, the objects will be further away from each other than the diameter of the beam, so it is possible to discern two separate structures. Sonographers should be aware that lateral resolution is equal to the beam diameter and smaller values imply better lateral resolution. If the scan line density is increased, the lateral resolution will be enhanced. Values that are higher will reveal image quality with less detail.

IMPROVING THE FRAME RATE DURING A COLOR DOPPLER STUDY

Sonographers can adjust many controls on the system pertaining to the use of color Doppler and frame rate during an exam. In order to optimize the temporal resolution, the user needs to be aware of the size and location of the color box. The color box will allow the velocity information to be portrayed as an overlay of color on the traditional grayscale image. As the color box size increases, the frame rate or temporal resolution decreases as more information needs to be processed. This is especially important when considering the width of the color box. More scan lines are required with a wider color box, and more time is required by the system to process the acquired data. The sonographer should limit the size of the color box to the anatomy of interest. The location is also something to consider because a deeper location may actually produce aliasing of the color flow because the PRF is lower.

EFFECTS OF IMAGING DEPTH ON FRAME RATE

The frame rate refers to the capability of an ultrasound system to produce multiple frames per second. Temporal resolution, which shows how precisely an object in motion, is portrayed from one second to the next and is decided by the frame rate. The frame rate depends on the imaging depth because a reflector that is deeper in the body will result in a longer time of flight to return to the transducer. A structure that is deeper in the body results in a lower frame rate, which tends to degrade temporal resolution. If a structure is located more superficially or more shallow, the time of flight is shorter, which results in a higher frame rate and better temporal resolution. Depth can be controlled by the ultrasound user.

ELEVATIONAL RESOLUTION

Resolution refers to how precise an object is being portrayed during a scan. Elevational resolution takes into account the portion of the beam that is perpendicular to the ultrasound wave and is also referred to as the slice thickness. Slice thickness determines if the returning signals are actually located above or below the imaging plane because sometimes, they will look as if they are within the beam. Sonographers are aware that the ultrasound beam is not a uniform shape, but rather it varies with depth and takes the shape of an hourglass. Because of this shape, some echoes may be included in the return signal, but they are actually located either above or below the ultrasound beam. Blood vessels or cysts may appear as if they are filled in due to the wider slice thickness. This happens when tissues that surround the blood vessel or cyst are being included in the image being sent back to the display.

PHASED ARRAY WITH A CRYSTAL THAT IS DEFECTIVE

If a sonographer is using a convex phased-array transducer, the image will appear as a sector shape that is blunted at the top. If that probe has a defective element, the user will visualize a vertical band of dropout directly under the affected crystal. A convex (curvilinear) probe contains numerous (120–250) pieces of active elements arranged beside each other in a curved line. The PZT elements are activated in groups sending out beams that are straight ahead, but the arced shape creates beams that are sent out in various directions. Linear sequential arrays are always parallel to each other because of the flat shape of the probe. If a sonographer is using an annular phased-array transducer with one ring that is damaged, there will be a horizontal band of dropout across the ultrasound image.

IMAGE PRODUCED WHEN USING A TRANSDUCER THAT HAS MALFUNCTIONED

If a sonographer is using a linear sequential (switched) array transducer with a defective piezoelectric crystal, there will be vertical dropout on the screen beneath the active element that has been affected. Recall that the image created by a linear sequential probe is in the shape of a rectangle. The pulses sent into the body are fired in groups at different times, but at various locations along the transducer's footprint. These groups of pulses that are transmitted are sent out in a linear fashion and spaced evenly from each other, so the only part of the image that is affected stems from the scan lines created by the piezoelectric crystal that has been damaged. If a sonographer is using a convex phased array transducer the image will appear as a sector shape that is blunted at the top. If this probe has a defective element, the user will visualize a vertical band of dropout directly under the affected crystal.

MECHANICAL TRANSDUCER WITH A FAULTY CRYSTAL

If a sonographer is using a mechanical transducer, it should be known that there is only one active element used to create an image. The shape of an image formed by a mechanical transducer is a sector or fan-shaped image. The beam is steered mechanically and has fixed-beam focusing because this type of transducer only has one crystal; if the crystal is damaged the user will not see an image. In other words, the image, as a whole, is lost. Mechanical transducers have been replaced by more modern transducers in which multiple active elements arranged in either a straight or curved line to send out pulses into the body. In these transducers a defective element will create either a vertical (curvilinear or linear sequential) or horizontal (annular phased array) band of dropout.

LOW-Q TRANSDUCERS

Low-Q-factor transducers are used for diagnostic pulsed-wave ultrasound because they offer improved axial resolution. Low-Q transducers contain backing material that controls the amount of ringing that takes place. By restricting the amount of ringing, shorter pulses are created. Shorter pulses will designate better axial resolution and, therefore, improved image quality. The fact that the pulses are shorter with axial resolution means that the majority of the ultrasound beam's energy will dissipate after the first couple of oscillations. Another advantage of low-Q transducers is their ability to offer multiple frequencies because of their wide bandwidth. Axial resolution offers the most accurate image in modern transducers and imaging systems. Recall that the accuracy of axial resolution is not affected by the depth of the image whereas elevational and lateral resolution is affected.

BANDWIDTH AND Q-FACTOR OF NONIMAGING AND IMAGING TRANSDUCERS

Nonimaging transducers are not capable of producing an ultrasound image. Examples of nonimaging transducers are continuous-wave Doppler that can be used to determine blood flow. Therapeutic ultrasound is another application that doesn't provide an image during use. These transducers do not contain backing material; therefore, they create long pulses. Long pulses, in this situation, refer to the length of the pulse as well as the amount of time that the crystal is excited. The lack of backing material also allows smaller reflectors to be converted more easily into electrical signals as they return to the transducer. Nonimaging transducers are considered to have a high Q-factor (quality factor), because the bandwidth tends to be narrow. Imaging transducers contain a layer of backing material. This is used to create short pulses by inhibiting the amount of time the piezoelectric crystals are vibrating. Remember that short pulses create diagnostic-quality images, but the layer of backing material tends to lessen the sensitivity. Probes that are capable of producing diagnostic-quality exams are referred to as low Q-factor and have a wide bandwidth.

FREQUENCY OF CONTINUOUS-WAVE TRANSDUCERS

The frequency of ultrasound transducers relies on how the active element is activated. These can either be determined by continuous- or pulsed-wave principles. Pulsed-wave ultrasound will send short electrical impulses that travel from the system to excite the piezoelectric lead zirconate titanate (PZT) element in the probe. In contrast, ultrasound transducers that are considered to be continuous wave tend to steadily induce an electrical impulse that activates the probe's active element. The following equation can be used to formulate the frequency:

$$\text{electrical frequency} = \text{acoustic frequency}$$

For example, if the voltage is 12 MHz, this is the electrical frequency. Therefore, the frequency of the sound beam would also be equal to 12 MHz.

PRESSURE

Pressure is an acoustic variable that helps determine which types of waves are ultrasound waves. Pressure is the amount of force within a particular area, and it can be measured in units of pascals. Pressure is directly related to intensity; therefore, if the pressure increases so will the intensity. Ultrasound is a longitudinal wave that must travel through a material in order to propagate because it is unable to travel in a vacuum. Ultrasound waves are created when an object in motion oscillates. These vibrations produce a difference in pressure or density. Compressions occur when there is an increase in pressure or density, and rarefactions take place when there is a decrease in pressure or density. Pressure energy is synonymous with potential energy in the body, and it is the principal type of energy that is present in the cardiovascular system as blood is being pumped from the heart into the blood vessels.

X-AXIS IN A B-MODE IMAGE

Recall that B-mode imaging is also referred to as brightness mode imaging. This refers to a series of dots that are processed by the machine in which the amplitude of the reflector corresponds to a white or gray dot on the image display. The x-axis is the horizontal axis, which correlates to the depth of the reflector signal that is being returned to the probe. This information is determined by the time of flight. In soft tissue, the depth can be calculated with precision when the time of flight is known. The 13-microsecond rule also applies when the ultrasound beam travels in soft tissue. It is known that it takes 13 μs for sound to travel 1 cm. If the time of flight is 26 μs, the depth of the object being imaged is 2 cm.

Most Basic Form of Real-Time or Gray-Scale Imaging

The most basic form of real-time or gray-scale imaging is known as brightness mode. This method is more commonly referred to as B-mode imaging. B-mode was the first gray-scale imaging method available. During B-mode, pulses are sent into the body and when the signal returns it appears as a dot on the screen. The amplitude or strength of the reflectors will be visualized as dots. Higher amplitudes will appear as bright-white areas on the screen. The areas that return weaker signals will be discerned as a gray dot on the image display. Even when color mode is used, the underlying image showing the actual anatomy of the patient is represented by gray-scale imaging.

M-mode Ultrasound

M-mode ultrasound refers to motion mode. The data acquired are considered to be axial with regard to the location of the transducer because these data are collected along one line of sight within the ultrasound beam. M-mode also offers information pertaining to time, which is represented by the x-axis. As the reflectors move across the screen, they are visualized as the activity is taking place at that specific instant. As the structures move from left to right across the screen, they may shift up or down. This demonstrates whether the object is moving toward or away from the transducer. The y-axis represents the depth of the objects that are in the path of the ultrasound beam. Amplitude is also reflected because some objects will have stronger returning signals than others.

X- and Y-Axes

Motion mode (M-mode) is represented by an x-axis and a y-axis. The x-axis is the horizontal portion of the display that equates to time. The vertical axis is the y-axis, and it correlates to the depth of the reflectors. The go-return time is a way to calculate the depth of the reflector. A higher go-return time correlates to structures that are deeper in the body, and smaller time-of-flight values are the result of signals that are shallower. Moving from right to left, if the tracing moves up, this indicates that the object is closer to the probe. A line that is moving down means that it is moving away from the probe. If the line is a horizontal tracing, it means that the reflector is not in motion.

Disadvantage of Pulsed-Wave Doppler

One major disadvantage of pulsed-wave Doppler is the inability to accurately measure high-velocity blood flow. When incorrectly portrayed, high-velocity flow will appear to wrap around the spectral window and look as if it is moving in the wrong direction. This phenomenon is known as aliasing and is a misrepresentation that is frequently seen with pulsed-wave Doppler. While using pulsed-wave Doppler, the sonographer should be aware of steps to take in order to eliminate aliasing. These include setting the scale as high as possible, adjusting the baseline, selecting a lower frequency, and finding a window that will be in a more shallow location. Also, it is important to note that aliasing will never take place when using continuous-wave Doppler.

PRF

The velocity scale (also referred to as the pulse repetition frequency [PRF]) is a control that sonographers are familiar with during color and pulsed-wave Doppler imaging. The PRF controls how rapidly data sampling takes place, and it will allow the ultrasound system to increase or decrease the Doppler shifts that are displayed. A high PRF enables more sampling to take place because there is less listening time between the pulses that are being transmitted into the body. It is important to have the PRF set correctly during both modalities so that aliasing does not occur. Color Doppler enables ultrasound users to determine the direction of flow when present, and it

49

requires 8 pulses/scan line. Spectral analysis allows operators to measure velocities as well as provide information about the direction and presence of flow, but it requires more effort at 256 pulses/scan line.

COLOR DOPPLER EXAM WITH A PATIENT WITH ANEMIA

If a patient is anemic, he or she has a lower than normal amount of red blood cells circulating in the blood. Some patients may be anemic because they do not have enough hemoglobin in their blood. Hemoglobin is a protein that contains iron, which transports oxygen from the lungs to all of the body's cells. A patient with anemia will still have a sufficient amount of red blood cells in their circulatory system to be able to successfully perform a color Doppler exam. For diagnostic ultrasound imaging, the main reflectors that provide information pertaining to Doppler frequencies are the red blood cells. Because the blood is constantly being transported throughout the heart and blood vessels, even a patient that is considered to be anemic will have a sufficient amount of red blood cells for a successful Doppler exam.

WHAT TO CHECK IF COLOR IS NOT DISPLAYED WITHIN A VESSEL AFTER TURNING ON COLOR DOPPLER

If color is not displayed within a vessel after turning on color Doppler, the sonographer should immediately consider the angle of the incident beam with regard to the flow angle. If the incident beam is 90 degrees to the blood vessel being interrogated, then the color will not be visualized. According to the Doppler equation, the cosine of 90 is zero; therefore, no color can be visualized. The next thing that a sonographer can do in order to improve visualization of color Doppler is to angle the color box so that the incident beam is not 90 degrees. Yet another adjustment that an ultrasound user can make is to increase the scale and the color gain in order to increase the amount of blood visualized in the vessel.

COLOR FLOW IMAGING APPLICATIONS

Red blood cells make up roughly 45% of the blood in the human circulatory system. Red blood cells supply all of the cells in the body with the necessary oxygen so they can carry out their functions. If color Doppler is applied, the reflections that are visualized are the movement of the red blood cells within the heart and blood vessels. In low-flow states, the moving blood may even be seen without turning on color Doppler. It is imperative that the user pays close attention to the color map because it will provide information pertaining to the direction the blood is moving and the velocity. If red is displayed at the top of the color map, it represents blood moving toward the transducer. If blue is on the bottom, it represents blood traveling in a direction away from the transducer.

PACKET SIZE WHEN USING COLOR DOPPLER

When sonographers are using color Doppler and are trying to decide if the packet size should be adjusted, he or she should be aware that the packet size can, in fact, be changed. The velocity of blood flow can be more true to form if the packet size is increased, but the frame rate may suffer as a result. Color Doppler requires every scan line to be pulsed more than once. The packet size (ensemble length or shots per line) represents these numerous pulses sent out for each scan line. The level of the packet size can be raised when trying to image smaller vessels that are within the venous system because the ultrasound machine will be able to detect low-flow states more readily.

PULSED-WAVE DOPPLER

Pulsed-wave Doppler is used to calculate the velocity of red blood cells that are moving within various blood vessels. From these calculations, the peak systole, end diastole, pulsatility index, and resistive index can be calculated; they provide useful information to clinicians pertaining to any pathology. The ultrasound user can choose the exact location where the measurements should be taken by placing the gate within the lumen of the vessel. The gate size can be adjusted if necessary, to get a more precise measurement. Aliasing may be a concern when using pulsed-wave Doppler, so the user may need to adjust the scale or depth of the anatomical structure being imaged, switch to a transducer with a lower frequency, or switch to continuous-wave Doppler. If the velocities are too high to be accurately measured, then the user should switch to continuous-wave Doppler to obtain the maximum velocity.

MEASUREMENT OF BLOOD FLOW VELOCITY

Spectral analysis is the technique used during pulsed Doppler to provide information pertaining to the various velocities obtained in the blood vessel or organ. Blood doesn't travel in the same direction or speed even when contained in the same sample volume. The spectral analysis window will allow clinicians to examine how the frequency shifts are dispersed within the Doppler signal. Two types of spectral analysis that are used are the fast Fourier transform (FFT) and autocorrelation. FFT is the method used to operate the spectral analysis during pulsed-wave and continuous-wave Doppler. This method can determine if the flow pattern is turbulent or if it is normal (laminar) flow. Autocorrelation is only used during color Doppler, but it is faster than the FFT method. The gate can be moved until it is where the user wants to perform a spectral analysis. The size of the gate can be changed so that it is only within the vessel that is being examined. For example, if one is sampling the carotid artery, but the spectral display is also showing venous flow, the technician will reduce the size of the gate and reposition it so only the artery is being interrogated.

ADVANTAGES AND DISADVANTAGES OF POWER DOPPLER

Power Doppler (also referred to as energy mode or color angio) is a form of color Doppler that does not display the speed of blood flow or any directional information. Rather, it only determines that a Doppler shift has taken place and shows the amplitude of the moving blood. If there are more red blood cells in one area, the signals will be brighter. Vessels represented with power Doppler will all be identical colors on the display. Advantages of power Doppler include the fact that aliasing does not occur because the speed and direction of blood flow is not applicable. Power Doppler picks up blood flow in smaller vessels and slow blood flow because of its increase in sensitivity. There is an increase in sensitivity because power Doppler is not altered by the Doppler angle. A disadvantage of power Doppler is that, due to the increased sensitivity, flash artifact may be visualized when the patient moves or breathes. Power Doppler does not evaluate the direction or velocity of blood flow. When compared to color Doppler, the temporal resolution is greatly reduced.

ULTRASOUND PHANTOMS

A phantom is a structure that contains one or more substitutes for human tissue. It is used to simulate ultrasound interactions in various parts the human body. Phantoms are used to perform numerous tasks on ultrasound equipment such as testing sensitivity, contrast resolution, axial resolution, and lateral resolution. This also includes teaching ultrasound techniques, and servicing the equipment. The most important aspect of a phantom used for ultrasound is that the speed of sound in the test object (phantom) is equal to the speed of sound in the target human tissue.

RELATIONSHIP BETWEEN DENSITY AND PROPAGATION SPEED OF SOUND IN SOFT TISSUE

Propagation speed describes how fast an ultrasound wave can travel through the body. The propagation speed depends on the medium; ultrasound waves cannot travel in a vacuum, so they must travel through tissue in order to propagate. The speed is associated with the density and the stiffness of the tissue being evaluated. The concentration of tissue within a volumetric area is referred to as the density. Density can be thought of as the weight of the medium, and tissues within the body have varying densities. There is an inverse relationship between the density of the medium and the propagation speed. This means that the denser a medium is, the slower the ultrasound wave will travel through the tissue. The speed of sound in soft tissue is about 1540 m/s.

EFFECTS OF STIFFNESS OF A MEDIUM ON PROPAGATION OF ULTRASOUND WAVE

The speed of sound is affected by the density and stiffness of a medium as it passes through a particular substance. Stiffness is also referred to as bulk modulus, and it determines how a particular medium will react when pressure is applied to it. As the stiffness of a medium increases, the velocity of sound waves moving through that material also increases. When the bulk modulus of the medium decreases; the speed of sound will be slower. Conversely, if the density increases, the speed of sound in the tissue tends to be faster. Stiffness can be thought of as a resistance to compress, and these substances are typically objects that are denser. There is a direct relationship between the stiffness of an object and the speed of propagation.

CALCULATING THE DEPTH OF AN OBJECT

Ultrasound systems can determine the depth of an object by calculating the time of flight. This time refers to the transducer sending out a pulse, and once the reflector has been identified, the signal is returned back to the transducer. The round trip of the pulse is calculated by the range equation and allows for a very precise calculation: $d = 1ct$, where d is the depth, c is the speed of sound in soft tissue, and t is the time of flight. The ultrasound system is designed to recognize the speed of sound in soft issue as 1540 m/s (1.54 mm/μs). Sonographers should realize that the time of flight is directly associated with the depth. If an object being imaged is shallow, the time of flight is short. On the other hand, if the reflector is deeper, the time of flight is greater.

HOW MUCH OF A BEAM'S INTENSITY IS TRANSMITTED IF TWO MEDIA HAVE IDENTICAL IMPEDANCE AND NORMAL INCIDENCE

Recall that incident intensity is the intensity of a sound beam prior to coming into contact with a boundary. The transmitted intensity is the forward propagation of the intensity of the incident beam after hitting that boundary. Normal incidence is when the incident sound beam comes into contact with the boundary at a 90-degree angle. Note that a reflection will only occur if the two types of tissue have different impedances; otherwise, transmission occurs. During diagnostic imaging, there is very little difference in the impedance of soft-tissue boundaries; therefore, greater than 99% of the incident beam will be transmitted. To summarize, with normal incidence (90 degrees) and identical impedance of the media, all of the incident beam's intensity will be transmitted. Keep in mind that the incident and transmitted intensities must always equal 100%.

CLEANING UP LOW-LEVEL REFLECTIONS IN THE NEAR FIELD OF A WELL-DISTENDED URINARY BLADDER

When a sonographer notices low-level reflections within the near field of a well-distended urinary bladder and would like to clean them up, he or she may do so using the reject control on the ultrasound system. On some machines, this may be known as rejection, threshold, or suppression, and it can be used to exclude weakened echoes from appearing on the ultrasound screen. Electronic noise produces low-level reflections, so the reject control can be used to reduce this noise. Because every echo must have a set minimum amplitude in order to be displayed, this control determines what that value is so that the signals are not processed, thus eliminating the noise.

IMPEDANCE WHEN DENSITY AND SPEED INCREASE

Impedance can be defined as the obstruction of the transmission of sound as it attempts to move through tissue. Impedance is the product of a medium's density and propagation speed of the medium, so if the density and speed increase, impedance will also increase. Acoustic impedance is a calculation that has an impact on the amount of reflection that occurs. If two tissue types have the same impedance, then all of the sound will be transmitted. If two tissue types have vastly different impedances, then the majority of the sound will be reflected. For example, sonographers cannot easily image an adult brain because very little sound will be transmitted through the skull. If a sonographer is imaging a soft tissue and bone interface, almost all of the sound will be reflected from the bone. In the example of an ultrasound of the adult brain, a low-frequency transducer would have to be used, which will provide images with poor detail.

INTENSITY OF THE SOUND BEAM IF DECREASED FROM THE ORIGINAL INTENSITY BY 3 dB

Decibels (dB) are a logarithmic ratio between the amplitude, power, and intensity of the ultrasound beam. Decibels are calculated by dividing the most recent intensity measurement by the original intensity measurement. A positive change in decibels indicates that the intensity of the wave is becoming larger or increasing. When there is a +3 dB change, the intensity of the wave is twice as large. A +10 dB change indicates that the intensity is 10 times greater. A negative decibel change represents a signal that is becoming weaker or decreasing. In the example above, a –3 dB indicates a reduction of the signal by half of the original intensity. If there is a change of –10 dB, it represents a reduction of the original beam by one-tenth.

SOURCES OF ARTIFACTS

Sources of artifacts:

- Acoustic interactions within tissues
- Instrumental factors (failures)
- Implanted devices
- Operator induced

Most tissue artifacts are well understood and taken into account for diagnoses.

ATTENUATION
EFFECTS OF DISTANCE

Attenuation is measured in decibels and is defined as a decrease in amplitude, power, and intensity as sound travels in the body. In soft tissue, two components that influence attenuation are the distance traveled and the frequency of the ultrasound beam. There is a direct correlation between attenuation and the distance that the sound beam navigates. There is a direct relationship between the frequency of the beam and attenuation. In other words, sound beams that are required to travel a longer distance will demonstrate greater amounts of attenuation and become weaker. Using higher frequencies will also cause greater attenuation of the ultrasound beam. A sound beam that travels a short distance will have a lesser degree of attenuation than a beam that is stronger. Lower frequency transducers will create a beam with less attenuation.

RATE OF ATTENUATION IN BONE, LUNG, AND SOFT TISSUE

Attenuation refers to the weakening of sound waves traveling through tissue. As sound travels, there will be a reduction in the intensity of the wave. When comparing the attenuation rates of tissue within the body, soft tissue will fall in the middle range. Examples of soft tissue are structures such as the liver, spleen, brain, and kidneys. The media that have the lowest rate of attenuation are bodily fluids such urine, amniotic fluid in pregnant women, and blood. Water has no attenuation when examined with low-frequency transducers. Bone tends to absorb a large portion of the ultrasound beam, which allows for a high rate of attenuation when compared to soft tissue. In the lungs, air tends to allow for the absorption of the sound wave; therefore, air is considered to have the highest attenuation rate.

COMPONENTS

Recall that as sound beams pass through the body, the intensity is diminished (as are the amplitude and power). Three components contribute to the attenuation of a sound beam: reflection, scattering, and absorption. Reflection occurs if a part of the sound beam is sent back toward the transducer. There are two types of reflection: specular and diffuse. Specular reflection takes place when there is a smooth boundary. This portion of the beam, however, does not return directly back to the transducer, but at an angle. Diffuse reflections take place at a boundary that is not smooth and tends to reflect in various directions known as backscatter. Scattering is the second component of attenuation and occurs when the energy tends to travel in many directions. One cannot predict where scattering will take place. Absorption is the third component of attenuation, and this is when the energy of the ultrasound wave is converted to heat.

RELATIONSHIP BETWEEN SCATTERING AND FREQUENCY

The correlation between scattering and frequency is a direct relationship. Lower frequency sound waves tend to result in less scatter than higher frequency waves. Higher frequency waves will scatter more than those waves that have a lower frequency. Scattering is a process that can be described as either a random or an organized modification of the direction of the sound beam. An example of organized scatter is Rayleigh scattering. This process tends to alter the direction of the sound wave 360 degrees. Rayleigh scattering also has a direct relationship with the frequency of the sound beam and can be represented by taking the frequency to the fourth power. For example, if the frequency triples, the Rayleigh scattering can be calculated by taking the frequency to the fourth power: $(3 \times 3 \times 3 \times 3) = 81$.

HALF-VALUE LAYER THICKNESS

The half-value layer thickness refers to how far sound is transmitted in order for the intensity of the wave to be reduced to half of the original intensity. The half-value layer is also known as the penetration depth or half boundary layer and describes attenuation. It can be calculated by the following formula:

$$\text{Penetration depth} = \frac{3}{\text{attenuation coefficient}}$$

Intensity is measured in decibels, so it can also be thought of as the distance that ultrasound will travel in tissue to reduce the original intensity by 3 dB. For diagnostic imaging, the range of the half-value layer is 0.25 to 1.0 cm. This thickness depends on the of the sound as well as the medium it is transmitted in. Half-value layers tend to be smaller for sound traveling at a higher frequency and those tissues that have higher attenuation rates. The half-value layer is greater for lower frequency sound and tissues that have a lower attenuation rate.

RAYLEIGH SCATTERING

Recall that scattering is an erratic, unsystematic diversion of the ultrasound beam in multiple directions. Rayleigh scattering is just one type of scattering, but instead of being erratic, the sound wave is directed in 360 degrees in an organized manner. Rayleigh scattering takes place because the actual size of the target is much smaller than the wavelength of the ultrasound beam. For example, if a sonographer can visualize blood flow in hepatic vessels without color flow Doppler, it is due to Rayleigh scattering. The red blood cells are the target of the ultrasound system, but the image may be misinterpreted because without color flow, the vessels may appear as if they are clotted. If the user decreases the frequency, then the signal amplitude of what may appear as a clot in the hepatic vessels should be less apparent. Rayleigh scattering is proportional to the frequency to the fourth power.

Intensity Limit in Which Bioeffects Are Not Developed

During an exam, the sonographer must keep the range of output intensity (or the energy of the ultrasound beam) within an acceptable level to reduce the chances of bioeffects. During an ultrasound study, the sonographer must be aware of the output intensity (or energy) of the ultrasound beam in order to reduce the chances of bioeffects to the patient. This intensity is called the spatial peak temporal average (SPTA), and it is the most pertinent intensity with regard to tissue heating. If an unfocused ultrasound beam is used, there must be a lower intensity limit set versus if a focused transducer is used. An unfocused beam is wider, and it allows more ultrasound energy to reach a greater cross-sectional area of tissue. Therefore, to compensate for the wide beam exposure to the patient, 100 mW/cm^2 is used for the intensity threshold of an unfocused beam. A focused beam intensity limit, which exposes less tissue to the energy of the ultrasound beam, is safely set at 1 W/cm^2 or 1,000 mW/cm^2.

ALARA Principle to Make an Entire Image Darker

Sonographers should always keep the as low as reasonably achievable (ALARA) principle in mind during all diagnostic imaging exams. This principle is followed in order to reduce the possibility of bioeffects during an ultrasound exam. Two controls on the machine will make an entire image darker or brighter as the result of adjusting the knob. In this example, the entire image is too bright, and the user wants to darken it. The sonographer may want to decrease the amount of receiver gain in order to darken the image. However, this is not the best step to take in order to demonstrate knowledge of the ALARA principle. Receiver gain will allow an image to become darker (or brighter), but using this control has no effect on the exposure to the patient. If one needs to darken an image while lessening patient exposure, the user should decrease the output (acoustic) power. This will result in a lower patient exposure because the strength of the voltage applied to the PZT crystals is weaker.

Thermal Index

Ultrasound should only be used for clinical exams in which the benefits outweigh the risks. One risk during an exam is an elevation of temperature in tissues exposed to the ultrasound beam. The thermal index (TI) will be highest during an exam with a high-frequency, high-intensity beam. This heating depends on exposure time and temperature. Typically, the greatest increase in temperature is witnessed with spectral Doppler exams. Pulsed-wave Doppler requires more energy than B-mode or gray-scale imaging. Ideally, the TI should be 1.0 or less and the time should be minimized to prevent tissue heating. If the TI is 1.0, it means that there is a possibility that the temperature of tissue will increase by 1 degree. TI is expressed by the soft-tissue thermal index (TIS), bone thermal index (TIB), and cranial bone thermal index (TIC).

Grayscale Imaging for Lowest Levels of Tissue Heating

It is no surprise that the lowest level of tissue heating occurs when the output intensity of the equipment being used is at its lowest numerical value. Generally, grayscale imaging is the method in which tissue heating will be the lowest. It is typically the highest when pulsed Doppler is being used. M-mode and color flow Doppler tend to fall in the middle of these intensities. One way to determine the numerical values of these intensities is to evaluate the sound wave by using a hydrophone. A hydrophone may be used by engineers to measure the output intensities as well as other characteristics of an ultrasound wave as well. The hydrophone is actually a transducer that is about the size of a needle that provides accurate values because of its compact size.

CAVITATION

The two types of cavitation that exist when the force and frequency from an ultrasound beam are applied to tissues are known as stable cavitation and transient cavitation. The mechanical index (MI) reading on the machine alerts the sonographer to the possibility that cavitation will create dangerous bioeffects within the tissue being imaged. A smaller MI number indicates that stable cavitation will occur. Stable cavitation is the increasing, decreasing, and vibration of gas bubbles located within tissue when it is exposed to variations in pressure of the sound wave. These bubbles tend to acquire much of the energy of the sound wave, but they do not rupture. Transient (normal, inertial) cavitation occurs with higher MI readings. In this situation, the microbubbles tend to rupture, creating increased pressure and temperature measurements.

HIGHLY FOCUSED BEAMS AND GREATER HEATING OF INTERNAL TISSUE

A highly focused ultrasound beam can produce a greater degree of internal tissue heating because the energy of the beam is condensed into a thin region, especially at the focus where the beam diameter is already the smallest. Although this has a positive effect on image resolution, it may increase the internal temperature of tissue. Tissue heating relates to the spatial peak temporal average (SPTA) intensity. This is a value that should be watched closely by the operator, especially during fetal scans because bioeffects must be taken into consideration. When compared to an unfocused beam, a focused beam is allowed to have a higher SPTA limit because less tissue is being exposed. The intensity limit of a focused beam is set at 1 W/cm^2 or 1,000 mW/cm^2.

APPLYING THE ALARA PRINCIPLE TO DECREASE PATIENT EXPOSURE

The as low as reasonably achievable (ALARA) principle is associated with radiation, but it is also an important rule for sonographers as well. For example, if an entire image is too bright, the most effective way to decrease patient exposure is to decrease the output power (also known as the acoustic power). By lowering the power, there is a decrease in the voltage applied to the ultrasound transducer, which, in turn, decreases the amount of energy that the patient is exposed to. A sonographer could also turn down the overall gain to prevent an image from being too bright but understand that gain has no effect on patient exposure. However, if an image is too dark, the best choice for adhering to the ALARA principle is to increase the gain because it does not affect the energy imparted to the patient.

HIGH PIXEL DENSITY FOR BETTER RESOLUTION

A pixel refers to all of the tiny boxes that will each have their own gray shade in order to make up a digital image. In order to gain an image with greater resolution, a higher pixel density is required. Pixel density is the number of boxes per inch on the display. A high pixel density will offer better resolution because there will be more pixels found in every inch of the image. This, in turn, requires the pixels to be smaller which is what is desired when trying to improve the spatial resolution. If an image has a lower number of pixels, the pixels will be larger, so the spatial resolution will not be as great. This is considered to be a low-pixel-density image.

PARAMETERS INCREASED WHEN INCREASING THE OUTPUT POWER

Increasing the output power will have an impact on many parameters. One impact is that the sonographer will be afforded the opportunity to penetrate deeper in the body of the patient. Another parameter that is adjusted is the brightness of the image. When the output power is increased, the image becomes brighter throughout the entire display. If the output power is decreased, the overall image becomes darker. Increasing the output power will force the pulser component of the ultrasound machine to increase the amount of voltage that the PZT crystals receive in the transducers. This will create stronger pulses that are sent into the tissue, which in turn, creates an image that is brighter because of the amplified signals. It is important to note that output power is also referred to as acoustic power or output gain.

13-MICROSECOND RULE

Ultrasound machines are designed to calculate the speed of the ultrasound wave in soft tissue as 1.54 mm/μs. The time of flight refers to the time it takes for a pulse to leave the transducer, hit a reflector, and return back to the transducer. The depth of the reflector can be calculated as being 1 cm when the time of flight equals 13 μs. Using this rule, if a target is 2 cm deep, the time of flight will be twice as long, equating to 26 μs. If the time of flight is 39 μs, the depth of the reflector will be 3 cm. Sonographers should be aware of the reflector depth and the total distance traveled. For example, if a question states that the time of flight was 13 μs, and it is asked what the total distance traveled is, the answer would be 2 cm. At 13 μs, the depth would only be 1 cm, but the total distance would be $1\ cm + 1\ cm = 2\ cm$.

NOISE

A sonographer should be aware of various spectral Doppler artifacts so that the results are not misconstrued. The parameters on the ultrasound machine should be understood and set correctly so that information is not lost or added to the image. Noise is one such artifact that can degrade the quality of the spectral waveform. Noise can typically be identified easily by the user and can be alleviated by reducing the amount of the pulsed Doppler gain. Noise may appear similar to spectral broadening, which could cause the interpreting physician to incorrectly diagnose it as turbulent flow. The user should turn down the gain so that the spectral window is clear, but the systolic and diastolic components can easily be visualized along with forward flow patterns.

REGIONS OF A TGC CURVE

A time gain compensation (TGC) curve has an x-axis as well as a y-axis. The horizontal x-axis refers to how much compensation is necessary for the depth of the object being imaged (y-axis). The top of the y-axis represents the patient's skin, and as it moves down, it refers to tissues that are located deeper in the body. The near gain is located superficially near the skin's surface. At this location, the structures being imaged need very little TGC because not much attenuation occurs. The slope is the middle portion of the TGC curve in which more compensation is necessary because of the greater depths. The knee is located at the distal portion of the slope and demonstrates where the most compensation will occur. The region of the far gain is distal to the knee at an ever-greater depth that also designates that the greatest amount of compensation has been offered by the machine.

OVERALL GAIN

Overall gain can also be referred to as receiver gain or the amplification of the ultrasound beam. It is a control on the ultrasound system that is used to produce a brighter or darker image. This control will affect the entire image. One should always keep the as low as reasonably achievable (ALARA) principle in mind because a sonographer can lessen the exposure to a patient if an image needs to be brightened by increasing the gain instead of the output power.

MEASURING COMPENSATION

Sonographers are aware of the term amplification. This refers to the brightness of an ultrasound signal. Amplification can be measured in decibels (dB). Compensation is a type of amplification, so it is also measured in dB. Amplification is the first process that takes place in the receiver. It will differentiate the strength of the beam as it enters and exits the receiver of the ultrasound system. The normal range for amplification of an image ranges from 60 to 100 dB. Changing only the amplification is not enough to create an image that is the same level of brightness throughout. The user must also consider adjusting the compensation. Compensation is the second process in the receiver and can be used in conjunction with amplification to create an image that demonstrates uniform brightness.

Fundamental Frequency and Harmonic Frequency

The fundamental frequency is the actual frequency that is being imparted from the ultrasound transducer and passed into the patient. This is also known as the transmitted frequency. Sometimes the ultrasound beam is altered and creates exams that are not of diagnostic quality. Modern ultrasound systems offer harmonic imaging to help increase diagnostic confidence in those difficult studies. If a sonographer uses harmonic ultrasound, the harmonic frequency used is two times higher than the fundamental (transmitted) frequency. The sound beam is altered less, and the harmonic ultrasound beam helps improve diagnostic capabilities. Tissue and contrast harmonics are two examples of the types of harmonic ultrasound used today.

Spatial Compounding Reduces Shadowing and Speckle Artifacts

Spatial compounding is a technique that requires processing to average data that are obtained from multiple angles of interrogation. This method has proven to be successful in eliminating artifacts such as shadowing and speckle. Speckle artifacts are created when the ultrasound beam is scattered after interacting with various tissues. Noise that results from speckle artifacts will make the image appear grainy, but spatial compounding improves the signal-to-noise ratio, helping to eliminate some of the noise. Spatial compounding may also suppress the amount of shadowing that is apparent in an image. This is corrected because a single transducer is able to steer the frames from multiple directions and many angles will be perpendicular to the structures, decreasing the amount of shadowing.

Reject

Reject is the last process that takes place in the receiver. This function is typically offered in two forms: one that takes place automatically and one that can be controlled by the operator. The reject function enables the user to decide if low-level echoes should be displayed within the image. Sometimes, weaker signals will offer important data for a diagnosis, but clinicians do not want noise to be present on the image. Stronger signals are not affected by reject. Some ultrasound manufactures will have other names for reject, such as suppression or threshold. Reject can decrease the amount of electronic noise that may be visualized while imaging the gallbladder or urinary bladder.

Avoiding Range Ambiguity When the Imaging Depth Is Increased

Range ambiguity is an imaging error in which the echoes have not yet been returned to the transducer before the next pulse is transmitted. If the pulse repetition frequency (PRF) is too high while scanning a structure deep in the body, range ambiguity may occur. If this happens, the system will incorrectly place the received reflections closer to the probe than their actual depth. PRF represents the number of pulses sent into the body every second, and it is presented in units of hertz (Hz). The normal range of PRF or imaging systems is 1,000–10,000 Hz. If a sonographer increases the imaging depth, the system automatically decreases the PRF in order to avoid range ambiguity. In other words, the PRF is inversely related to the imaging depth; therefore, if the scan depth is twice as deep, the ultrasound system will automatically reduce the PRF by one-half.

Contrast and Dynamic Range

The dynamic range is a ratio between the largest to smallest of intensities that can accurately be displayed by the ultrasound system. The units of dynamic range are decibels. If an ultrasound system produces an image that displays numerous shades of gray (more information), the image would be considered to have a wide dynamic range. An image with numerous shades of gray is considered to be of low contrast. On the other hand, if the system produces an image that is considered to have a narrow dynamic range, it will tend to be more black and white, and it will have fewer shades of gray. This is a high-contrast image.

IMPROVING SPATIAL RESOLUTION

Regarding improving spatial resolution, should a sonographer choose a 2000 × 2000 analog display or a 400 × 400 digital display?

Pixel stands for picture element. A pixel is the smallest portion of an image that is in a digital format. For example, a picture taken with a digital camera is made up of thousands of picture elements. Each pixel will consist of one color. Spatial resolution is a term that sonographers are familiar with, and this also applies to other digital technology. Pixel density refers to the number of pixels contained in every inch of the image. The more pixels that an image contains, the higher the spatial resolution will be. A high pixel density will dramatically improve an image whether it is on a digital camera, flat-screen TV, or ultrasound display. In this example, the terms "analog display" and "digital display" are added as additional information to throw the reader off, but if better spatial resolution is desired, the user must choose the 2000 × 2000 analog displays because of the higher pixel count.

ANALOG-TO-DIGITAL CONVERSION

There are many components of an ultrasound system that are necessary to create an image. In order, the processes that take place are the pulser, beam former, receiver, memory, and image display screen. The pulser applies voltages to the transducer in order to excite the active elements within the probe. The functions of the pulser will take place during transmission of the ultrasound beam. The beam former controls the time delays when phased array technology is used. The receiver collects the returning signals from objects being imaged so that the data can, as an end result, be viewed on the image display screen. Memory is where the information is kept until it can be displayed on the ultrasound monitor. The analog-to-digital conversion has to take place between the transducer and the memory (also known as the scan converter). The analog signals received from the transducer must be digitized before they reach the memory of the system. A computer mouse is an example of an analog-to-digital conversion.

DIGITAL-TO-ANALOG CONVERSION

There are many components of an ultrasound system that are necessary to create an image. In order, the processes that take place are the pulser, beam former, receiver, memory, and image display screen. The pulser applies voltages to the transducer in order to excite the active elements within the probe. The functions of the pulser will take place during transmission of the ultrasound beam. The beam former controls the time delays when phased-array technology is used. The receiver collects the returning signals from objects being imaged so that the data can, as an end result, be viewed on the image display screen. Memory is where the information is kept until it can be displayed on the ultrasound monitor. The digital-to-analog conversion has to take place between the memory and the image display because the signal in the memory has to be changed into an analog signal to be displayed on the television monitor. An example of a digital-to-analog conversion is an iPod.

HIGH CONTRAST

If the image displayed on an ultrasound system has a high amount of contrast, this means that the pixels are either black or white. In ultrasound images that are considered to be high contrast, very few shades of gray are visible. Sonographers should be familiar with the term dynamic range. This controls how the intensity of the signals is transformed into various shades of gray. This will either increase or limit the different shades of gray. In this example, if only black and white are created, then there is a narrow dynamic range. A dynamic range that shows many shades of gray would be considered a wide dynamic range. These images will be considered to be of low contrast. The dynamic range can be changed on the ultrasound system. If the user believes that the image is grainy, the dynamic range can be increased. If the image is too smooth, the user can increase the dynamic range.

WRITE MAGNIFICATION

The type of magnification that is preferred because it offers improved spatial resolution is write magnification. Write magnification takes place before the data are stored in the scan converter. With this process of magnification, the area identified in the region of interest (ROI) is rescanned and the old data are ignored to obtain new information. This type of zoom increases the number of pixels when compared to the first image, which automatically increases the amount of spatial resolution. That is why this magnification process is the preferred method to zoom an image. Because it is completed before the data are stored in the scan converter, it cannot be performed after the image is frozen and is considered to be a preprocessing technique. Once rescanned, the temporal resolution may be improved if the new image is shallower than the original data.

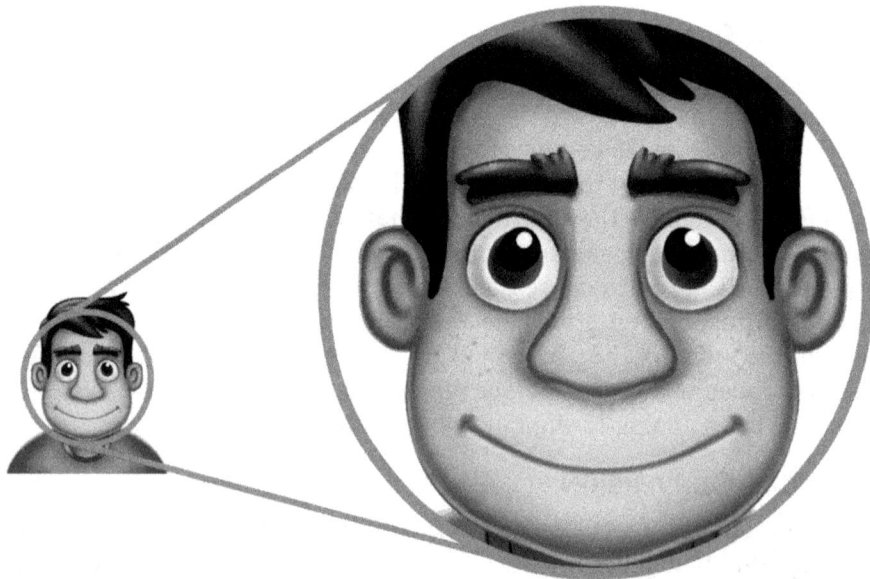

FREQUENCY COMPOUNDING

Frequency compounding is one method to reduce the amount of speckle in an ultrasound image. Ultrasound images, of course, are filled with speckle, but it is important that a reduction takes place in order to discern objects that demonstrate low contrast. Targets that are smaller may not be visualized if the amount of speckle is not reduced. Frequency compounding is an averaging method that tends to take the speckle patterns of multiple images into consideration to reduce the noise and speckle artifact that are present.

EDGE ENHANCEMENT

If a sonographer wants to improve the sharpness of a mass located within the liver, edge enhancement can be applied. This is a technique that allows better delineation of the border of structures by sharpening the edges of a mass. Often, it is difficult to discern the differences in tissue types. Raising the image contrast at the interface of these tissues will enhance the change that may not be as obvious without edge enhancement. At the boundary between two or more tissue types, various shades of gray are displayed, and edge enhancement will produce edges that are more reflective to help the mass stand out against normal liver tissue. Edge enhancement can also be helpful when imaging uterine fibroids or masses within the thyroid.

READ MAGNIFICATION

Magnification allows users to zoom in or increase the size of a region of interest. Read magnification is performed after an image has already been stored in the scan converter; it allows for postprocessing function because it can enlarge an image that has been frozen, but the spatial resolution tends to stay the same because the magnified image still contains the same number of pixels as the original image. The image is not reconstructed by the system; the pixels are just larger than they were in the first image. This function has no effect on the frame rate (temporal resolution) because the image will be located at the same depth as the original information. Because the spatial resolution is not any better than the original image, this is not the preferred method of magnification.

3D RENDERING

Postprocessing allows ultrasound users to manage information after it has been stored in the ultrasound system's scan converter. For example, anything that a sonographer does to a frozen image is a postprocessing technique. All postprocessing applications can be undone because the original data are saved. The 3D rendering is one example of a postprocessing technique. The data are required, and the image is either reconstructed on the ultrasound system or it is sent to an offline workstation that is equipped with special software to manipulate and analyze the images. Other examples of postprocessing would be to adjust the gain after an image is frozen or to magnify the image after it has been frozen.

FUSION IMAGING

Fusion imaging (also known as hybrid imaging) is a technique that provides sonographers and clinicians with greater diagnostic confidence when following up lesions discovered on previous computed tomography (CT) or magnetic resonance imaging (MRI) studies. Fusion imaging also reduces the amount of radiation that a patient is exposed to because ultrasound does not use radiation. Still another advantage is greater dynamic monitoring during invasive procedures. Real-time virtual sonography is one example of hybrid imaging that allows gray-scale, color Doppler, or the use of contrast harmonics and CT or MRI images to be displayed simultaneously. The CT or MRI images must be sent to the ultrasound system so that the same cross-sectional image can be recreated with sonography. Fusion imaging requires a sensor that is attached to the transducer that determines the probe location during the scan as well as a transmitter that is attached to the patient.so the sonographer knows the suspicious lesion is being evaluated.

VISUALIZING AS MUCH OF THE ABDOMINAL AORTA AS POSSIBLE

If the radiologist would like to visualize as much of the abdominal aorta as possible, the sonographer could use the extended field of view control on the ultrasound system. This panoramic image is available on most modern ultrasound equipment and replaces the split-screen method of demonstrating objects that are longer than the transducer face. By acquiring various volume data, the system will stitch the information together in order to display one image. This single image will offer clinicians the ability to visualize the structure at the same time. This application can be used when interrogating the abdominal aorta, and it may provide additional information regarding the exact location of aneurysms that may be encountered. Often, anatomical structures are enlarged, and it may be difficult to obtain measurements from them. These include the thyroid, testes, polycystic kidneys, musculoskeletal exams, as well as some breast lesions.

3D Ultrasound Technology

Three- and four-dimensional (3D and 4D) ultrasound exams are performed with a 2D array transducer. This is also referred to as volume imaging because once a good 2D image is created, the transducer will allow volume data acquisition when turning on 3D or 4D. These transducers are able to obtain volume data with the complex arrangement of the active elements. Thousands of active elements are arranged across the transducer face. They are not only situated vertically, but also in a horizontal line across the transducer. The 2D array probes allow for the sound beams to be electronically steered and focused beams. This design in the arrangement of the crystals will result in extremely thin slices of the sound beam when compared to traditional transducers. The thin slices enable better contrast resolution because the beam is not wider than the structure being interrogated. Contrast resolution is augmented due to diminished volume averaging.

2D Transducers

Two-dimensional transducers (2D arrays) offer a fairly recent technology that is continuing to be developed and improved. These 2D transducers are used to create 3D and 4D images. These probes contain thousands of piezoelectric elements arranged in what can be compared to the shape of a checkerboard. These beams are electronically focused and steered in order to obtain volume data. A 3D rendering can then be performed on the data collected to create the 3D images. This 3D technique is considered to be postprocessing because the computer-generated images are manipulated. This technology is used in obstetrical ultrasound as well as diagnostic imaging for various diseases and disorders on nonpregnant populations. For example, 3D and 4D have proved useful during pelvic ultrasounds looking at the uterus and the ovaries. They can also be applied to abdominal exams to better discern liver, renal, or adrenal masses.

Most Basic Form of Grayscale Imaging

The most basic form of real-time or grayscale imaging is known as brightness mode. This method is more commonly referred to as B-mode imaging. B-mode was the first gray-scale imaging method available. During B-mode, pulses are sent into the body and when the signal returns, it appears as a dot on the screen. The amplitude or strength of the reflectors will be visualized as dots. Higher amplitudes will appear as bright-white areas on the screen. The areas that return weaker signals will be seen as gray dots on the image display. Even when color mode is used, the underlying image showing the actual anatomy of the patient is represented by grayscale imaging.

Adjusting for Echoes That Are Too Bright 4 cm from the Surface

Sonographers are able to visualize the depth of every reflector because there will be a scale on one side of the image that correlates to how deep the reflectors are located in the body. Every dot typically represents 1 cm. Counting down 4 cm from the top will locate the reflector that is appearing too bright on the monitor. In order to adjust for the increased echogenicity of the structure, the sonographer can find the time gain compensation (TGC) slide pod that correlates to that location and move the slider to the user's left (or toward the right of the ultrasound system). TCG can be used in conjunction with the receiver gain (amplification) in order to provide an image that has a brightness that is the same throughout the image.

Echotextures

Various organs, tissues, glands, cysts, and masses can be interrogated with ultrasound technology, and they will display a typical echotexture. Radiologists will comment on the size and echotextures of these structures in their reports to give the ordering physician additional information to help reach a diagnosis. Common ultrasound terms associated with echotexture include cystic, solid, complex, homogeneous, and heterogeneous. Ultrasound is often used when a mass is felt or suspected to determine if it is cystic (fluid-filled), solid (not cystic), or complex (containing cystic and solid components). Other common terms used when describing organs and glands are homogeneous (uniform echo pattern) and heterogeneous (uneven echo patterns). Some diseases, such as cirrhosis of the liver, will change the normal echotexture of the liver and be referred to as a coarse echotexture. In this case, the typical smooth appearance is no longer evident.

VARIANCE MODE MAP

A variance mode map gives the sonographer information not only about the direction and velocity of red blood cells in the sample, but also about the flow pattern of the blood. Similar to velocity mode maps, variance mode maps have a black line that represents where no Doppler shift occurs. Above this black line is flow moving toward the probe, and below the black line is flow moving away from the probe. However, the boxes above and below the black line contain different colors on each side. Recall that normal flow in a vessel is considered laminar flow, which is represented by flow on the left of the color map. Turbulent flow is the opposite of laminar flow and is found on the right side of the color map. An example of turbulent flow may be the result of blood flow moving through a stenotic vessel.

ALIASING

Aliasing is an imaging error that occurs when a sonographer is interrogating a structure with Doppler ultrasound. Although power Doppler imaging (PDI) is a special form of color Doppler, it only indicates that a Doppler shift has taken place. It does not examine the velocity (speed and direction) of the moving blood cells, but rather the strength of the signal (amplitude). Because there are not any data pertaining to the velocity, aliasing will not occur. This is just one advantage of the use of PDI. PDI is more sensitive than color Doppler, so it is often used to visualize blood flow within smaller vessels or areas of venous (low) flow.

TYPE OF FLOW VISUALIZED DURING AN ECHOCARDIOGRAM

An echocardiogram is an ultrasound exam that evaluates various structures of the heart. The movement of blood flow as it travels through the heart is also observed, and measurements can be taken. Hemodynamics refers to the observation of blood flow as it courses through the heart and blood vessels. During an echocardiogram, the ultrasound user would expect to visualize blood flow that is pulsatile. The heart is constantly contracting and relaxing, which will create velocities of blood flow that will fluctuate because of the movement of the heart wall. Pulsatile flow is also visualized in the arterial system because blood is moving at a greater velocity than it is in the venous system.

INCREASING PRF TO HELP VISUALIZE RAPIDLY MOVING FLOW IN VESSELS

Correct optimization of color flow is always the goal when examining vessels while using color Doppler. In order to get the entire vessel to fill in properly, one of the first steps that the sonographer can perform after turning on the color flow is to adjust the pulse repetition frequency (PRF). The PRF is often referred to as the color scale when color Doppler is activated. In this example, the blood flow is moving at a rapid pace, and it is likely in an artery, so the ultrasound user would want to increase the PRF. This raises the Nyquist limit of the machine, which will help avoid aliasing. Aliasing can occur in color Doppler imaging and will appear as a variety of colors within the lumen of the blood vessel. The next step the sonographer may take is to increase the color gain if the vessel is not completely filled with color.

HIGH SENSITIVITY WITH CW TRANSDUCERS

Dedicated continuous-wave (CW) transducers cannot produce an ultrasound image, but they have a heightened sensitivity to blood flow. The reason that they are more prone to signals that are weaker within the body is because these probes do not contain backing (damping) material. Backing material inhibits the amount of ringing of the crystals during the transmitting and receiving phases, which makes them less receptive to receiving returning signals that tend to be smaller. If these tiny signals are not recognized by the transducer, then the ultrasound system cannot convert them into electrical signals to be visualized on the screen. Dedicated continuous-wave probes are great tools to detect tiny Doppler shifts such as blood flow in the foot. Matching layers are, however, present in dedicated continuous-wave probes to allow for the propagation of sound in and out of the body more readily.

MULTIPLE SPECKLED COLORS IN THE COLOR BOX

If a sonographer visualizes multiple speckled colors throughout the color box after turning on color Doppler, the first step that he or she can take to correct this noise is to turn the color gain down. Color gain that is set correctly is adjusted so that the amplitude is set at the highest level without displaying color speckles. Aliasing, color Doppler gain that is set too high, and turbulent flow all have different appearances, so ultrasound users should be able to discern what is taking place. Some are artifacts and can be corrected with the adjustment of parameters on the ultrasound machine.

LAMINAR FLOW

Laminar flow is the type of flow that is exhibited in normal anatomical structures. If a clinician listens to the blood moving through a vessel with laminar flow, it will not be heard. This flow is layered, smooth, and travels parallel along the length of the vessel. There are two configurations regarding laminar flow. The first is plug flow, which will have the same velocity in all layers present. A parabolic pattern tends to have velocities that are higher in the middle of the vessel and lower velocity flow along the walls. The shape that is created with a parabolic flow pattern is similar to a bullet. A blood vessel that contains laminar flow will produce a Reynolds number of less than 1,500. The Reynolds number is a way to forecast if the flow will be laminar or turbulent. Turbulent flow will have a Reynolds number that is greater than 2,000.

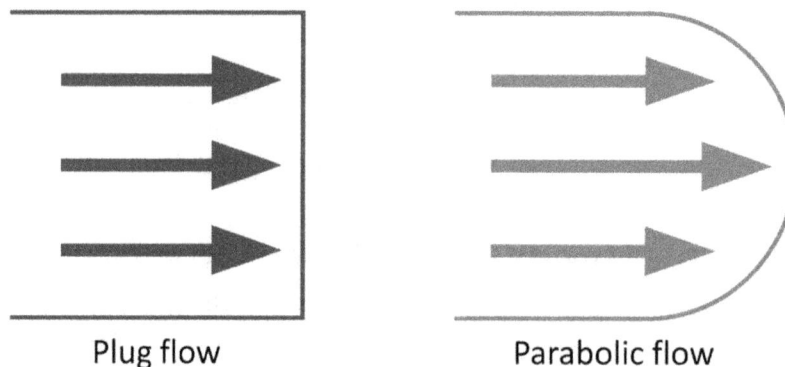

Plug flow   Parabolic flow

ADVANTAGES AND DISADVANTAGES OF A LARGER PACKET SIZE

Packet size should be carefully evaluated so that color Doppler velocities can be interrogated more accurately. The advantages of a larger packet size include a heightened receptiveness to blood vessels that have blood flow that is moving at a slower velocity. Another advantage is that when the packet size is larger, more pulses are sent out for every scan line that is available, and in turn the velocity measurements of the blood flow tend to be more precise. The disadvantages are that because more pulses are required for larger packet sizes, the frame rate and temporal resolution will be degraded because more processing time is required by the system.

DISADVANTAGE OF PERSISTENCE

Persistence (also called temporal averaging or temporal compounding) is a method that can be used during grayscale or color Doppler imaging. By overlapping information obtained from older frames onto more recent images obtained, the machine can produce an ultrasound image with greater detail that has less noise, is smoother, and has a higher signal-to-noise ratio. If the signal-to-noise ratio is higher than the noise, the system will get rid of the noise signals. Although the image detail improves with the use of temporal compounding, the temporal resolution is degraded because of the additional processing. This makes imaging structures that are moving rapidly very difficult because there will be a lag as the temporal resolution is decreased. Persistence is best used with structures that demonstrate slow motion.

CRYSTALS REQUIRED IN TRANSDUCERS THAT OFFER PULSED-WAVE DOPPLER

Pulsed-wave Doppler only requires one active element. This lead zirconate titanate (PZT) crystal is able to transmit the pulse into the body as well as listen for the returning signals. Only one PZT crystal is necessary because the sonographer places the sample volume (gate) in exactly the position at which a sample velocity is necessary. Once the probe transmits a pulse into the body, it listens for it to return to the transducer. This is known as the time of flight (go-return time). Transducers that allow pulsed Doppler are also able to create a grayscale image. This is referred to as duplex/triplex imaging. A duplex/triplex exam consists of gray scale, color Doppler, and pulsed-wave Doppler. In contrast, a continuous-wave transducer will consist of two crystals. One active element serves as a transmitter that introduces pulses into the body at a constant rate. The second active element acts as a receiver for the returning echoes.

RANGE RESOLUTION

Range resolution allows ultrasound users to select the exact region where a pulsed-wave Doppler sample should take place. Range resolution is also called range specificity because a specific location is chosen. Perhaps this area is where a stenosis is visualized on grayscale images, so the sonographer must obtain a measurement within the stenotic portion of the vessel as well as check for turbulence distal to this location. When pulsed-wave Doppler is activated, the gate (sample volume) will appear on the screen and it can be quickly moved to the location of interest. Continuous-wave Doppler does not offer range resolution because the sample is being obtained from every vessel that is in the path of the ultrasound wave. This is superior to pulsed-wave Doppler when measuring vessels that have an extremely high velocity, but range ambiguity occurs with continuous-wave Doppler.

RANGE AMBIGUITY WHEN THE PRF IS TOO HIGH FOR THE SCANNING DEPTH

Recall that range ambiguity artifact (also known as range specificity or range resolution) is typically prevented when an ultrasound operator uses pulsed-wave Doppler. During these exams, a sample volume is used to determine the exact location in which a velocity measurement should be obtained. However, in this example, if the pulse repetition frequency (PRF) (scale) is set too high for the depth of the reflector being interrogated, range ambiguity will exist because the system will be directed to send out pulses before the earlier pulses have been returned. If the echoes are not returned in the order that they are transmitted, the system will incorrectly determine the depth of the object being scanned because this is assumed by the ultrasound system. In this case, aliasing will occur, which can be corrected by increasing the scale.

RELATIONSHIP BETWEEN THE PRF AND THE NYQUIST LIMIT TO ELIMINATE ALIASING

Sonographers should recognize the Nyquist limit as the greatest velocity of blood flow that can be measured just before aliasing occurs. Aliasing is when the color or spectral Doppler patterns wind around the display. The pulse repetition frequency (PRF) can be referred to as the velocity scale, and it plays an important role in eliminating aliasing. When the sonographer modifies the PRF, the Nyquist limit automatically changes as well. There is a direct relationship between the PRF and the Nyquist limit. When the PRF scale is as high as it can go, the likelihood of aliasing occurring is slim. A scale that is set low will have a lower Nyquist limit with a greater chance of aliasing.

DIRECTION OF BLOOD FLOW IN SECTOR-SHAPED IMAGE WITH VESSEL THAT IS IN A HORIZONTAL DIRECTION

Sonographers should remember that color flow in a sector-shaped image cannot be steered as it can be with a linear transducer. Only the size and location can be adjusted. In the example given in which a sector-shaped image contains a vessel that is in a horizontal direction, it is first important to find the color map to decide what color represents flow moving toward the transducer (above the black line). The user will also notice that the color beneath the black line on the color map refers to blood moving away from the transducer. The user can then decide if the blood flow is moving from left to right (or right to left) by tracking the blood flow from the top color to the bottom color. This will make the direction of blood flow more apparent.

ADVANTAGE OF CONTINUOUS-WAVE DOPPLER

The main advantage of using continuous-wave Doppler on an ultrasound system is that precise velocity measurements can be obtained because two crystals are used instead of one. The crystals are constantly and simultaneously transmitting an ultrasound pulse while one is always listening or receiving a signal. When using a nonimaging continuous-wave probe, the sensitivity is increased because this probe can detect very small Doppler frequencies because it doesn't contain a dampening (backing) layer. Both of these types of continuous-wave devices have a matching layer to make them more proficient in sending and receiving pulses. Continuous-wave Doppler will never display aliasing because only pulsed-wave Doppler will alias. One major disadvantage is that there isn't a sample gate, so the precise location of where the velocities are located is not known.

DOPPLER PRINCIPLE

The method used to measure the velocity of blood flow within the body is called the Doppler principle. The frequency of sound varies as the distance between the transmitted frequency and receiver change positions. If the distance between the sound source and receiver stays the same, the frequency will not be altered. An alteration of the frequency is called a Doppler shift or Doppler frequency. The Doppler shift is directly related to the velocity of blood within the circulatory system. Keep in mind that the velocity includes the speed (magnitude) and direction of blood flow. Slower velocities will cause a lower Doppler frequency. A higher velocity will create a greater Doppler shift. Blood flow velocities are reported in units of meters per second (m/s).

RANGES OF REYNOLDS NUMBERS FOR LAMINAR AND TURBULENT FLOW

The Reynolds number is a value that predicts the onset of flow that is turbulent. The Reynolds number is a unitless value that is calculated from the following equation:

$$\text{Reynolds number} = \frac{\text{average flow speed} \times \text{vessel diameter} \times \text{density}}{\text{viscosity}}$$

If the calculated value is less than 1,500, laminar flow will be present. If the value is more than 2,000, it is predicted that a turbulent flow will be visualized. Disturbed flow will fall between the 1,500 and 2,000 range. From the above equation, if there is an increased speed of flow, there will be a higher Reynolds number. If the diameter of the vessel is larger, the Reynolds number will also be greater. Density has the same effect on the Reynolds number. The Reynolds number has an indirect relationship with the viscosity of the blood.

PHASIC AND STEADY FLOW

Three types of blood flow that are witnessed in the circulatory systems of humans are phasic, pulsatile, and steady flow. Phasic flow is the typical flow pattern seen in veins. Phasic flow will exhibit velocity changes associated with breathing that causes red blood cells to speed up or slow down. Steady flow is constantly present in the venous system, and it takes place when the patient holds their breath. Steady flow does not vary in velocity, but rather it moves at the same speed. No acceleration or deceleration is present due to the contraction of the heart.

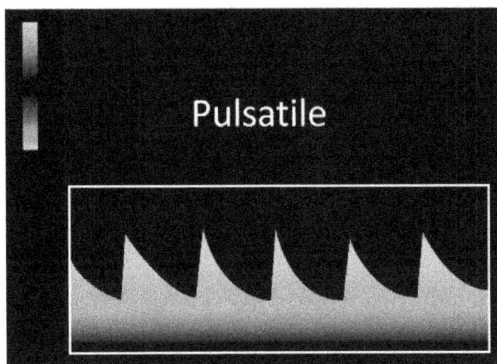

Pulsatile — High fluctutation

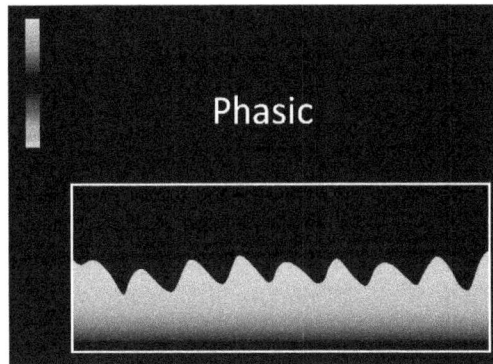

Phasic — Low fluctutation

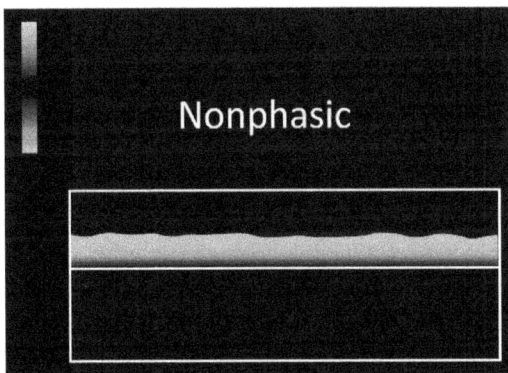

Nonphasic — No fluctutation

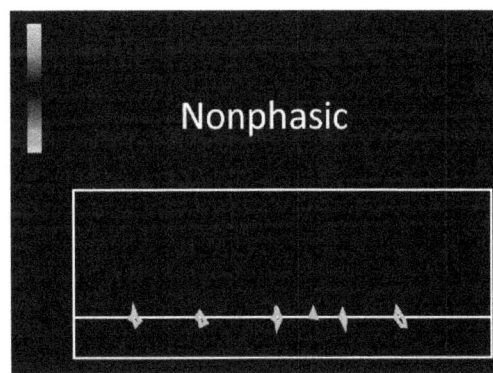

Nonphasic — No flow

RANGE IN WHICH A DOPPLER SHIFT TAKES PLACE

When using ultrasound for diagnostic purposes, the frequency of the transducers used during a Doppler exam ranges from approximately 2 to 10 MHz. This question asks about the range in which a Doppler shift takes place. This falls in the audible range in which sound can actually be heard, which is anywhere between 20 Hz and 20,000 Hz. The formula to calculate a Doppler shift is as follows:

$$\text{Doppler shift} = \text{reflected frequency} - \text{transmtted frequency.}$$

Remember that Doppler shift is often referred to as Doppler frequency, and it provides information pertaining to velocity.

COLOR FLOW IMAGING

Blood is composed of many components including red blood cells (erythrocytes), white blood cells (leukocytes), platelets (thrombocytes), and plasma. Roughly 45 percent of the blood that travels throughout the circulatory system (heart, arteries, capillaries, and veins) is comprised of red blood cells. Red blood cells supply oxygen to all of the cells in the body and are the most numerous type of cell in whole blood. The life span of red blood cells is about 120 days, but they are constantly being replenished with new red blood cells. Because red blood cells are traveling in the heart and blood vessels, they create the reflections that are seen by the human eye when color Doppler is turned on (sometimes the blood flow can be seen, especially in low-flow states without color Doppler). Color Doppler should also be used when scanning a mass to demonstrate if the flow pattern is within or around the perimeter of the lesion.

ANGLES THAT PROVIDE THE GREATEST AMOUNT OF DOPPLER SHIFT

If a sonographer is using pulsed-wave Doppler in order to determine the peak velocity of blood flow in a vessel, the operator must remember that when the red blood cells are moving along the same path of the ultrasound beam, the most accurate measurements will be obtained. Thus, the Doppler shift (otherwise known as the Doppler frequency) will be highest at 0 or 180 degrees. This parallel movement can be either toward or away from the transducer, but in this case the entire velocity of the moving particles will be measured with 100% certainty. If the angle between the target and reflector is anything other than 0 or 180 degrees, the velocity is less precise. If an operator tries to interrogate a structure at a 90-degree angle with pulsed-wave Doppler, no Doppler shift will take place because it is calculated to be zero.

DIFFERENTIATING BETWEEN FLOW REVERSAL AND ALIASING DURING AN EXAM USING COLOR DOPPLER

It is important for sonographers to realize that aliasing can occur not only with spectral Doppler analysis, but also with color flow Doppler. The user must be able to discern between aliasing and the reversal of flow (bidirectional flow). In order to determine if aliasing is present, the user must pay close attention to the color map located on the side of the image. If the colors on the map tend to wrap from the top around the outside and to the bottom of the map, then users may assume that aliasing is present. If the colors on the middle of the color map communicate with each other, then bidirectional flow is present. The best step that an ultrasound user can take in order to remove an aliasing artifacts from a color Doppler exam is to increase the level of the velocity scale.

SAMPLING VELOCITIES AT A CHOSEN LOCATION DURING A PULSED-WAVE DOPPLER EXAM

When performing a pulsed-wave Doppler exam, the user is able to determine exactly where a velocity measurement should be taken within a vessel. Once the sonographer has the grayscale image optimized, color Doppler can be activated to better visualize the blood vessels. Then, one can bring up the cursor for pulsed-wave Doppler and a line that is intersected by two dashes close together will be visualized. This is the gate (sample volume). The gate can be moved with the trackball until it is right where the user wants to perform a spectral analysis. The size of the gate can be changed so that it is only within the vessel that is being examined. For example, if one is

68

sampling the carotid artery but the spectral display is also showing venous flow, reduce the size of the gate and reposition it so that only the artery is being interrogated.

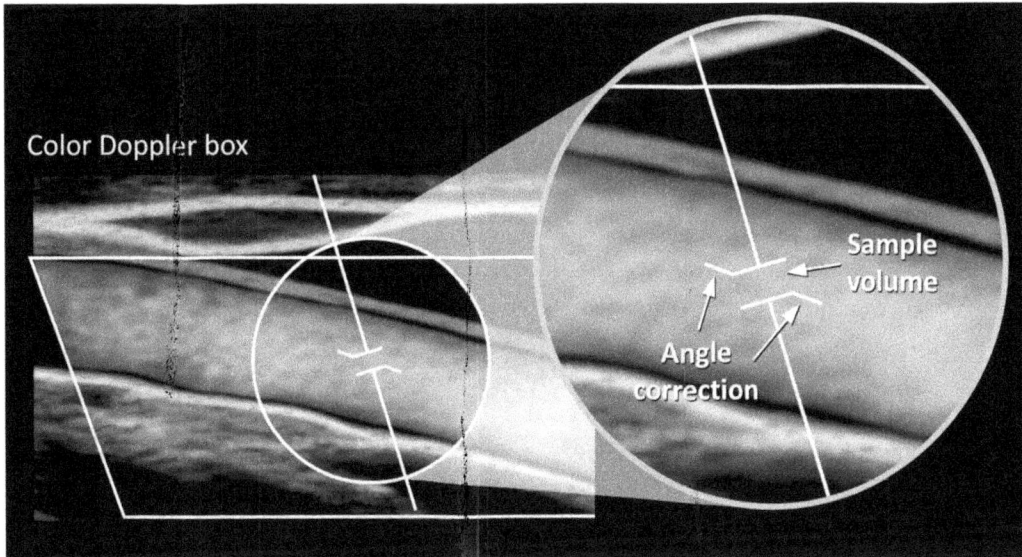

SPECTRAL BROADENING

A spectral Doppler waveform represents all of the many velocities found in a sample of a blood vessel. Two types of flow can be ascertained in the sample. They are normal or laminar flow, in which the spectral window is clear and the red blood cells are traveling at almost the same velocities. Turbulent flow shows flow that is disorganized because the blood is traveling at different speeds and various directions. Instead of a clear spectral window as seen in laminar flow, it appears to be filled in, which represents spectral broadening. Spectral broadening is a display of a broad range of Doppler shifts that are apparent within the sample of blood flow taken in a vessel. This may happen due to a stenosis or tortuous vessel.

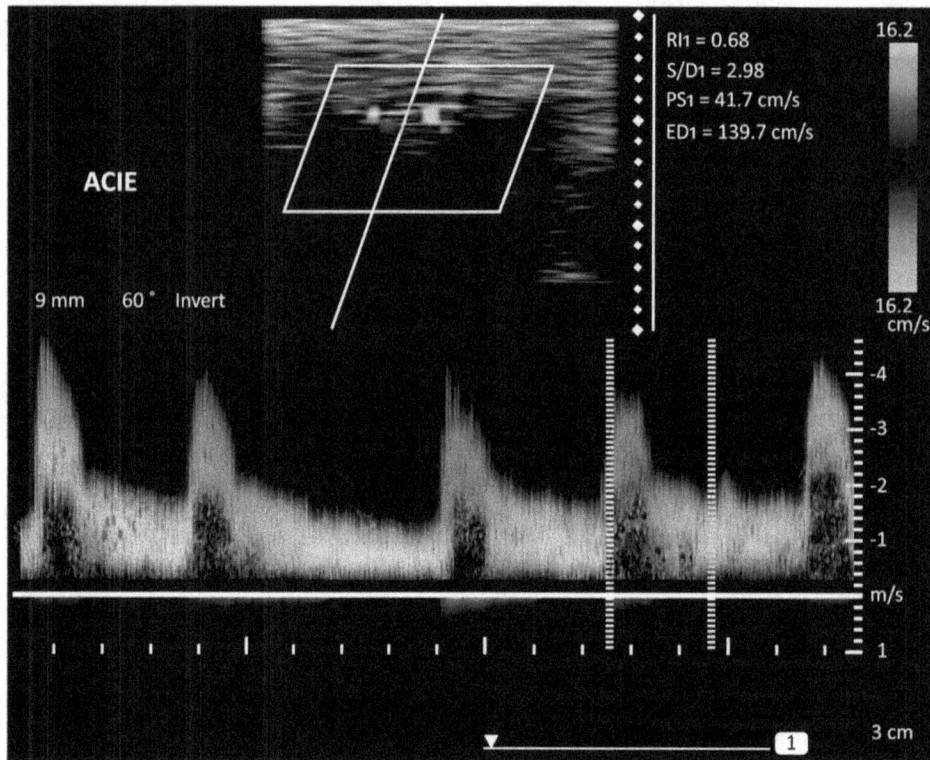

ADJUSTING SPECTRAL DOPPLER GAIN IF SPECTRAL DISPLAY CAN BARELY BE VISUALIZED

Pulsed-wave Doppler provides important information that can be used to diagnose many disorders in patients. Correct Doppler settings are crucial, and sonographers must have a strong understanding of not only anatomy, but also ultrasound physics. If the machine is not set properly, an artifact can occur that may limit the amount of diagnostic information present. If a sonographer turns on the pulsed-wave Doppler, but the spectral display can barely be visualized, then the next step will be to turn up the pulsed-wave Doppler's gain. If the gain is turned up too high, then noise may appear in the spectral display. One can increase the gain by turning it up until noise appears. At this point, the gain may be slowly reduced until the noise disappears.

RI

Recall that arteries are the blood vessels that supply organs with oxygenated blood. These arteries are able to direct the flow of blood to the organs that require more blood such as the brain, liver, kidneys, and gonads. These arteries can control the resistance of the blood flow so that it is routed to those organs. The term RI refers to the resistance (or resistivity) index, and it is a number that can be calculated by today's ultrasound machines to measure this resistance to blood flow. Low-resistance flow is seen in arteries that supply organs that need a constant source of blood flow such as the internal carotid, hepatic, and renal arteries. High arterial resistance demonstrates arterioles that have constricted and created a channeling to reroute the blood flow elsewhere. Examples of high-resistance vessels include the external carotid arteries, mesenteric arteries in a patient that is fasting, and arteries that supply the limbs. Sonographers should be aware that the normal value for RI will be different from one artery to the next, but anything above or below the typical values may be an abnormal finding.

Spectral Analysis

Spectral analysis is the method that provides information pertaining to the individual velocities of blood cells that are contained within a specific sample. Spectral analysis is a tool that simplifies the many Doppler shifts that are produced when blood travels through the body. Blood does not travel in a uniform fashion, and because of this, spectral analysis is necessary to provide data that can offer diagnostic information in order to correctly diagnosis patients that suffer from vascular disease. Sonographers realize that even within the same blood vessel that is free of any pathology, the blood moves at different speeds. When pathology is present, or the vessels change shapes and sizes, the flow patterns can change dramatically. Spectral analysis is a great tool that allows users to visually sort out all of this information along with measuring various velocities.

Correlation of Velocity of Blood to Spectral Broadening

Spectral analysis with pulsed-wave Doppler allows users to see, hear, and measure various blood flow velocities. The spectral window is the clear, black region between the baseline and the spectral line. When this area is filled in and there is widening of the line, spectral broadening is indicated. Spectral broadening is typical when turbulent (high-velocity) blood flow is sampled. This turbulence comprises many areas of flow reversal and various velocities, and flow may be seen beneath the baseline. If a carotid artery is being interrogated and the sonographer can visualize a tight stenosis, there may be spectral broadening. This may also be present when small vessels are being investigated or if a sample is obtained where a vessel bifurcates.

Raising the Nyquist Limit to Prevent Aliasing During Pulsed Doppler Exam

The Nyquist limit can be calculated by dividing the pulse repetition frequency (PRF) by 2. Aliasing will be apparent if the Doppler frequency is higher than the Nyquist limit. Therefore, in order to prevent aliasing, the sonographer should raise the Nyquist limit. This can be done by raising the PRF (also known as the scale); if the PRF is increased, so is the Nyquist limit. One may also raise the Nyquist limit by finding a new sonographic window that is at a shallower location. The PRF is determined by the depth of the reflector. If the depth is deeper in the body, the PRF will be low, as will the Nyquist limit. This decreased value makes the ultrasound system more susceptible to aliasing.

Wall Filter

The wall filter is an important tool that sonographers can use in order to remove Doppler shifts below a certain set frequency during spectral and color Doppler interrogations. In other words, this control will help remove the lower frequency Doppler signals that may arise from the motion that anatomical structures such as the heart or blood vessels create. Wall filters are also referred to as high-pass filters and do not play a role in higher Doppler shifts such as those created from the movement of blood cells in the circulatory system. Sonographers should remember that blood that is moving slower will create a lower frequency Doppler shift. The system is less likely to detect blood that is moving slowly when the wall filter is set at a higher level.

Adjustments If Picking up Velocities from an Artery and a Vein

Pulsed-wave Doppler provides range resolution, which provides users with knowing precisely where the velocity measurements are being taken. When pulsed-wave Doppler is selected on the machine, the user will move the gate to the blood vessel that is to be interrogated. The size of the gate, also known as the sample volume, can be adjusted so that the user is sampling a good portion of the blood vessel. Sometimes, the sonographer will notice that blood flow from arteries and veins is being displayed. If this happens, the user can adjust the size of the gate in order to only obtain data from the vessel of interest. One may also have to adjust the location because perhaps the gate was accidently moved into a different vessel. Modern systems will have a triplex function that allows the user to display gray-scale, color Doppler, and spectral Doppler at the same time. If the user is picking up flow from two different vessels, he or she updates the triplex image and moves the sample volume into the vessel that is under investigation.

VELOCITIES BELOW THE BASELINE

When using spectral analysis to determine the velocity of blood flow and flow velocities are below the baseline, this represents blood cells that are traveling in a direction away from the transducer. Aliasing is an error in imaging that can represent high-velocity flows to wrap around the baseline and appear as if they are moving in the opposite direction. An advantage of pulsed Doppler is that the user knows exactly where the blood flow velocity is being sampled because of the gate. Color flow Doppler allows information pertaining to the velocities to be superimposed on a grayscale image. Color flow Doppler also allows users to determine in which direction the blood is traveling.

RING-DOWN ARTIFACTS AND COMET-TAIL ARTIFACTS

A ring-down artifact is indicative of abdominal gas pockets such as those seen in pneumobilia (the presence of gas in the biliary ducts). It appears as a solid streak (or parallel bands) radiating away from the gas pocket itself.

The comet-tail artifact appears as multiple, small, white streaks running parallel to the target structure. It is caused by the reflection of the ultrasound beam off of small, spherical, reflective objects (such as gas bubbles or stones).

REFRACTION ARTIFACTS AND REVERBERATION ARTIFACTS

Refraction is ultrasound beam bending that occurs when the incident beam is not perpendicular to the target structure. It commonly occurs where bone meets soft tissue. Refraction may produce images that are not viewed in their correct positions on the ultrasound monitor. This may result in an inability to accurately measure characteristics such as length or depth. Reverberation occurs when the ultrasound beam reflects off of tissues that have different levels of acoustic impedance (resistance to vibration). Reverberations appear as equally spaced, bright rings that decrease in brightness as the transducer face moves away.

MIRROR ARTIFACT

A mirror artifact will always be visualized at a depth greater than that of the actual structure being imaged. It is known as a mirror artifact because a very strong reflector tends to redirect the sound waves as it strikes the mirror. This mirror will appear between the actual object being imaged and the second copy of the structure. The second copy will be equidistant from the reflector as the object, but it will be at a greater depth. This artifact can appear not only in grayscale imaging, but also during color Doppler interrogation. In this case, a second vessel may appear deeper than the actual vessel, but it is actually a mirror artifact. When imaging the abdomen, a common mirror imaging artifact visualized is lung tissue on either side of the diaphragm, which is seen as a bright reflector.

ENHANCEMENT AND SHADOWING ARTIFACTS

Clinicians may use ultrasound artifacts as a tool to increase diagnostic confidence. For example, if a structure is fluid filled, posterior enhancement should be visualized posterior to the cyst. Anything that is filled with fluid will appear anechoic because it has a lower attenuation rate. The surrounding tissue that is below anything that is fluid filled will appear brighter and is known as an enhancement artifact. While evaluating the ovaries, the enhancement artifact helps clinicians discern that the structure is fluid filled. Shadowing is the opposite of an enhancement artifact; this is a hypoechoic area posterior to a highly attenuating structure. This hypoechoic area prevents users from being able to see any underlying anatomy to these objects, but it provides clues of stones or calcifications. Sonographers may visualize small calcifications within the ovary, artery, or even within blood vessels.

REFRACTION

Refraction is the bending of a sound beam when it travels from one medium to another. Two conditions must occur in order for refraction to take place in a clinical setting: (1) There must be an oblique incidence, and (2) the two media must be traveling at different speeds because refraction cannot take place if they have identical speeds. Clinically, an ultrasound beam will only bend slightly at various tissue interfaces. Bone tends to create larger refraction angles because the speed of ultrasound in bone is faster than the speed of sound in soft tissues. Snell's law is used to calculate refraction, and the following equation may be used:

$$\frac{\sin(\text{angle of transmission})}{\sin(\text{angle of incidence})} = \frac{\text{speed of medium 2}}{\text{speed of medium 1}}$$

EDGE SHADOWING

When a sonographer visualizes a shadow protruding from the edge of a curved structure that is parallel to the axis of the ultrasound beam, it may be referred to as an edge shadow. These artifacts are portrayed as thin, hypoechoic structures that may actually prevent a user from visualizing underlying anatomical structures. These artifacts are created from a decrease in intensity as a sound beam refracts and diverges at the same time after making contact with a curved reflector. Refraction will take place when the propagation speeds are different in the presence of oblique incidence. These artifacts are often seen when performing an ultrasound of a cyst or during a testicular scan. Other examples may include a transverse image of the gallbladder or fetal head due to the curvature of these structures.

ENHANCEMENT ARTIFACTS

While imaging a structure that is fluid filled, for example, a cyst or the gallbladder, the tissue that is visualized posterior to these structures often appears extremely echogenic. The artifact that is the opposite of shadowing is known as an enhancement artifact. These fluid-filled structures visualized are the result of a lower rate of attenuation than the tissue that surrounds them, so structures below them may appear brighter. Shadowing produces a hypoechoic area behind an object that is highly attenuating, and it can prohibit visualization of the structures that extend underneath these structures. Enhancement can be of diagnostic value because radiologists rely on this enhancement artifact to reassure them that a structure is cystic.

ARTIFACTS ENCOUNTERED DURING ABDOMINAL OR SMALL-PARTS EXAMS

Shadowing is visualized when a highly attenuating structure is situated just above this artifact. Shadowing artifacts can often prevent the user from seeing underlying anatomical structures, but they may also serve as a helpful diagnostic indicator during ultrasound exams. A shadowing artifact appears as a hypoechoic or anechoic area deep to the structure that is highly attenuating. Sonographers may notice shadowing posterior to calcifications such as kidney stones and gallstones to aid the radiologist in making a correct diagnosis. The artifact that appears completely different than those characteristics of a shadowing artifact is known as enhancement. Enhancement also provides diagnostic value because radiologists rely on this enhancement artifact to reassure them that a structure is cystic. In this case, a hyperechoic region appears deep to a structure that is weakly attenuating. For example, while imaging a cyst or the gallbladder, the tissue that is visualized posterior to these structures often appears extremely echogenic. Artifacts often seen

73

during a testicular scan or while imaging cysts are edge shadows. They are the result of a decrease in intensity as a sound beam refracts and diverges at the same time after making contact with a curved reflector.

ARTIFACTS VISUALIZED DUE TO PATIENT MOTION WHEN USING PDI

A disadvantage of power Doppler imaging (PDI) is that the study may suffer because of flash artifact. Flash artifact occurs not because of the motion of the red blood cells, but rather it is a burst of color visualized when there is motion taking place outside of the blood vessels. Often, this motion is caused by patient motion. Examples of patient motion may be that the patient is actually moving on the exam table, but it may also be involuntary motion such as movement of the heart or lungs during respiration. Flash artifact may also appear because of motion caused by the transducer as the sonographer is moving it on the patient or even motion caused from the pressure that the transducer places on soft-tissue structures. Flash artifact may appear as a randomized burst of color, occurring outside of the vessels.

ROLE OF INTERMITTENT SAMPLING IN PULSED-WAVE DOPPLER ALIASING ARTIFACTS

Aliasing is common during pulsed-wave Doppler exams due to intermittent sampling. Intermittent sampling occurs if the Doppler frequency is not evaluated correctly. When the Doppler frequency is larger than the Nyquist limit, which is equal to half of the pulse repetition frequency (PRF), then aliasing will take place. Aliasing is when the blood flow direction is incorrectly portrayed either above or below the baseline; it will wind around the entire spectral window and appear to move in the opposite direction. Aliasing can also arise when color flow Doppler is being used, so ultrasound users should be able to identify if it is present. Aliasing will never occur with continuous-wave Doppler because it can only be the result of pulsed ultrasound technology.

ALIASING IN COLOR DOPPLER EXAMS

Color Doppler uses grayscale imaging to locate the anatomical structures, and when activated, a color box will be layered on top of the B-mode image. This information includes data about the mean velocity of blood moving through various structures instead of peak velocity as measured by pulsed-wave and continuous-wave Doppler. Color Doppler does provide information regarding the direction of blood flow, and it is prone to aliasing. Ultrasound users should be able to tell the difference between color Doppler that is aliasing and flow that is moving in the reverse direction. The operator must pay close attention to the color map displayed on the screen. Just as pulsed-wave Doppler that is aliasing tends to wrap around the spectral window, color Doppler that is aliasing winds around the top of the color box around to the bottom.

ADJUSTING THE BASELINE TO ELIMINATE ALIASING

During a spectral display, the system can document flow that is moving in opposite directions. Flow that is visualized above the baseline demonstrates flow that is moving toward the transducer. Flow below the baseline signifies blood flow traveling away from the transducer. If the user notices that flow is wrapping around the baseline, this is an aliasing artifact. Sonographers can take many steps to eliminate aliasing. One such corrective measure that can be done is to adjust the baseline. If the flow is above the baseline but aliasing occurs, the user can move the baseline lower so that the entire waveform is going in one direction. This allows for extremely high velocity flow to be shown moving in the correct direction and still allows for an accurate measurement.

CORRECTING AN ALIASING ARTIFACT DURING A CAROTID DUPLEX EXAM IMAGED AT 35 DEGREES WITH A 10 MHZ TRANSDUCER

Spectral Doppler waveforms can provide clinicians with a lot of insight pertaining to blood flowing throughout the body. Blood does not necessarily travel in the same speed or direction, even within the same blood vessel. Spectral analysis is a tool that identifies every velocity obtained within the signal that is reflected. However, when there are aliasing errors in the spectral waveform, the interpreting physician may mistake that data as true information. This could lead to a misdiagnosis. In this example, a 10 MHz transducer is creating an aliasing artifact so the sonographer may try to reduce the transducer's Doppler frequency. The PRF scale could also be increased to raise the Nyquist limit, and the baseline could be moved down. If that doesn't work, the user could increase the angle of incidence or switch to continuous-wave Doppler.

ARTIFACTS ENCOUNTERED WHEN COLOR DOPPLER IMAGING IS USED

Doppler gain artifacts must be corrected so that data are not lost or misinterpreted. In order to get the entire vessel to fill in properly, one of the first steps that the sonographer can perform after turning on color flow is to adjust the pulse repetition frequency (PRF), which is often referred to as the color scale when color Doppler is activated. In arteries, the blood is flowing rapidly, so the ultrasound user would want to increase the PRF. This raises the Nyquist limit of the machine, which will help avoid aliasing. Aliasing can occur in color Doppler imaging and will appear as a variety of colors within the lumen of the blood vessel. The next step the sonographer may take is to increase the color gain if the vessel is not completely filled with color. Color Doppler is often used during venous duplex exams of the extremities. In this example, the sonographer is trying to optimize color flow in the smaller vessels of a patient's lower leg. If color flow is not immediately visualized after turning on color Doppler, the sonographer should adjust the PRF, otherwise known as the color scale.

ALIASING ARTIFACT AND CORRECTIVE MEASURES TO TAKE WHEN USING SPECTRAL DOPPLER

Spectral analysis is a tool that identifies every velocity obtained within the signal that is reflected. However, when there are aliasing errors in the spectral waveform, the interpreting physician may mistake the data as true information, which could lead to a misdiagnosis. Aliasing is considered an artifact that demonstrates an error in imaging because the waveform tends to wrap around the baseline. There are many steps that can be taken to eliminate signals that display aliasing. The first step a sonographer should try is to adjust the pulse repetition frequency (PRF) (velocity scale). In arteries, the blood flow is moving rapidly so increasing the PRF may help unwrap the spectral display. This step increases the Nyquist limit, which is also known as the aliasing frequency and is equal to half of the PRF. If this alone does not take care of aliasing, the baseline may be adjusted accordingly. Another helpful tip to eliminate aliasing is to switch to a lower frequency transducer or even find a window that is at a shallower location. The angle of incidence could also be increased to help eliminate aliasing. If that still doesn't work, then the user could switch to continuous-wave Doppler.

EFFECTS OF OPERATOR CONTROLS ON FRAME RATE

Many of the parameters that a sonographer can adjust will have an effect on the frame rate. The frame rate controls temporal resolution, which is the ability of the system to accurately track the location of structures with regard to time. If a system tends to "lag" or have a low frame rate, this will result in poor temporal resolution. Temporal resolution is considered optimal when there are several frames per second. Controls that a sonographer can alter to affect frame rate include changing the scanning depth. If a system is imaging a structure that is deep in the body, the temporal resolution will be poorer because there is more listening time, which results in a lower frame rate. Changes that the sonographer can make to alter the number of pulses sent into the body are changing the number of focal zones, adjusting the field of view (sector size), and changing the line density.

EFFECTS OF ADDING MULTIPLE FOCAL ZONES ON TEMPORAL RESOLUTION

Modern imaging systems have the capability to operate while using multiple focal zones. Using multiple foci will greatly improve the detail of an image, but users must balance detail and the time required for the study. If a sonographer is looking at an object using a single focus, the temporal resolution will be superior because the frame rate is higher. If additional focal zones are added, not only are more pulses required, but extra pulses are also needed in each scan line. This will degrade the temporal resolution because the frame rate is slower. A multifocus sound beam will greatly improve the lateral resolution of an image because the beam is narrowed over many depths, but the temporal resolution will suffer.

USE OF PERSISTENCE TO IMPROVE COLOR DOPPLER IMAGES

Persistence is an averaging technique that will combine images from older frames with those of newer data. In gray-scale imaging, persistence can be used to smooth out an image or reduce the amount of noise present. Persistence is also found to be useful in color Doppler imaging, especially if the vessels to be visualized are deeper in the body, to identify vessels that contain slow-moving blood, or if there is an obstruction of a vessel. Smaller vessels can also be identified more readily than with methods that do not implement persistence. Users should know that the temporal resolution is often decreased when persistence is applied to an image.

INTERROGATING A VESSEL THAT DISPLAYS SLOW FLOW

PRF stands for pulse repetition frequency, but it is also referred to as the scale while pulsed Doppler is being used. In this example, the vessel being interrogated displays blood flow that is moving slowly. If color is not optimized after turning on color Doppler, the sonographer would decrease the PRF so that the ultrasound system is more receptive in picking up slower blood flow signals. Blood that is within the venous portion of the circulatory system is often where slow flow will be visualized. If this step alone does not improve color Doppler visualization of the vessel, the sonographer may need to increase the color gain. If the operator chooses to increase the PRF scale, he or she may notice a decreased sensitivity to slow flow states. However, if one is interrogating a vessel with higher velocity flow, the PRF should be set higher in order to raise the Nyquist limit and prevent or eliminate aliasing.

OPTIMIZING THE TEMPORAL RESOLUTION WHEN IMAGING THE GALLBLADDER

Ultrasound operators should be aware that a high frame rate is ideal during an exam. If a sonographer would like to optimize the temporal resolution during a gallbladder exam, he or she could, of course, decrease the depth. However, if additional steps need to be taken to further improve (increase) the frame rate, the operator could decrease the field of view (the width of the sector). When the field of view is smaller, there are fewer pulses necessary to create the image, which takes less time. The frame rate (temporal resolution) is inversely proportional to the sector size of the image. A gallbladder can typically fit in a smaller sector size, especially when imaging in the transverse plane, so this is one step that can quickly be taken to improve the temporal resolution. Also, the operator should find out how many focal zones are being used. Reducing the amount of focusing may also improve temporal resolution.

ADVANTAGES OF LASER DISCS OR COMPACT DISCS FOR STORAGE

Modern ultrasound machines produce high-resolution images of anatomical structures, but the exams create very large files. Many facilities today archive studies on a picture archiving and communications system (PACS), but some prefer to have a backup of the patient's exams. One affordable way that centers may choose to do this is to save the exams on optical media such as laser discs or compact discs. The advantages of these devices tend to be that they are economical, they have large storage capacities, and they will not be erased if exposed to a magnetic field. They do, however, require a browser in order to view the images on a computer. It is also necessary to decide where these discs will be stored so that they can be retrieved, if necessary.

PACS

The picture archiving and communications system (PACS) allows users of digital imaging to electronically share and archive images so that they can be viewed on a network. Clinicians and other medical personnel can also access diagnostic imaging reports because they can be stored on PACS. PACS has been used to replace film for facilities that have converted to digital imaging systems. This not only saves storage space for the film and chemicals used to process film within imaging departments, but it also allows more than one user to visualize studies at the same time as well as grants instantaneous access to the stored images. If a patient comes into the emergency department (ED) with an abdominal aortic aneurysm, not only can an ED physician view the images, but a surgeon can also see the images in the operating room. Over time, film studies tend to deteriorate, and this will not occur with studies that are archived with PACS.

DISADVANTAGES

A picture archiving and communications system (PACS) offers storage and sharing capabilities for facilities that provide imaging services. Whether this facility is part of a hospital or outpatient center, referring physicians and specialists can access the patient's imaging studies along with their reports. This is a huge advantage of having PACS, but the disadvantages are the initial cost of the system and the necessary equipment. Because it is a computerized system, it requires a team of exclusive information technology professionals to manage it. Protocols must be in place in case PACS is not accessible. End-user training is required for all employees and providers that will need access to PACS. Referring physicians located off site must have the system installed on their computers and be granted access to use PACS.

DISADVANTAGE OF STORAGE THAT REQUIRES CHEMICALS TO PROCESS FILM

There are disadvantages any time that chemicals are used to process film. First, a darkroom is required, which can take up a large amount of space within an imaging department. An adequate supply of film must be on hand. Second, a processor is necessary in conjunction with the darkroom. A processor requires chemicals and periodic maintenance and cleaning. Next, chemicals must be purchased, stored, and refilled when exhausted. Films must be stored, which also takes massive amounts of space. The films must be organized so that they can be found with ease. Artifacts can occur with films, especially if they are not stored under proper conditions (temperature and humidity). Processing artifacts can also occur if the chemicals are contaminated or the processor is not working properly. Some departments have laser film printers, which do not require the use of a darkroom or chemicals, but these films must also be stored under proper conditions.

CINE LOOP STORAGE

Ultrasound is an imaging modality that relies heavily on the skills of the sonographer. The interpreting physician typically reads the study by only reviewing still images, so it is important that the images presented for review are not blurry. Many years ago, unless an entire exam was videotaped, the ultrasound operator was the only person to see the dynamic study. Modern ultrasound systems offer cine loop storage, in which the operator can send short, live clips to the interpreting physician. These clips can also be stored on the PACS and on CDs so that surgeons can view the exams in real time. This can increase diagnostic confidence during exams that require compression or Valsalva maneuvers, pediatric imaging such as pyloric stenosis studies, and renal exams. The cine loop can also be useful if a patient is unable to hold their breath. A sonographer can use cine to capture images in which there isn't patient motion in order to freeze an image that could be of diagnostic value.

DICOM

Digital Imaging and Computers in Medicine (DICOM) can be thought of as the link between the ultrasound machine (or any other digital imaging system) and the PACS system. DICOM allows for the integration of the networks, printing devices, workstations, and PACS that may have been purchased (often from multiple vendors). These protocols allow the ultrasound machine to send the images to the PACS network for archiving purposes. In contrast to JPEG images, DICOM images are extremely large, and one cannot just load these images onto their computer. DICOM data are not recognized by Windows, so users cannot just double-click on an image to load it. A DICOM browser is necessary so that the images can be viewed on various computers, workstations, or even a CD.

BASIC POSITIONING OF PATIENT FOR BASIC ULTRASOUND EXAMS

The sonographer progresses through very extensive training to learn techniques and positioning of both the patient, the transducers, and the sound beams when doing an ultrasound examination. The patient must be correctly positioned for each individual examination for the best acoustic window and to gain the best images of a specific organ or tissue. There are common positions for routine scans. The supine or dorsal recumbent position is the position where the patient lies on his or her back looking straight up. Sometimes a pillow can be placed under the knees or the head for comfort. This is used to examine the abdomen, ribs, and pelvis. A side-lying position, known as the lateral position, may allow the patient to elevate the dependent arm above the head. One leg is straight and one bent for comfort and support. The prone position is lying on the abdomen with arms flexed at each side. The feet may extend off the examination table and a small pillow may be used for comfort for the head.

Abdominal Procedures

SKILLS NEEDED TO MASTER PROPER SONOGRAPHIC TECHNIQUES

It is understood that the sonographer has basic knowledge of anatomy, sonographic data, and disease processes. The technician must also do more than just know the basics of the equipment, the transducers, and the way to record the images. The sonographer today must have a vast knowledge of the disease process, the understanding of conditions that require a special technique or unique view to be conclusive, and how to prepare the patient in the case of any special last minute scanning procedures to ensure a proper diagnosis. They must be able to compile clinical data, review charts, obtain a patient history, and to put all of that together to help form the clinical picture. Then the sonographer must use critical thinking to help get the best images from each individual patient to make the right diagnosis. Each patient differs in body make, weight, age, and the technician must put it all together to make the best use of the scan to get the best images.

DESCRIBING MEASUREMENTS OF TISSUES IN PRELIMINARY REPORTS

The measurements of organs, tissues, masses, or cysts should be documented in length and width of each in established normal measurements. The kidney should be measured in the longest length, the perpendicular anteroposterior length, and width. The common bile duct is measured in a sagittal plane and done from where the duct crosses to the main portal vein and hepatic artery. These examples show how the normal accepted anatomy is used to set the standards for measurement. The normal measurements then are used to determine what is abnormal or pathologic. All organs can be measured in length and width. All solid masses or cysts should be measured for size by width and length.

DIFFICULTIES WITH SCANS FOR ABSCESSES

It can be difficult to determine bowels versus an abscess. The image must be done for several minutes over the worrisome area. Sometimes it helps to let the patient drink which fills the stomach and bladder with fluid. When repeating the scan over an area, make certain to duplicate the exact scan plane with every image. A water enema can also help when scanning the intestines to help differentiate a persistent bowel gas pattern from a gossypiboma. It may be necessary to rescan in a day or two to see if there is a significant change. Fat deposits also make imaging difficult and fatty areas may resemble an abscess. Ascites can be misinterpreted for an abscess but it may be helpful to place the patient in an erect or decubitus position to see if the fluid will shift. The mirror reverberations of the sound waves may show a collection of abscesses to appear as an artifact. It may help the image to scan through a different part of the bladder.

IDENTIFYING ORGANS, TISSUE, AND VESSELS

It is important for the sonographer to know the anatomy of the area being scanned in order to recognize both the normal and abnormal tissue in the patient. Understanding how the blood flows from arteries and veins throughout the circulatory system will help to identify stenosis, abnormalities in the vessels, and blood filled organs. Some vascular structures can be seen in the mid-abdominal scan in a transverse section. Understanding locations of each organ in the abdomen will guide in imaging the area. It is important to remember that the bowel can have a different appearance depending on its contents. The small bowel is more difficult to visualize than the larger bowel, and air and gas can cause shadows on scanning and may give a mottled appearance. Bowel filled with fecal material will look distended and may be misrepresented as pathology.

IMPORTANCE OF OBTAINING WRITTEN CONSENT AND LABS PRIOR TO ULTRASOUND

Ultrasound operators must be certain to obtain a consent form from every patient that is scanned (either on paper or electronically). State and federal regulations require proof of this record, and proper documentation demonstrates that the patient was provided a sufficient amount of information about the exam to be performed. The written consent form is not only for the procedural steps of the exam, but that the benefits, any associated risks, and other options for treatment were communicated to the patient. Patients should always speak to the physician performing the exam to make sure that all of his or her questions or concerns are addressed. It is, of course, the patient's prerogative to opt out of any procedure whether it is prior to or during an exam. Lab values should always be obtained prior to any procedure because these results may offer the provider ample amounts of data pertaining to the patient's health. For example, it is important to know that the patient's liver or kidneys are functioning normally or if their blood clots properly.

TECHNIQUES AND NORMAL VALUES WHEN MEASURING ORGANS DURING ABDOMINAL ULTRASOUNDS

Ultrasound systems allow operators to quickly measure organs to provide useful diagnostic information pertaining to the size of the organs. The various lobes of the liver may vary in size and shape, but the left lobe is smaller than the right lobe. The liver is measured from the diaphragm to the inferior tip of the right lobe in a sagittal plane at the midclavicular line. This measurement should not exceed 15.5 cm and is often less than 13 cm. The kidneys should be measured in two planes; they are typically 12 cm long, 5 cm wide, and 2.5 cm thick. The spleen is also measured in order to diagnose splenomegaly. A splenic index is typically calculated and should fall in the 120–480 cm^3 range. If the length of the spleen alone is used as an indicator, it should be less than 13 cm in healthy adults. The pancreas is not typically measured, but it is about 2 cm thick. The pancreatic duct, when seen, should not be more than 2 mm.

REGULAR DUTIES OF ULTRASOUND TECHNICIANS

The technician must do routine quality assurance tests to make certain the ultrasound lab is being run efficiently. They must clean and prepare all transducers after each examination and be prepared for the next patient. Someone in the department is responsible for ordering equipment and supplies and someone is responsible for checking the orders for the next day, scheduling patients, and preparing those patients for their exams. A technician is responsible for recording and generating images, storing those images or transmitting them to the appropriate physicians, and for archiving all of the images for future reference. There is someone responsible for clean linen in the department, having gels and extra supplies in each ultrasound room, and for providing the patient with gowns, towels, and sterile trays for possible procedures each day.

PHYSICAL FINDINGS TO BE AWARE OF DURING A SCAN

The ultrasound technician must understand how to assess a patient during an ultrasound examination. The technician should look at the color of the patient and the way the patient is breathing. The technician should be able to take a pulse, assess heart rate and respiratory rate, call for assistance in the case of an emergency, and tell how the patient is tolerating the procedure. If a patient is on a cardiac monitor, the technician should be familiar with the normal way the heart rate appears on the monitor screen and be able to pick up on changes a patient may be experiencing during the procedure. The technician should have a basic understanding that an adult heart rate is normally between 60-100 beats per minute and that a child's rate can be between 100-120 beats per minute. An infant or neonate can have a heart rate even higher. Understanding normal heart and respiratory rates helps the sonographer recognize when a patient is experiencing distress.

APPLICATIONS OF HARMONIC IMAGING DURING ABDOMINAL ULTRASOUNDS

Tissue harmonics are not contained within the ultrasound beam that is emitted from the transducer. Tissue harmonics are produced when the sound beam interacts with tissues that are deeper in the body in a nonlinear fashion. With this being said, tissue harmonics do not occur when the scanning depth is shallow. These sound beams that are being transmitted must be strong; weak sound waves will not produce any tissue harmonics at all. With strong beams, the harmonics are created within the main line of the ultrasound wave. Tissue harmonics will only emerge from this main axis and will create very few imaging errors because of the strength of the beam. Harmonic frequencies allow the sonographer to scan patients at higher frequencies that will improve not only the axial resolution, but the lateral resolution as well. The lateral resolution tends to improve because the wave is more narrow (higher frequency beams produce a narrower beam). Harmonics are enabling sonographers to see organs that are deeper in the body, as well as eliminating reverberation artifacts in organs such as the gallbladder. The reverberation artifacts can mimic sludge within the gallbladder.

EVALUATING URINARY SYSTEM FOR VASCULAR ABNORMALITIES USING DOPPLER ULTRASOUND METHODS

Renal artery stenosis occurs when there is stenosis (narrowing) of the renal arteries. This is typically caused by atherosclerosis, and if left untreated it may cause hypertension or renal failure. A renal artery duplex exam may be ordered to determine the cause of uncontrolled or sudden-onset hypertension, determine the cause of an abdominal bruit, follow up from abnormal lab values or prior imaging studies, or if an aneurysm is suspected. A renal artery duplex includes gray-scale, color, and spectral Doppler interrogation of the abdominal aorta, kidneys, renal arteries, and veins, as well as the smaller vessels within the kidneys. These arteries include the segmental, interlobar, arcuate, and interlobular arteries. The direction of blood flow and turbulence should be documented along with the measurement of peak and end diastolic velocities, resistive index, and pulsatile index.

STANDARD RIGHT AND LEFT UPPER QUADRANT ABDOMINAL EXAMINATION

The longitudinal (sagittal) views should be used with the left and right upper quadrants. The scan should include the aorta and the distal aorta especially in patients over the age of 55. The scan should include the inferior vena cava, the main lobar fissure, and the gallbladder. Always include the head of the pancreas, the right and left kidneys, and the side aspect of the liver so the diaphragm and pleural spaces can be seen. Scans should include images of the spleen, the adrenal glands, and any abnormalities seen. Color Doppler can be used to view the main portal vein which will point out blood flow. Transverse views can include the levels of the portal veins, the common duct, the hepatic artery, and the neck, body, and fundus of the gallbladder, as well as the pancreatic region.

ULTRASOUND SYSTEMS THAT ENABLE VISUALIZATION OF ORGAN PERFUSION

The supply of blood to an organ is also known as organ perfusion. Ultrasound systems that have color Doppler capabilities provide users with a visual representation of blood moving through the body. The colors represent the directional flow of the red blood cells. Power Doppler can also be used, but instead of showing the direction of flow within blood vessels, it represents the presence of blood flow. Power Doppler is more sensitive than color Doppler. Some newer ultrasound systems can provide end users with an even greater ability to look at the smallest vessels — even those that display low flow velocities. This can be used when performing renal artery stenosis studies because the arteries that branch within the kidneys are quite small. These include the segmental, interlobar, arcuate, and interlobular arteries.

ABDOMINAL VASCULATURE

The arterial anatomy of the abdomen contains many major arteries including the aorta. The function of the vascular system is to transport oxygenated blood to the organs and tissue and to return the unoxygenated blood back to the lungs. The venous anatomy includes major vessels as well. Types of pathology pertaining to the abdominal vasculature have the potential to be life threatening and careful examination with ultrasound is essential. Aneurysm is the weakening of an arterial wall and rupture can be devastating. Accurate imaging and documentation of an abdominal aortic aneurysm must be monitored for growth and should not exceed two mm/year. Other arterial pathology may include arterial stenosis, arteriosclerosis, atherosclerosis, and pseudoaneurysm. Color Doppler may be used to demonstrate opposite flow directions particularly in a dissecting aneurysm.

TRANSDUCERS USED BY CARDIAC SONOGRAPHERS

Cardiac sonographers gravitate toward linear phased-array transducers. With these transducers, the beam is steered electronically, which allows more coverage without having any parts in motion. When performing echocardiograms, optimal temporal resolution must be exhibited in order to examine the heart in motion. Phased-array technology enables frame rates to be higher. The beam is also focused electronically, which allows for additional focusing should the technologist find it necessary to add more focal zones. The focal depth can be adjusted so that images deeper in the body can be seen with greater detail resolution. One of the main reasons that a cardiac sonographer may choose a linear phased array is that the footprint is rather small. This lets the sonographer image via the intercostal spaces so the heart can be visualized without rib shadowing.

MIRROR IMAGE ARTIFACT OF THE WAVEFORM DURING ABDOMINAL AORTIC DOPPLER EXAM

During a spectral Doppler exam, if flow is visualized above and below the baseline, the sonographer may want to double-check with color Doppler to see if the flow is moving in more than one direction. If it truly is unidirectional flow, this bidirectional flow is an artifact. Crosstalk is a mirror artifact that will only occur during a spectral Doppler study and will show an exact replica of the flow velocity on both sides of the spectral baseline. This can occur if the sonographer is attempting to obtain a velocity, but the incident angle of the ultrasound wave is perpendicular to the motion of the red blood cells. Electronic mirror imaging associated with crosstalk may occur if the Doppler gain is set too high.

AORTIC DISSECTION

An aortic dissection is a life-threatening condition in which the innermost layer of the aorta tears and allows blood to pool between the inner and middle layers of the arterial wall. Although dissections are a fairly uncommon occurrence, they can be difficult to diagnose without medical imaging because the symptoms can mimic a heart attack. Patients may complain of sudden, excruciating chest or abdominal pain that radiates to the back or down the leg and shortness of breath. The quicker that the diagnosis can be made, the better the chances of survival for the patient. Bedside sonography can provide a quick, noninvasive look at the aorta. If an intimal flap is seen within the lumen of the abdominal aorta, a dissection is assumed, and the patient must be sent to surgery immediately. If the outer layer of the aorta ruptures because of the pooling of blood, the patient will typically die.

ABDOMINAL AORTIC ANEURYSM

Ultrasound is often the first modality chosen in the detection of abnormalities of the retroperitoneum due to the low cost and the fact that it does not use ionizing radiation. Ultrasound exams can provide a quick method for detecting an abdominal aortic aneurysm (AAA). The abdominal aorta can be examined by gray-scale, color, and spectral Doppler in patients that are experiencing abdominal or flank pain, when a pulsatile mass is detected in the abdomen, or if a clinician hears an abdominal bruit. Ultrasound is typically the method of choice to follow up an AAA when detected by previous imaging exams or modalities. Any measurement that is greater than or equal to 3 cm in diameter in the infrarenal portion of the aorta is considered to be aneurysmal. This region is also considered to be positive for an aneurysm when the diameter is 1.5 times greater than the segment that is proximal to the renal arteries; this is a great guideline to follow especially in patients that are smaller than average.

IMPORTANCE OF IDENTIFYING THE LOCATION OF THE LEFT RENAL VEIN

Ultrasound is a cost-effective modality to examine patients that present with symptoms such as fevers, hematuria, urinary tract infections, flank or inguinal pain, or varicoceles. Ultrasound is often the first step in diagnosing any abnormalities of the urinary system. Multiple congenital variations of the left renal vein may occur in which it is positioned behind the aorta and in front of the spine. Although a rare phenomenon, this is known as a retroaortic left renal vein, and symptoms arise because compression increases the pressure of the renal vein. Symptoms such as hematuria are often exasperated by physical activity. Color Doppler is helpful in tracking the renal vein from the kidney to the inferior vena cava, and sonographers may notice that the left renal vein tends to have a smaller diameter when it courses anteriorly to the spine. It is important to note this finding in symptomatic patients or those that are having any type of renal surgery.

ADVANTAGE OF USING ULTRASOUND TO DETERMINE A THROMBUS IN THE IVC

Ultrasound is a cost-effective and noninvasive tool that can be used to quickly diagnose medical emergencies. Ultrasound can be performed bedside so that the patient does not have to be taken to the radiology department. The inferior vena cava (IVC) is located to the right of the abdominal aorta, and it returns blood from the lower body to the right atrium of the heart. The IVC is formed when the right and left common iliac veins join within the retroperitoneum. A thrombus (blood clot) may be readily identified in the IVC because it appears as an echogenic filling defect within the lumen of the IVC; a blood clot within the IVC is life-threatening. Color Doppler can also be used to demonstrate the incomplete saturation of color within the vessel. A thrombus in the IVC is typically the result of a deep vein thrombosis of the legs. An IVC filter may be placed in patients that cannot take anticoagulants to prevent emboli from lodging within the lungs or heart.

DIAPHRAGMATIC CRURA

The diaphragmatic crura begin as tendinous fibers forming two "legs" (crura) along the spine. The right crus "leg" is longer, larger, and more lobular. The right renal artery runs in front of the right diaphragmatic crus and in back of the inferior vena cava (IVC). The left diaphragmatic crus runs along the anterior lumbar vertebral bodies in a superior direction and inserts into the central tendon of the diaphragm. Additionally, the diaphragmatic crura of children appear large, relative to body size since crural width does not increase significantly with age.

LIVER'S PORTAL AND HEPATIC VEINS

The portal vein drains blood from the digestive system (including the associated glands). The union of the splenic and superior mesenteric veins forms the portal vein. It divides into the left portal vein and the right portal vein before entering the liver. The left portal vein is smaller and located towards the front and top of the liver. The right portal vein is larger and located towards the back and bottom of the liver. The hepatic veins are all of the veins that carry the blood from the liver. These veins terminate into three large veins (the right hepatic vein, the middle hepatic vein, and the left hepatic vein) that open into the inferior vena cava (IVC). The right hepatic vein is the largest and joins the IVC at the right side. The middle hepatic vein joins the IVC towards the front. The left hepatic vein is the smallest and joins the IVC towards the front.

VASCULAR AND DUCTAL LANDMARKS OF THE PANCREAS

The following vascular and ductal landmarks are found on or near the pancreas:

- Portal vein and its offshoots: These are located behind the neck of pancreas at the point where the superior-mesenteric vein and the splenic vein meet.
- Splenic artery: This artery runs along the top edge of the pancreas (slightly above and behind the splenic vein).
- Common hepatic artery: This artery runs along the top of the duodenum and then splits into two branches (the proper hepatic artery and the gastroduodenal artery).
- Superior Mesenteric Artery: This artery branches off the aorta (at the lower body) and runs to the front of the duodenum and enters the small bowel's attachment to the back wall of the abdomen.
- Common Bile Duct: The common bile duct crosses in front of the portal vein and to the right of the proper hepatic artery.

EFFECTS OF PORTAL HYPERTENSION ON THE SPLEEN

Portal hypertension is the buildup of pressure in the portal vein (the vein connecting the intestines and the liver). Normally, the pressure is low compared with the arterial pressure, but slightly above the pressure in the other veins of the body. The most common cause of portal hypertension is liver disease (such as cirrhosis). Portal hypertension usually causes moderate splenomegaly and dilated, tortuous blood vessels at the splenic hilum. It also causes dilation of the portal vein itself. If portal hypertension is suspected, the liver and portal vein should be examined along with the spleen.

SCANNING TRANSPLANTED KIDNEYS

Select a transducer with the highest frequency for depth penetration, usually a 5-MHz one is adequate. A curved transducer gives a large field allowing for accurate length measurements of the entire kidney. Using the postoperative scar helps to locate the transplanted kidney. Long axis views of the kidney will appear along the axis of the scar and the transverse view of the kidney will be at a right angle to the scar. The urinary bladder will be scanned. If the bladder is full of urine, voiding may make what appears as hydronephrosis disappear when scanned again. Color Doppler may be helpful to image flow of blood to and from the transplanted kidney.

ULTRASOUND EXAMINATION OF RENAL TRANSPLANT PATIENTS

The following conditions should be looked for:

- Any swelling of the kidney due to the back up of urine (hydronephrosis).
- Fluid collections (such as lymphocele). Lymphoceles are the most common fluid collections in the transplant population (occurring in five to fifteen percent of patients). They are most frequently associated with obstruction of the urethra. On ultrasound, these collections may appear heavily septated and large.
- Any bleeding (hemorrhage). Perinephric hematomas account for twenty-five to thirty percent of all complications. While most are small and do not require additional therapy, haematomas may occasionally compress the ureter and produce hydronephrosis.
- Any signs of acute (or diffuse) infection and acute tubular necrosis (ATN).
- Any signs of rejection (increased size, prominent hypoechoic medullary pyramids, obliteration of the renal sinus fat, or thickening of the renal pelvis).

PRE- AND POST-SURGICAL ULTRASOUND EXAMINATION FOR LIVER TRANSPLANT

Ultrasound is a very useful tool in the pre and post operative evaluation of the liver patient. Prior to surgery ultrasound is used to evaluate:

- The health of liver tissue (hepatocytes).
- Identify lesions.
- Determine the openness and size of the portal vein, hepatic veins, and the inferior vena cava (IVC).
- Assess the biliary system for dialation.

After surgery, blood clot formation in the hepatic artery (thrombosis) is the most dangerous complication. Ultrasound is used to monitor the health of the hepatic vascular structures after surgery. Thrombosis of the hepatic artery or portal vein may lead to massive death of liver cells (hepatic necrosis). The presence of air in the hepatic parenchyma (functional cells of the liver) shows up as shadowing on the sonogram. Gangrene of the liver is also apparent in the hepatic texture. Some other things to monitor for are portal vein thrombosis and any blockages of the IVC and hepatic veins.

TRANSVERSE SCAN SONOGRAM

Transverse scanning is used to image structures that lie transversely (sideways) within the body (such as the pancreas). The transverse plane divides the body into upper and lower portions and extends from side to side.

The correct orientation of a transverse scan sonogram is as follows:

- For a transverse scan through the left thyroid, the patient's right side is on the left of the sonogram
- For a transverse scan of the gallbladder, the patient's left side is on the right of the sonogram
- For a transverse scan of the left kidney, the top of the sonogram represents the anterior

BILE

Bile is made up of:

- Bile Salts (cholates, chenodeoxycholate, deoxycholate): The liver produces bile salts by breaking down cholesterol. They function in a detergent-like way that breaks down dietary fats. This allows the fats to be dissolved and absorbed by the body.
- Cholesterol and Phospholipids: Four percent of bile is in the form of cholesterol. The secretion of cholesterol into bile is the major way that cholesterol is eliminated from the body. Phospholipids (a major component of cellular membranes) assist with the ability of bile salts to dissolve cholesterol.
- Bilirubin: Bilirubin is an end product of the body's metabolism of hemoglobin (the component of red blood cells that allows oxygen to be carried). This component also gives bile its characteristic yellow-green color.
- Protein: Bile proteins may play a role in regulating the intensity of bile production.

SOURCE AND RE-CIRCULATION

The functional liver cells (hepatocytes) excrete bile into the canaliculi (spaces between the liver cells). The bile drains into the right hepatic duct and the left hepatic duct that join together to form the common hepatic duct. A portion of bile travels to the gallbladder through the cystic duct. The gallbladder has a capacity to hold five tablespoons of bile. The gallbladder makes the bile ten times stronger by removing water during fasting. When a person eats a meal, the gallbladder is stimulated to contract and release the concentrated bile to the small intestine through the opening of the sphincter of Oddi (the muscle opening that controls the flow of bile and pancreatic enzymes). The liver produces about one to two liters of bile every day. Ninety five percent of the bile that enters the small intestine is recovered and returned to the liver through the terminal ileum (located at the end of the small intestine).

CHOLEDOCHTAL CYSTS

Abdominal ultrasound is the preferred method for examining choledochal cysts. It does however, have limitations such as an inability to differentiate the cysts from other structures (such as the gallbladder). It may also have a decreased sensitivity due to overlying bowel gas and the presence of inflammatory diseases (such as cholangitis).

Sonographic features:

- The cyst may appear as a true cyst due to the presence of accumulated bile.
- The location of the cyst will be in the upper right quadrant of the liver region.

Choledochal cysts are put into four classifications based on their anatomy:

I. A localized widening of the common bile duct.

II. An offshoot with a pouch (connected to the common bile duct). This may resemble the cystic duct and gallbladder.

III. A widening of the common bile duct which folds into the duodenum.

IV. A widening of the common bile duct plus a widening of the common hepatic duct.

BILIARY OBSTRUCTION
PROXIMAL TO THE CYSTIC DUCT

Biliary obstructions proximal to the cystic duct are usually caused by carcinoma of the common bile duct (Sonographically viewed as a tubular branching of the hepatic ducts.) or metastases originating in the porta hepatis. The patient typically shows signs of jaundice and an overall itching of the body (pruritus). Alkaline phosphatase and direct bilirubin levels are also elevated. The gallbladder itself does not enlarge even after a full meal is consumed.

Distal TO THE Cystic Duct

Biliary obstructions distal to the cystic duct are usually caused by gallstones. Symptoms of gallstones include; upper right quadrant pain, jaundice, and itching (pruritus). Alkaline phosphatase and direct bilirubin levels are also elevated. The gallbladder itself appears small in size. The presence of gallstones appears (on the sonograph) as hyperechoic lesions along the bottom of the gallbladder. The common hepatic duct may also show the presence of gallstones.

COMPOSITION OF GALLSTONES AND UPPER NORMAL LIMITS FOR BILIARY DUCTS

Ultrasound is the imaging modality of choice when a patient presents with abdominal pain (with or without jaundice) in which biliary obstruction is suspected. Biliary obstruction may be the result of cholelithiasis (gallstones), choledocholithiasis (gallstones present in the bile ducts) or masses that are compressing the bile ducts. Bile is produced in the liver, but the gallbladder is a pouch that collects bile until it is released into the small intestine to aid in digestion, such as when a fatty meal is consumed. If there is too much cholesterol (as in the majority of cases in the United States) or bilirubin in the bile, gallstones may develop. In addition to the gallbladder, the liver, bile ducts, and pancreas should also be evaluated to determine the cause of biliary obstruction. Intrahepatic ducts measuring greater than 2 mm are considered to be the cutoff normal limit. There are two hepatic ducts (right and left) that combine to form the common hepatic duct, and they typically measure less than 4 mm. The common hepatic duct merges with the cystic duct to become the common bile duct (CBD). The CBD should not measure greater than 6 mm unless the patient is elderly or has had his or her gallbladder removed.

ACOUSTIC SHADOWING IN PATIENT WITH GALLSTONES WHEN USING A 3.5 MHZ MULTIFREQUENCY PROBE

A sonographer can improve the resolution in what appears to be gallstones by two methods. If gallstones are suspected, but distal acoustic shadowing is not clearly identified with a 3.5 MHz probe, a sonographer can increase the frequency as high as it will go. Higher frequency transducers will create an ultrasound beam that is narrower. If the ultrasound wave is wider than the gallstone, the beam picks up signals from either side of the stone and the shadow may not be visualized as well or at all. In this case, perhaps the operator can bump the frequency all the way up to 5 MHz. Another parameter that a sonographer can adjust to create a narrow beam is to place the focal point so it is at the depth of the gallstones.

USEFULNESS OF HARMONICS WHEN IMAGING THE GALLBLADDER

The gallbladder is an organ that is subject to image artifact during an ultrasound. It can be difficult to discern if reflectors visualized within are real. Tissue harmonics is a concept that has helped clinicians and operators gain diagnostic confidence because it tends to eliminate some signals that are not pathological. Harmonic frequencies allow the sonographer to scan patients at higher frequencies that will not only improve axial resolution but will improve the lateral resolution as well. The lateral resolution tends to improve because the wave is more narrow (higher frequency beams produce a narrower beam). Gallbladders that are imaged with harmonics have seen a decrease in improved signal-to-noise ratios, being able to see those organs that are deeper in the body, as well as eliminating reverberation artifacts. The reverberation artifacts can mimic sludge within the gallbladder.

FALSE-POSITIVE RESULTS OF ULTRASOUND GALLSTONE EXAMINATIONS

False-positive results for a gallstone examination are possibly due to:

- Polyps within the gallbladder.
- Adenomyosis (the cells that normally line the gallbladder grow into the tissue of the gallbladder wall).
- The presence of gas in the small intestine (duodenum).
- The presence of air in the biliary tree.
- Porcelain gallbladder (calcium encrustation of the gallbladder wall)

FALSE-NEGATIVE RESULTS OF ULTRASOUND GALLSTONE EXAMINATIONS

False-negative results for a gallstone examination are possibly due to:

- The gallbladder is in its contracted state (emptied of bile).
- The cystic duct obscures the view of Hartmann's pouch (the part of the gallbladder (near the neck) where gallstones tend to collect).
- The gallstone is hidden in the fundal (bottom) cap of the gallbladder.

CHOLECYSTECTOMY AND POST-SURGICAL FUNCTION OF THE BILIARY TREE

Cholecystectomy is the surgical removal of the gallbladder. It is most commonly performed when a patient has gallstones that are causing chronic symptoms. Each year, about five hundred thousand Americans undergo this surgery. The major complications of this surgery are due to injury to the bile ducts. This may allow bile to leak (called a biliary fistula) into the abdominal cavity (causing a potential for infection). Also, bile duct strictures (contraction of the duct) can occur impeding the flow of bile through the biliary tree. Ultrasound examinations (before and after surgery) can help to detect complications and their source. With the gallbladder removed the sphincter of Oddi remains relaxed (loss of tonus) and the overall pressure of bile within the biliary tree drops. The flow of bile continues irrespective of fasting or eating.

PREPARING A PATIENT FOR A GALLBLADDER ULTRASOUND

The patient should fast for 8-12 hours before a scan to offer a better window for the imaging. It allows for less air in the stomach and gives room for water if needed to get a clearer image. Use a transducer with a high frequency and set the focal zone to the back wall of the gallbladder where stones collect. The frequency must be strong enough to go through the entire organ but may be changed when scanning the liver to avoid subtle shadowing. Harmonic imaging may help clear artifacts. Start with positioning the patient in a supine position. It is also advisable to get left lateral decubitus views, oblique, and prone views so not to miss scanning a gallbladder stone. The upright position is an awkward position for the patient but may be helpful if the liver is small or high in the quadrant. A standing position for this upright scan is often better and offers an acoustic window which enhances the view of the gallbladder.

LABORATORY TESTS TO DIAGNOSE DISEASES OF THE GALLBLADDER AND BILIARY TREE

The following liver function tests are used to diagnose diseases of the gallbladder and biliary tree:

1. Lactate dehydrogenase (LDH). LDH is an enzyme that is present in many body tissues, especially the heart, liver, kidney, skeletal muscle, brain, blood cells, and lungs. When these tissues are damaged, LDH is released to the blood.
2. Alk Phos (alkaline phosphatase) and GGT (gamma-glutamyltranspeptidase). Alk Phos and GGT bloodstream levels are elevated in a number of disorders that affect the drainage of bile (such as a gallstone, cyst or tumor blocking the common bile duct). Since alkaline phosphatase is also found in other organs, GGT is utilized as a confirmatory test to be sure that the elevation of alkaline phosphatase is indeed coming from the liver or the biliary tree.
3. Serum glutamic oxaloacetic transaminase (SGOT) or aspartate aminotransferase (AST). This is an enzyme that is normally present in liver and heart cells. It is released into the blood when there is damage to the heart (such as occurs with a heart attack) or to the liver (such as occurs with cirrhosis).
4. Serum glutamic pyruvic transaminase (SGPT) or alanine aminotransferase (ALT). Similar to SGOT, this is another enzyme that is released to the blood when heart or liver cells are damaged. This enzyme is more specific to liver cell damage than SGOT.

The blood levels of these enzymes rise and then fall back to normal for acute disorders and remain elevated for chronic disorders.

ANATOMY OF THE GALLBLADDER AND BILIARY TREE

The gallbladder is about three inches long and located beneath the liver. It is shaped like a small sack. The gallbladder stores and concentrates bile (a bitter, alkaline, yellow-colored liquid that is produced by the liver and aids in the absorption and digestion of food, especially fats). The gallbladder delivers the concentrated bile to the first part of the small intestine (called the duodenum). The gallbladder is connected to the liver and the duodenum by a series of ducts called the biliary tree. Beginning at the liver, the right hepatic duct and the left hepatic duct join to form the common hepatic duct. The gallbladder is connected to the common hepatic duct by the cystic duct to form the common bile duct. The pancreatic duct finally joins the common bile duct and the entire biliary tree ends at the duodenum (at the hepaticopancreatic ampulla or the sphincter of Oddi).

CHOLECYSTITIS

Cholecystitis is an acute inflammation of the gallbladder. Ninety percent of the time gallstones (inside the gallbladder) cause the problem. Bile becomes trapped within the gallbladder causing irritation and pressure. Untreated, the condition may develop into a bacterial infection and ultimately perforation of the gallbladder. The primary symptom is abdominal pain (especially following a fatty meal).

CHOLANGITIS

Cholangitis is a condition where there is an infection present in the common bile duct. The infection commonly causes inflammation of the common bile duct resulting in symptoms of fever, chills, and pain in the right upper quadrant of the liver. It typically occurs when the common bile duct becomes clogged by a gallstone or tumor. If left untreated, serious life-threatening problems may develop (such as the spread of infection to the liver and pus-filled abscesses).

SYMPTOMS, CLINICAL CORRELATION, AND COMPLICATIONS FOR GALLBLADDER AND BILIARY TREE DISEASES

Disruption of the production, flow and re-circulation of bile cause most of the common symptoms of gallbladder and biliary tree disease. Patients typically develop diarrhea because the body loses the ability to digest and absorb fat (called steratorra). They may also develop deficiencies of the fat-soluble vitamins (Vitamin A, D, E, and K). The body may lose the ability to properly eliminate cholesterol, resulting in the elevation of blood cholesterol to dangerous levels. This increases the patient's risk for vascular diseases such as heart attack and stroke. The body may lose the ability to properly eliminate bilirubin. The bilirubin levels can then build-up, causing a yellowing of the skin and eyes (jaundice). Bile production and re-circulation is the major path for elimination of waste from the liver. Physical blockages of the gallbladder and biliary tree (caused by gallstones, injuries or tumors) may cause abnormal liver function test values, abdominal pain, and fever.

GALLBLADDER ADENOMYOMATOSIS

Adenomyomatosis is the most common cause of thickening of the gallbladder wall. It is caused by a benign tumor called an adenoma. It is usually without any symptoms and is discovered incidentally (through imaging or surgery). The tumor takes the form of firm, rubbery, well-defined nodule. It is located at the bottom (fundic) end of the gallbladder. It is more commonly found in women and those over thirty-five years of age. It is also a condition associated with gallstones and cholesterolosis.

GALLBLADDER CHOLESTEROLOSIS

Cholesterosis (strawberry gallbladder) occurs frequently when gallstones are present. It is a chronic inflammatory condition that results in the formation of cholesterol polyps. The interior of the gallbladder appears as a strawberry. The cholesterol crystals form the background with little yellow specks of cholesterol esters making up the "seeds". The cholesterol crystals may detach from the wall of the gallbladder and form the beginning of a cholesterol stone.

CARCINOMA OF THE GALLBLADDER

Carcinoma of the gallbladder is the most common source of carcinoma of the liver and biliary tree. Its frequency is three cases per one hundred thousand persons. It is most commonly seen in older adults (primarily women over sixty years old) with gallstones. The exact cause is unknown however it is thought to occur through years of irritation and repair cycles of the gallbladder mucosa due to gallstones. The tumor is typically made up of columnar cell adenocarcinoma.

Ultrasound features include:

- The shape of the mass is similar to the shape of the gallbladder itself.
- The echotexture is heterogeneous, solid and semi-solid.
- The gallbladder wall has been thickened.
- The adjacent liver tissue usually appears heterogeneous due to the spread of the cancer.
- The dilated biliary duct appears as a "shotgun-sign".

PAPILLOMAS

Papilloma is a benign epithelial (made up of a layer of cells) tumor. It does not develop into cancer. There may be a single or multiple scattered tumors present.

ULTRASOUND FEATURES OF BENIGN MASSES OF THE GALLBLADDER

Ultrasound features of benign tumors:

- Typically show up as small attached lumps (elevations) on the interior surface (lumen) of the gallbladder.
- Adneomyomatosis is indicated if there is reduced or no flow of bile to and from the interior of the gallbladder (through the cystic duct).
- Sometimes mistaken for a tumor (or gallstones) is a condition called Phrygian cap in which the gallbladder fundus (bottom) is abnormally tilted and a partial septum exists.

There are several other benign masses that may be observed including mucosal hyperplasia, inflammatory polyps, mucous cysts, and granulomata (caused by parasites).

CHOLELITHIASIS

Cholelithiasis is the presence of gallstones within in the gallbladder (or biliary tree). Gallstones are formed when the concentrations of bile pigments and salts (both calcium and cholesterol based) become unbalanced. The gallstones themselves may very tiny or as large as one inch in diameter. In most cases, they do not cause any symptoms and are discovered incidentally. They are most likely to be found in the part of the gallbladder nearest to the opening of the cystic duct (called Hartmann's pouch).

CHOLEDOCHOLITHIASIS

Choledocholithiasis is the presence of gallstones in the common bile duct. About fifteen percent of patients with gallstones develop choledocholithiasis. Symptoms only occur if the flow of bile through the bile ducts becomes obstructed. This may lead to infection of the biliary tree and (if the pancreatic duct is also obstructed) pancreatitis. Typical symptoms may include pain (that worsens after a fatty meal), nausea, vomiting, fever and jaundice.

TUMORS ARISING FROM EXTRAHEPATIC BILE DUCTS AND INTRAHEPATIC BILE DUCTS

Malignant tumors that originate in the extrahepatic bile ducts (usually the common bile duct) show the same ultrasound features as pancreatic tumors. They show a distinctive pattern of the tumor bulging against a dilated common bile duct. When these tumors appear in the left and right hepatic ducts, the cancer primarily affects the ductal walls without showing signs of dilation (bulging). There is a level of difficulty in imaging these tumors since the tumor itself is not seen. The only sign is a bulging (dilation) of the duct above the tumor itself. Malignant tumors that originate in the intrahepatic bile ducts show the same ultrasound features as primary tumors of the liver. The tumors also show a pattern of dilation to the intrahepatic ducts.

DUPLEX COLLECTING SYSTEM

In a normal urinary tract, each kidney is connected to one ureter that drains urine into the bladder. Patients with a duplex collecting system will have two ureters for one kidney that drain independently into the bladder. This condition often occurs with the distal ureter ballooning at its opening into the bladder, forming a sack-like pouch (called a ureterocele). When a patient has an ureterocele, the portion of the ureter closest to the bladder typically becomes enlarged because the ureter opening is very tiny and obstructs urine outflow. As the urine flow is obstructed, urine backs up in the ureter tube. In a duplex collecting system, the ureter with the ureterocele generally drains the top half of the kidney while the duplicate may drain the lower half. An isolated duplex collecting system may be a completely benign condition and may not require therapy.

POLYCYSTIC RENAL DISEASE

The most common of these is inherited polycystic renal disease (or PRD). PRD is marked by the formation of fluid-filled cysts in the kidney tubules. These cysts compress functioning kidney tissue, eventually replacing it. In the more common type (autosomal dominant PRD), almost half of the patients develop chronic kidney failure between the ages of 40 and 60. The rare form (autosomal recessive PRD) causes kidney failure in early childhood. Renal cystic disease consists of inflammatory or necrotic cysts. In most cases of renal cystic disease both kidneys typically show enlargement. Patients may experience back (or flank) pain, red blood cells in the urine (hematuria), white blood cells (leukocytes) in the urine, and excess protein in the urine (proteinuria).

NEPHRITIS

Inflammation of the kidneys (nephritis) is the primary characteristic of several kidney diseases. In the most common type, glomerulonephritis (also known as Bright's disease), the glomerulus (the filtering part of the kidney) becomes inflamed and scarred. The kidneys slowly lose their ability to remove wastes and excess water from the blood to make urine. Diseases such as diabetes and lupus can cause glomerulonephritis. The disease may be acute or chronic in nature. Abscesses and bacterial infections are also common causes of nephritis. Typical symptoms include back (or flank) pain, fever, elevated white blood cell (leukocyte) count, and pus in the urine (pyuria). In some cases, there is also an increase in blood urea nitrogen (BUN), albumen, and total plasma protein levels.

FUNCTIONS OF THE KIDNEYS AND URINARY TRACT

Following are the major functions of the kidneys and urinary tract:

- Toxin Removal: The human body is constantly accumulating toxins either from food digestion or waste products produced by cells. These toxins need to be removed quickly or they will build up to dangerous levels in the blood. The kidneys filter the toxins out of the blood and safely eliminate them for the body in the form of urine.
- Drug Removal: Many drugs are eliminated in the urine after being metabolized.
- Maintaining a proper fluid balance: The body is constantly gaining fluid (from the diet) and losing it (evaporation, urine, stool). The kidneys regulate the body's fluid balance to keep it from swelling up or becoming dehydrated.

91

- Electrolyte Balance: In order for cells to function properly, the concentrations of electrolytes in the blood need to be tightly controlled. The kidneys regulate this process. Here are the most important electrolytes and the organs that are sensitive to their changes:
  o Sodium – Brain and nerves
  o Potassium, Magnesium – Heart, muscle, and nerves
  o Calcium – Heart, muscle, nerves, and bone
  o Phosphorus – Muscle and bone
- Acid-Base Balance: The body's processing of proteins is sensitive to changes in acid concentration of blood. The kidneys remove excess acid to maintain the proper pH balance.
- Blood Pressure Control: The kidneys play a role in regulating blood pressure by balancing fluid and salt levels in the blood.
- Hormone Production: The kidneys produce erythropoietin (affects the bone marrow to make more red blood cells) and calcitriol (active form of vitamin D for bone health)

KIDNEY STONES

Kidney stones (renal calculi) are solid crystals made up of dissolved minerals that occur in urine. They are typically found inside the kidneys or ureters. The size of the stone can be as large as a golf ball. Tiny kidney stones usually leave the body in the urine stream unnoticed. The larger stones can cause an obstruction of a ureter. This in turn causes the ureter to swell with urine and causes moderate to severe pain. The pain is most commonly felt in the back (flank), lower abdomen, and groin. The most common composition of kidney stones is calcium oxalate. Clinical symptoms of kidney stones include intermittent back (flank) pain, vomiting, red blood cells in the urine (hematuria), infection, and an elevated white blood cell (leukocyte) count.

TECHNIQUE FOR KIDNEY ULTRASOUND

The right kidney is best seen if the sonographer has the patient lie supine and the transducer is angled obliquely. The liver acts as the window for the sound beam. A coronal and a lateral approach are also possible. It is often helpful to have the patient roll to a right-side-up position and the transducer used at a lateral approach. To scan the left kidney, have the patient left-side up. The patient raises the arm above his head and the technician uses the coronal approach to scan through the spleen. Using the transducer at a decubitus and oblique position look for the clearest image of the left kidney with the highest frequency available. Use pillows under the patient to eliminate the cavity between the ribs and the hip bone.

SONOGRAPHIC RENAL MEASUREMENTS

A renal ultrasound is a common test ordered when a patient's laboratory results suggest chronic kidney disease. Ultrasound can provide volumetric data of the kidneys as well as measurements of the cortical thickness and images that display the echogenicity. The echogenicity of the kidneys should be compared to the liver and the spleen. Obtaining a renal volume can be a challenge because the kidneys are not elliptical in shape, and it may take experience to get a good volume. This can be difficult when follow-up studies are requested because experience is required, so some clinicians prefer to use the length of the kidney. Another important measurement that may indicate renal disease is cortical thickness. Some studies have shown this as a more accurate indicator of renal function than the length of the kidney. Chronic renal disease will present as kidneys that are smaller than normal with a loss of cortical thickness.

TUBEROUS SCLEROSIS

Tuberous sclerosis (Bourneville's disease) is a congenital disease that causes multiple renal cysts. Typically, there are also multiple renal angiomyolipomas (benign tumors composed of fatty (adipose) tissue, muscle cells, and vascular structures). The typical patient afflicted with this disease has a history of seizures, mental deficiency, and skin tumors.

ACQUIRED CYSTIC DISEASE OF DIALYSIS

Patients that require long-term dialysis have a greater chance of developing renal cysts. Up to ninety percent of dialysis patients show some signs of renal cystic disease after two to three years of treatment. These cysts sometimes bleed (hemorrhage). These patients also have an increased incidence of renal adenomas and cancer (up to seven times greater than the general population).

BERTIN'S COLUMNS

Bertin's columns are "sheath-like" indentations of the kidney's outer surface (renal cortex) that penetrate the renal medulla to various depths. This is a completely normal feature of the renal cortex. Patients that have any duplication in the renal sinus show the greatest number and size of Bertin's columns. Following are the renal-mass-effect features of kidneys affected by hypertrophied Bertin's columns:

- A lateral indentation of the renal sinus.
- A clear definition from the renal sinus.
- A maximum depth that does not exceed one inch.
- The columns are contiguous with the renal cortex.
- The echogenicity resembles the renal parenchyma.
- The presence of two distinct groups of renal sinus echoes (the "split sinus" sign).
- The renal surface contour appears normal.

NORMAL RENAL PARENCHYMA

When the patient in the supine position (lying down face-up), three segments of the kidney can be observed. They are:

- A hypoechoic renal medulla zone (made up of many anechoic triangle-shaped renal pyramids).
- A renal cortex that is moderately echoic.
- A highly echoic central renal sinus.

RENAL MEDULLA

The renal medulla shows up as hypoechoic pyramid shapes that are uniformly spaced. The pyramids are separated by linear barriers that extend to the renal sinus. The shapes are similarly sized and appear as regularly-spaced triangles. The tip of pyramid points towards the renal sinus and the base sits next to the renal cortex. The bow-shaped blood vessels are located at the base of the pyramids.

RENAL BLOOD VESSELS

The renal arteries are best observed when the patient is in the supine position (flat on their back) or lying on their left side (left lateral decubitus (LLD)) position. The right renal artery (RRA) and the left renal artery (LRA) originate at the aorta and run to the central renal sinus. The RRA and the LRA appear as circular tubular structures in back of the inferior vena cava (IVC). The right renal vein (RRV) and the left renal vein (LRV) run from the central renal sinus to the inferior vena cava (IVC). The renal arteries have a hypoechoic central lumen with strongly echogenic borders. The renal arteries are positioned underneath the renal veins and can be found by following their connections to the aorta. The "nutcracker" phenomenon results from compression of the left renal vein between the superior mesenteric artery and the aorta.

ANATOMY OF RENAL NEPHRONS

The renal nephrons (also known as tubules) are the functional internal parts of the kidneys. Each kidney has up to five hundred thousand nephrons. Each nephron is about one half inch long. It has very thin walls made up of cells that function to filter blood and eliminate waste (in the form of urine). The nephron has one open end and one closed end. The closed end is a cup-shaped structure called Bowman's capsule. Blood (that needs to be filtered) enters Bowman's capsule and flows through a tightly wadded network of capillaries (called the glomerulus). The blood is filtered through the glomerulus and ultimately returns to the body through the renal vein. The filtrate drains towards the open end of the nephron and is further processed (for salt, water, and electrolyte balance), through the proximal convoluted tubule, Henle's loop, and the distal convoluted tubule. Any leftover waste products are then eliminated from the body in the form of urine.

EXTRARENAL PELVIS

The renal pelvis is the expansion on the upper end of the ureter into which the renal calices open. The renal pelvis is normally situated entirely within the renal sinus. In the case of an extrarenal pelvis, a large part of the renal pelvis lies outside the kidney. The kidney itself will appear longer than normal. In most case this is a benign condition, however, an extrarenal pelvis could indicate that an obstruction of the junction between the ureter and the pelvis is present.

The following ultrasound features are present:

- The extrarenal pelvis will appear as a central cystic area that lies outside of the kidney proper.
- A transverse view should be used to observe the connection of the extrarenal pelvis with the renal sinus.

SOLITARY KIDNEY

A solitary kidney is a rare condition. It occurs when only one kidney is formed (instead of two) during embryonic development due to agenesis (the absence or failed development of a body part). The solitary functioning kidney is typically enlarged, and the remaining "empty" kidney location should be examined for the presence of a small, non-functional kidney.

PELVIC KIDNEY

If a kidney is not observed in its normal location, the patient's retroperitoneum and pelvis should be scanned. In most cases the "lost" kidney will be found in the patient's bony pelvis region. Pelvic kidney is a developmental abnormality in which the kidney (or kidneys) is located in pelvis instead of normal abdominal lumbar position in the renal fossa.

DETAILED ANATOMY OF THE KIDNEYS

The detailed anatomy of the kidneys is described below:

- Blood is supplied to the kidneys by the renal artery. The renal artery originates from the aorta.
- The renal artery splits into three branches as it enters the kidney through the hilus. Two of these branches are located in front of the ureter and one is located behind the pelvis of the ureter.
- A total of five to six veins join together to form the renal vein. The renal vein exits the hilus directly in front of the renal artery and drains into the inferior vena cava (IVC).

- The lymph vessels run along the renal artery and join the lateral aortic lymph nodes (near the origin of the renal artery).
- Nerves line the branches of the renal vessels and begin in the renal sympathetic plexus.

HORSESHOE KIDNEY

Horseshoe kidney is an anomaly of the kidney included in a group of called fusion anomalies, in which both kidneys are fused together in early embryonic life. Horseshoe kidney is the most common fusion anomaly. Horseshoe kidney refers to the appearance of the fused kidney, which results from fusion at one pole. In more than ninety percent of cases, fusion occurs along the lower pole. Specifically, the term horseshoe kidney is reserved for cases in which most of each kidney lies on one side of the spine. It includes:

- Symmetric horseshoe kidney (fusion along the midline).
- Asymmetric horseshoe kidney (or L-shaped kidney) when the fused part (the isthmus), lies slightly alongside the midline (lateral fusion).

GENERAL ANATOMY OF THE KIDNEYS AND URINARY TRACT

The kidneys are two dark-red bean-shaped organs located at the back of the abdominal cavity just below the ribs (one on each side of the spine). Each kidney is about four inches long and two inches thick. There is an adrenal gland located above each kidney. The kidneys lie under the peritoneum in a cushion of two types of fat (perirenal and pararenal). The right kidney typically lies lower than the left due to the presence of the liver. Blood is supplied to the kidneys via two renal arteries (that branch off of the abdominal aorta). Blood leaves the kidneys through the renal veins. The urinary tract is made up of a series of organs that produce, store, and eliminate urine. It is composed of two kidneys, two ureters, the urinary bladder, two sphincter muscles and the urethra.

ANATOMIC VARIANTS OR CONGENITAL ANOMALIES THAT MAY BE VISUALIZED WHEN PERFORMING A RENAL ULTRASOUND

Several anatomic variants or congenital anomalies may be visualized when performing a renal ultrasound. A dromedary hump is often seen on the lateral portion of the left kidney and should not be mistaken for a mass. This hump is created when the spleen (which is in the left upper quadrant) comes into contact with the left kidney and causes a bulging of the normal renal tissue. Horseshoe kidneys may also be identified on ultrasound, in which the poles of the kidney are joined, and a bridge of renal tissue is draped across the middle of the abdomen. Sometimes, the band of tissue may not be obvious, but if the shape of the kidneys is triangular or appears inverted, this alteration of the normal renal outline should be investigated further, and horseshoe kidneys should be considered. If a sonographer is not able to see both kidneys in the normal location, it is important to check for a pelvic kidney.

ANGIOMYOLIPOMA

Angiomyolipoma is a benign renal tumor (neoplasm) composed of fat, vascular, and smooth muscle. It is a rare tumor with an overall incidence of less than one percent. There are two types of this tumor:

- Isolated angiomyolipoma is usually a small and solitary tumor. It accounts for up to eighty percent of these tumors. The typical patient is a forty year old female. The right kidney is involved eighty percent of the time.

- Angiomyolipoma associated with tuberous sclerosis accounts for twenty percent of these tumors. The tumors are larger than isolated angiomyolipoma and there are usually multiple tumors present. Angiomyolipoma occurs in about eighty percent of patients with tuberous sclerosis.

Small angiomyolipoma tumors usually do not cause any symptoms. Larger tumors can result in a palpable mass, hematuria (blood in the urine), and bleeding (hemorrhage) within the tumor.

MULTILOCULAR CYSTIC NEPHROMA

Multilocular cystic Nephroma, is a rare benign cystic renal tumor. It is not hereditary, and the cause is not well understood. It most often occurs in boys up to four years old, and women who are over thirty years old. It typically affects only one kidney and appears as a solitary multiloculated cyst. The cyst is lined with epithelial cells and there are multiple cystic spaces within the tumor (that are separated by fibrous septa). The tumor does not communicate with the renal pelvis, however, it can bulge (herniated) into the renal pelvis. Hydronephrosis may occur due to compression of the renal collecting system. Up to ten percent of these cysts show calcification.

SINUS LIPOMATOSIS

Sinus lipomatosis is the accumulation of a moderate amount of fat in the kidney's sinus region. The kidney's normal sinus is composed of fibrous tissue, fat, lymphatic vessels and vascular structures. The degree of fat infiltration (in the form of fibrofatty tissue) varies by patient. The fibrofatty tissue may cause an enlargement of the sinus region. This condition is usually normal and benign. However, it has been associated with chronic renal infections, abscesses and kidney stones.

The following ultrasound features are present:

- The central sinus region may be enlarged and show an increase in echogenicity.
- In the normal kidney, the sinus region appears as a central bright area.

DROMEDARY HUMP

The dromedary hump appears as a distinct bulge-like shape along the side and above the border of the left kidney. In some cases, it may be large and prominent enough to be mistaken for a tumor. It is believed to form due to pressure by the spleen against the upper part of the left kidney during fetal development. The dromedary hump is a benign feature of the left kidney and is completely normal. This is confirmed by the presence of a uniform thickness of the renal parenchyma between the bulge and the underlying normal calyces.

The following ultrasound feature is present:

- The ultrasound echogenicity is very similar to the renal cortex.

RENAL ADENOMA AND ONCOCYTOMA

Renal adenoma and oncocytoma are relatively common, benign solid renal tumors. These tumors rarely cause symptoms and are most often incidentally detected through ultrasound and CT scans of the kidney. They appear as small renal masses that are not easily distinguished from renal cell carcinoma.

The following ultrasound features are present:

- An adenoma may show differing degrees of calcification.
- An oncocytoma appears as a central scar with surrounding "spokes of a wheel" patterns of enhancement.
- Since these tumors are considered pre-cancerous, the sonographer should look for evidence of spreading to the blood vessels and lymph nodes near the kidney. Any possibilities of malignancy should not be ruled out.

ATYPICAL CYSTS OF THE KIDNEYS AND URINARY TRACT

Atypical cysts are cysts that tend to show bleeding (hemorrhage). Ultrasound shows low-level echoes, multiple divisions (septae), and echoes within the cyst. Some (up to three percent) show mural nodules or rim-shaped calcification. Of these, up to twenty percent may be malignant.

PARA-PELVIC CYSTS OF THE KIDNEYS

Para-pelvic cysts show up in the renal hilum, but do not spread to the urine collecting system. Symptoms may include flank pain, high blood pressure (hypertension), and symptoms related to obstructions (such as acute renal failure). Ultrasound shows no divisions (septations). There may be irregular borders due to distortion of the renal sinus structures (caused by compression). The cyst may cause an obstruction of the renal system.

MEDULLARY CYSTIC KIDNEY

Medullary cystic kidney is a rare disease that causes chronic interstitial nephritis and fibrosis of the renal medulla. It is not hereditary and typically not seen in children. The renal collecting ducts and tubules can become obstructed due to fibrosis. Calcification occurs in up to eighty percent of affected patients. The cysts themselves are very small (about one twelfth of an inch). Urinary sediments are common (which is rare in cystic disease of the kidney). The condition may cause salt-wasting nephropathy in young adults.

The following ultrasound features are present:

- The kidneys appear smaller than normal.
- There is an increase in echogenicity (causes the renal pyramids to blend with sinus fat).

MULTI-CYSTIC DYSPLASTIC KIDNEY

Multi-cystic dysplastic kidney is the most common palpable mass found in neonates. It is a congenital condition that is not hereditary. Usually, only one kidney is involved. In infants, the kidney appears enlarged and is non-functioning. In adults, the affected kidney may appear smaller than normal with significant calcification. Large, multiple cysts are usually seen that cover the entire parenchyma. This results in a "cluster of grapes" appearance of the kidney. To rule out hydronephrosis, the sonographer must be able to show connection to the renal pelvis.

Some associated complications are:

- Urethral atresia (congenital unconnected, or absent, ureter).
- A non-functioning kidney.
- Atretic renal artery (congenital unconnected, or absent, renal artery).

SIMPLE RENAL CYSTS OF THE KIDNEYS AND URINARY TRACT

The exact causes of simple renal cysts are not well known. It is believed to develop after tubular obstruction, vascular occlusion, or focal inflammation. These cysts develop in up to fifty percent of adults over fifty years old.

The following ultrasound features are present:

- There are no internal echoes present.
- Acoustic enhancement occurs.
- There is a clear outline of the back wall of the cyst.
- The cyst is spherical or slightly ovoid in shape.

Low-level echoes originating from the cyst may be due to an artifact (sensitivity is set too high or a transducer frequency that is too low), infection, hemorrhage, a necrotic cystic tumor, or technique (a high amount of reverberation from the back wall of the cyst).

VON-HIPPEL-LINDAU CYSTS OF THE KIDNEYS AND URINARY TRACT

Von Hippel-Lindau syndrome is an inherited condition that manifests itself by forming fluid-filled cysts throughout the body. The cysts usually form during young adulthood, however, the signs and symptoms related to the presence of the cysts may occur at any age. Patients afflicted with this syndrome commonly develop cysts in the kidneys and pancreas. Renal adenomas can also form and may turn cancerous (renal adenocarcinoma). A unique tumor called a hemangioblastoma is characteristic of von Hippel-Lindau syndrome. The tumor is usually located in the brain (or eyes) and is composed of newly formed blood vessels. It is mostly non-cancerous; however it may cause complications depending on where the tumor is located within these organs.

HYDRONEPHROSIS

Hydronephrosis is any swelling of the kidney due to the back up of urine. The following ultrasound features are usually present:

- A dilated renal pelvis and calices.
- The renal sinus and tissue (parenchyma) become more and more compressed (as the urine backs up) until only tiny cyst-like spaces remain.
- Any congenital obstructions of the ureteropelvic junction (UPJ) can be observed.
- The ureters and bladder should be scanned in order determine if they are dilated. Dilation of these structures may indicate obstruction of the urethra or ureterovesical junction.
- If there is any localized hyronephrosis, it is usually due to stones (calculi), focal masses (tumors), or a duplex collecting system.
- Conducting the scan shortly after urination can help to eliminate false-positive errors due to over-hydration, under-hydration, extrarenal pelvis, and any previous urinary diversion procedures.

JUNCTIONAL PARENCHYMAL DEFECT

Using ultrasound, a junctional parenchymal defect is observed as a triangle-shaped echogenic area within the upper part (pole) of the kidney. It is best observed using a sagittal plane scan. The defect is formed by extensions of the renal sinus cavity in cases where there is a clear division between the upper and lower poles of the kidney. This division is the result of the way the kidney is formed in the fetus. Two masses of embryonic parenchymatous tissue (renunculi) fuse to form the kidney itself. When there is a partial fusion, the junctional parenchymal defects occur where the original two masses of renunculi joined together. This is an entirely normal and benign condition.

ACUTE INTERSTITIAL NEPHRITIS

Acute interstitial nephritis is inflammation the spaces between the tubules (interstitium). It is most often caused by infections (such as those caused by diphtheria and scarlet fever) or side effects of drugs (including allergic reactions). Common symptoms include uremia (accumulation of urea in the blood), proteinuria (excess protein in the urine), hematuria (blood in the urine), eosinophilia (elevation of allergy-fighting white blood cells), rash, and fever. The kidneys become enlarged and mottled, and their function is compromised.

The following ultrasound features are present:

- Renal cortical echogenicity is increased.
- If diffuse active disease is present, the increased cortical echogenicity is exaggerated.
- If diffuse scarring is present, the increased cortical echogenicity is subdued.

ALPORT'S SYNDROME

Alport's syndrome is a chronic nephritis that affects the cell membranes of the kidneys (and often the eyes and ears). This rare, inherited disorder damages the internal structures of the kidney (the glomeruli) and impairs their function by causing glomerulonephritis. Ultimately, this may lead to kidney failure. Alport's syndrome primarily affects males because the genetic defect is on the X chromosome. Typical symptoms include hematuria (blood in the urine), proteinuria (excessive protein in the urine), hypertension, hearing loss, and kidney failure.

The following ultrasound features are present:

- Renal cortical echogenicity is increased due to the presence of cellular infiltration and fibrosis in the open gaps and spaces within the kidney.
- The kidneys appear abnormally small.

ACUTE GLOMERULONEPHRITIS

In acute glomerulonephritis, the glomerular tissue becomes inflamed. This causes necrosis and excessive cellular growth within the glomeruli. It affects males more than females by a two to one margin. The age of onset is typically five to fifteen years old. Common symptoms include hematuria (blood in the urine), proteinuria (excessive protein in the urine), high blood pressure (hypertension), edema, and impaired renal function. Secondarily, the disease affects the renal vascular elements, tubules, and interstitium. Ultimately, the kidneys become enlarged (up to fifty percent larger than normal) and kidney function is compromised.

The following ultrasound features are present:

- There are increased cortical echoes.
- Depending on the source condition causing the glomerulonephritis (membraneous, idiopathic, membranoproliferative, rapidly progressive, or poststreptococcal) unique echo patterns emerge.

LUPUS NEPHRITIS

Lupus nephritis is an inflammation of the kidney caused by systemic lupus erythematosus. It is a disease of the immune system, and causes inflammation of the skin, joints, kidneys, and brain. The kidneys are affected in more than fifty percent of patients with systemic lupus erythematosus. The disease attacks the glomeruli within the kidney, ultimately causing kidney failure. It occurs in females (more than males) at around thirty years of age. Common symptoms include weight gain,

99

high blood pressure (hypertension), hematuria (blood in the urine), proteinuria (excessive protein in the urine), renal vein thrombosis, and general swelling of the body.

The following ultrasound features are present:

- Increased cortical echogenicity.
- Renal atrophy.

PAPILLARY NECROSIS

Renal papillary necrosis is a disease of the kidneys involving death of the renal papillae. The renal papillae are the areas of the kidney where the openings from the collecting ducts enter the renal pelvis. Necrosis (tissue death) of this area may make the kidney unable to concentrate the urine. This causes polyuria (the passing of an excessive quantity of urine) and nocturia (frequent urination at night). A complication is that the dead tissue may break off and cause an obstruction of the renal pelvis or ureter. Also, the presence of dead tissue in the urine may cause urinary tract infection. If enough of the renal papillae die, kidney failure will result. Some of the conditions that cause renal papillary necrosis are:

- Sickle cell anemia.
- Renal transplant rejection.
- Urinary tract obstruction.
- Diabetic nephropathy.

Ultrasound may reveal round or triangular cystic spaces at the corticomedullary junction.

SICKLE CELL NEPHROPATHY

Sickle cell nephropathy is a progressive renal disease resulting from red blood cells (in patients suffering from sickle cell anemia) sickling in the renal capillaries. This produces focal areas of bleeding (hemorrhage), necrosis, inflammation, fibrosis, and tubular atrophy. Symptoms may include those commonly tied to renal failure, including hematuria (blood in the urine), urinary tract infections, and polyuria (the passing of an excessive quantity of urine). These abnormalities lead to renal failure and may progress to end-stage renal disease. Similar abnormalities can occur (to a lesser extent) in patients with the sickle cell trait and occasionally lead to kidney failure.

The following ultrasound feature is present:

- If acute renal vein thrombosis is present, the kidneys appear enlarged with deceased echogenicity in the areas secondary to edema.

INTRINSIC RENAL DISEASE

There are two classes of diseases that constitute intrinsic renal disease. The first group produces an increase of cortical echoes due to their deposits of collagen and fibrous tissue. This first list includes:

- Interstitial nephritis: Nephritis in which the connective tissue between the cells is mostly affected.
- Acute tubular necrosis: Acute tubular necrosis is a disease involving the damage and death of the renal tubule cells. It is caused by a lack of oxygen to the kidney (ischemia).
- Amyloidosis: Damage of the kidney caused by deposits of amyloid (a waxy, translucent substance, composed primarily of protein fibers).

- Diabetic nephropathy: Disease of the kidney (caused by diabetes) in which the glomerulus thickens and allows abnormally high levels of protein to be eliminated in the urine.
- Systemic lupus erythematosus: an autoimmune inflammatory disease of the kidney's connective tissues.
- Myeloma: A malignant tumor formed by the cells of bone marrow.

The second group of diseases causes a loss of the ability to distinguish between the renal cortex and medullary regions. This second list includes:

- Chronic pyelonephritis: Long-term inflammation of both the lining of the pelvis and the parenchyma of the kidney.
- Renal tubular ectasia: Dilatation or distension of the renal tubules.
- Acute bacterial nephritis: Episodic inflammation of the kidney caused by a bacterial infection.

Renal atrophy is a common outcome of these diseases. The kidneys take on a highly echogenic enlarged appearance. The renal sinus is enlarged (and appears filled with fat) with a very thin cortical rim.

Accumulation of fluid within the kidney (edema) caused by renal vein thrombosis, pyelonephritis, or renal transplant rejection results in an increase in echogenicity and renal enlargement.

EFFECTS OF AIDS ON KIDNEYS

Acquired immune deficiency syndrome (AIDS) is a contagious disease passed through intimate contact with various bodily fluids (blood, semen, etc.). It is not passed through casual contact with an infected person. The virus destroys the body's immune defenses by destroying white blood cells (T-Cells). It then replicates widely in the infected person and causes serious damage to many organs. When it attacks the kidneys, uremia (a buildup of toxic urea in the blood) is a common symptom.

The following ultrasound features are present:

- There is typically an echogenic pattern in the parenchyma.
- There is an increase in echogenicity of the renal cortex.
- The kidneys appear to be of normal size to somewhat enlarged.

INFECTIONS OF KIDNEYS AND URINARY TRACT

Infection of the kidneys and urinary tract usually starts as pyelonephritis (the presence of pus in a renal system that has been obstructed for some time). It can then progress to focal bacterial nephritis, and finally turn in an abscess. Ultrasound reveals low-level echoes when there are significant fluid debris levels. Emphysematous pyelonephritis is an infection caused by the presence of air in the kidney parenchyma. It is a very serious condition related to complications from diabetes.

Xanthogranulomatous pyelonephritis is a somewhat rare infection related to long-standing urinary tract obstruction. The condition results in damage and destruction of the renal parenchyma. Typical symptoms include renal failure, and the presence of staghorn calculi (kidney stones that involve the renal pelvis and extend into at least 2 calyces). Ultrasound reveals the replacement of normal renal tissue with cystic spaces, diffuse/segmented wave forms, and an enlargement of the affected kidney.

URETERS

Each ureter is about ten inches long. The ureter shows a narrowing at three different points, they are:

- Where the pelvis-of-the-ureter joins the ureter itself.
- A kinked portion that crosses the pelvic brim.
- Where the ureter penetrates the bladder wall.

The pelvis-of-the-ureter is the flower-shaped, expanded portion within the hilus of the kidney. The major calices feed into the pelvis-of-the-ureter. The ureters run downward (parallel to the spine) along the psoas muscles that also provide a measure of protection from the bones of the spine. The ureters then run along the sides of the pelvic bone and then turn forward to connect with the bladder. Blood is supplied to the ureters from the renal, testicular (or ovarian), and superior-vesical arteries.

URETHRA

The urethra connects the urinary bladder to the outside of the body. The urethra has a function to allow urine to be expelled from of the body. It also serves a reproductive function in the male, as a path for semen during ejaculation. The external-sphincter is made up of a smooth muscle that is voluntarily controlled for urination. The internal-sphincter is also made up of a smooth muscle and is controlled involuntarily (opens when the bladder is full). The urethra is about one inch long in the female and about eight inches long in the male.

Following are medical terms related to the urethra:

- Stricture: Any closure of the urethra.
- Urethritis: Inflammation of the mucous membrane located in the urethra.
- Dysuria: Difficulty in urination.
- Cystitus: Inflammation of the bladder.
- Cystostomy: Open-bladder surgery.
- Cystectomy: Surgical removal of the bladder.

URINARY BLADDER

The urinary bladder continuously collects urine delivered by the kidneys (via the ureters). The urinary bladder expands until it is full; the collected urine is then expelled from the body through the urethra. The urinary bladder is a hollow, muscular and elastic (bag-shaped) organ that is located on the pelvic floor. Its capacity is about eighteen ounces of urine. The stimulus to urinate (produced by the bladder's nervous receptors) is usually experienced when it is about half full. The ureters enter the bladder along the side and back of the bladder. The urethra exits the bladder from the front. The detrusor muscle (made up of smooth muscle fibers) is a layer of the urinary bladder wall. When the detrusor muscle contracts, urine is pushed from the bladder. For the urine to finally exit the bladder, both the involuntary controlled internal-sphincter and the voluntarily controlled external-sphincter must be opened.

COLOR DOPPLER FOR EVALUATION

If a mass is visualized in the urinary bladder, it should be documented with gray-scale ultrasound, measurements should be performed, it should be characterized as a mobile or a nonmobile filling defect, and it should be examined with color Doppler. If a solid mass is present, it is helpful in reaching a diagnosis to determine the vascularity of the mass. Blood clots or fungal balls when visualized in the bladder will not demonstrate color flow. Color Doppler may also be useful when evaluating the ureteral jets. The ureteral jets show the urine entering the bladder from the ureters. They are not always visible with gray-scale, so they can be examined more closely with color Doppler for diagnostic confidence as the bladder is filling. If after several minutes one of the jets is not visualized, it may indicate an obstruction of the ureter on that side. If stones are identified within the bladder, it may be useful to determine if "twinkling artifacts" are present when color Doppler is used.

TRANSITIONAL CELL CARCINOMA

Transitional cell carcinoma is a type of malignant tumor that develops in the lining of the renal pelvis, ureter, or bladder. These tumors are mostly found in the bladder. It is also likely there will be multiple tumors present. Men are more likely to develop these tumors by a three to one ratio. The likelihood of developing transitional cell carcinoma increases with age (the peak age is sixty to seventy years old).

The following ultrasound features are present:

- If the tumor is located in the renal pelvis, a mass will be seen with low level echoes, a widening of central sinus echoes, and a hypoechoic central region.
- With this type of tumor, the sonographer may not be able to discern any significant abnormalities.

SPLEEN

The spleen is in the upper left of the abdomen. It is located behind the stomach and immediately below the diaphragm. It is about the size of a thick paperback book and weighs just over half a pound. It is made up of lymphoid tissue. The blood vessels are connected to the spleen by splenic sinuses (modified capillaries). The following peritoneal ligaments support the spleen:

- The gastrolienal ligament that connects the stomach to the spleen.
- The lienorenal ligament that connects the kidney to the spleen.
- The middle section of the phrenicocolic ligament (connects the left colic flexure to the thoracic diaphragm).

The main functions of the spleen are to filter unwanted materials from the blood (including old red blood cells) and to help fight infections. Up to ten percent of the population has one or more accessory spleens that tend to form at the hilum of the original spleen.

CALCULATING THE VOLUME OF A PATIENT'S SPLEEN

One of the advantages of sonography is quickly being able to measure organs or other anatomical structures within the body. These measurements are useful in the follow up treatment of many diseases. These measurements can be added to and displayed on a calculations worksheet for the physician that will be interpreting the results. When it is necessary to calculate the volume of an organ, the user will measure the spleen (in this example) in three planes using 2D ultrasound. Volume is displayed in any units of length cubed and is calculated by multiplying the length times the width times the height. Organs are typically measured in centimeters; therefore, the volume is in centimeters cubed (cm^3). Three-dimensional ultrasound is also used to calculate the volume of an organ. This method is actually considered to be superior to measurements obtained on 2D images, but it requires more time to perform.

SCANNING THE ABDOMEN WHEN SPLENOMEGALY IS APPARENT

Other areas to be scanned when the spleen is enlarged would be both the upper and lower quadrants of the abdomen, looking for liver enlargement or liver disease. The ultrasound technician should scan over the areas of the portal veins and the splenic vein. Look for nodes that may be enlarged or masses that may be present causing some kind of obstruction. Look around the area of the gallbladder and pancreas. Look for enlargement or shadows that may suggest or confirm lymphoma. Look at the kidneys and for any signs of hydronephrosis, pancreatitis, obstruction of the ureter, or, in female patients, the ovaries. When scanning one quadrant of the abdomen, it is likely that the sonographer will look around the four quadrants of the abdomen for abnormalities as well as anatomically correct focal points.

TRAUMA TO THE SPLEEN

Blunt abdominal trauma is the most common reason for injury to the spleen. Motor vehicle accidents are the primary cause (accounting for up to thirty percent of cases). Additionally, any of the diseases (such as portal hypertension) that cause splenic enlargement may cause the spleen to rupture. The affected patient usually presents with upper left quadrant pain. Hypotension and a decreased hemoglobin level may indicate internal bleeding.

The following ultrasound features are present:

- Splenomegaly with progressive enlargement and an irregular splenic border.
- Focal hematomas are represented by intrasplenic fluid collections.
- Sub-capsular hematomas show perispleic fluid collections.
- Blood exhibits various echo patterns (depending on the age of the injury).
- Focal areas show tiny lacerations that give rise to small collections of blood interspersed with disrupted pulp (contusion).
- When the spleen heals (and returns to normal) small, irregular foci may remain.

INFARCTION OF THE SPLEEN

Infarction of the spleen is usually caused by infection or a blood clot. Several conditions that may cause infarction of the spleen include pancreatitis, endocarditis, leukemia/lymphoma, and sickle cell anemia. Its ultrasound appearance is dependent on when the infarct occurs. A fresh infarct (hemorrhagic) appears hypoechoic. A healed infarct (with scarring) appears as an echogenic, wedge-shaped lesion. The affected patient will usually present with pain in the upper left quadrant of the abdomen. Additional symptoms may include fever, chills, nausea, vomiting, chest pain (upon breathing), and left shoulder pain. Splenic abscess may result, especially if the infarct was caused by an infection.

SPLENOMEGALY

Splenomegaly is an enlargement of the spleen. It is highly associated with hypersplenism (an enlarged spleen and a decrease in one or more types of blood cells). Any condition that causes a rapid breakdown of blood cells (such as any of the hemolytic anemias) can place a great strain on the spleen and make it enlarge. Other common causes include portal hypertension, acquired immune deficiency syndrome (AIDS), infiltration of the spleen by leukemia (or lymphoma), and infection. Symptoms of splenomegaly may include an inability to eat a large meal and pain in the upper left side of the abdomen.

HISTOPLASMOSIS

Histoplasmosis is a disease caused by the fungus histoplasma capsulatum (a common soil-based fungus found in the central and eastern US). The disease primarily affects the lungs (since the dry fungal spores are usually inhaled). The symptoms are similar to tuberculosis. It can, however affect other organs in the body. This form of the disease is called disseminated histoplasmosis, and it can be fatal (especially if left untreated). Disseminated histoplasmosis is more frequently seen in patients with cancer or AIDS. Using ultrasound, the affected spleen appears with multiple focal, bright, echogenic, granulomatous lesions throughout.

CYSTS OF THE SPLEEN

Eighty percent of all splenic cysts are pseudocysts (an abnormal structure that resembles a cyst but has no membranous lining). They are usually the result of prior trauma to the spleen. More rarely, they can also be caused by congenital conditions (epidermoid cysts) and parasites (echinococcal). Affected patients typically present with a symptom-free lower upper quadrant mass.

The following ultrasound features are present:

- Parasitic cysts appear as anechoic lesions (with possible calcification) or as solid masses (with fine internal echoes and poor distal enhancement).
- True (or primary cysts) are typically solitary and rarely calcified.
- Both types of cysts have well defined walls.

BENIGN TUMORS OF THE SPLEEN

There are three main types of benign tumors that affect the spleen. They are:

- Hamartomas: A common benign tumor of the spleen composed of splenic tissue that grows in a disorganized mass. They are usually asymptomatic. On ultrasound, they appear as well-defined hyperechoic solid masses.
- Cavernous hemangiomas: These tumors are made up jumbled growths of blood vessels fed by numerous tributary arteries. They typically go through a growth phase followed by a rest phase (during which they virtually disappear). They only cause symptoms if they bleed or increase the size of the spleen enough to affect other organs. On ultrasound, they usually appear as a large echogenic mass with small hypoechoic areas.
- Cystic lymphangiomas: A rare benign congenital tumor. It appears as a mass with extensive cystic replacement of the normal splenic tissue.

MALIGNANT TUMORS OF THE SPLEEN

There are three main types of cancerous tumors that affect the spleen. They are:

- Hemangiosarcoma: This is an aggressive form of cancer. It is a blood-fed sarcoma (the blood vessels grow directly into the tumor and it is typically filled with blood). A frequent cause of death is the rupture of the tumor (which causes severe bleeding). On ultrasound, the tumor has a mixed cystic pattern.
- Lymphoma: Any of the various malignant tumors (of lymphatic and reticuloendothelial tissues) that occur as circumscribed solid tumors. They are composed of cells that resemble lymphocytes, plasma cells, or histiocytes.
- Metastases: Cancer that has spread from other organs of the body. The spleen is the tenth most common site for this type of cancer. It appears (on ultrasound) as multiple, hyperechoic lesions.

ANATOMIC VARIANTS THAT MAY BE VISUALIZED WHEN SCANNING THE SPLEEN

If the sonographer visualizes a mass located in the splenic hilum, an accessory spleen must be considered. It is a common variant that is a congenital anomaly, and it can be identified as an oval or spherical "mass" that has the same appearance as the tissue found in the spleen. Although the typical location is within the splenic hilum, it may actually be visualized anywhere in the abdominal or pelvic cavity. A wandering spleen occurs when this organ is not in the usual left upper quadrant (LUQ) location. The ligaments that typically hold the spleen in place were not present at birth, which may allow the spleen to migrate from the LUQ. If this occurs, the vessels of the spleen may become twisted and cut off blood supply to it. Another variant includes the shape of the spleen, which can look different from patient to patient and not take on the typical elliptical shape with a concave border inferiorly.

PANCREAS

The pancreas is six to ten inches long in an adult and located at the back of the abdomen behind the stomach. It is a long, tapered organ. The wider (right) side is called the **head,** and the narrower (left) side is called the **tail**. The head lies near the **duodenum** (the first section of the small intestine), and the tail ends near the **spleen**. The body of the pancreas lies between the head and the tail. The pancreas is made up of exocrine and endocrine tissues. The **exocrine tissue** secretes digestive enzymes from a series of ducts that collectively form the main pancreatic duct (that runs the length of the pancreas). The **main pancreatic duct** connects to the common bile duct near the duodenum. The **endocrine tissue** secretes hormones (such as insulin) into the bloodstream. Blood is supplied to the pancreas from the splenic artery, gastroduodenal artery, and superior mesenteric artery.

ENDOCRINE FUNCTIONS OF THE PANCREAS

Located amongst the groupings of exocrine cells (acini) are groups of endocrine cells (called islets of Langerhans). The islets of Langerhans are primarily made up of insulin-producing beta cells (fifty to eighty percent of the total) and glucagon-releasing alpha cells. The major hormones produced by the pancreas are insulin and glucagon. The body uses insulin to control carbohydrate metabolism by lowering the amount of sugar (glucose) in the blood. Insulin also affects fat metabolism and can change the liver's ability to release stored fat. The body also uses glucagon to control carbohydrate metabolism. Glucagon has the opposite effect of insulin in that the body uses it to increase blood sugar (glucose) levels. The levels of insulin and glucagon are balanced to maintain the optimum level of blood sugar (glucose) throughout the day.

EXOCRINE FUNCTIONS OF THE PANCREAS

The pancreas assists in the digestion of foods by secreting enzymes (to the small intestine) that help to break down many foods, especially fats and proteins. The precursors to these enzymes (called zymogens) are produced by groups of exocrine cells (called acini). They are converted, through a chemical reaction in the gut, to the active enzymes (such as pancreatic lipase and amylase) once they enter the small intestine. The pancreas also secretes large amounts of sodium bicarbonate to neutralize the stomach acid that reaches the small intestine. The exocrine functions of the pancreas are controlled by hormones released by the stomach and small intestine (duodenum) when food is present. The exocrine secretions of the pancreas flow into the main pancreatic duct (Wirsung's duct) and are delivered to the duodenum through the pancreatic duct.

CONGENITAL ABNORMALITIES OF THE PANCREAS

Congenital abnormalities of the pancreas are very rare. In most cases, they are related to the non-development of the organ (agenesis) or the partial development of the organ (hypoplasia). There is a condition where the head of the pancreas encircles the duodenum (called annular pancreas). Congenital cysts are the result of malformed pancreatic ducts. There is usually more than one and they can range from less than a quarter inch to up to two inches in diameter. Cystic fibrosis is a congenital abnormality that affects one in every two thousand persons. It manifests itself in problems with the liver, biliary tree, and pancreas especially as a person ages. The exocrine glands secrete an abnormal thick, sticky mucous. Eventually, cysts form due to the coagulation of the normal secretions of the liver, biliary tree and pancreas. Ultrasound shows increased echoes due to the presence of excess fibrous connective tissue.

ULTRASOUND TECHNIQUE FOR AN EXAMINATION OF THE PANCREAS

The pancreas remains one of the more difficult organs to examine with ultrasound. The success of the technique depends on an accurate knowledge of the vascular structures of the pancreas and on correct adjustment of the ultrasound equipment. In preparation for examination, the patient must fast for six to eight hours. This assures that the gallbladder is dilated, the bile ducts are full, there is a minimum of bowel gas, and the stomach is empty. Real-time scanning allows the operator to view the peristalsis (contractions within the small intestine), duodenum (first part of the small intestine), and stomach. A three megahertz to five megahertz transducer works best for adults. In children, use a five megahertz to seven and a half megahertz transducer.

The patient should be in the supine position (lying down face up). The head, neck, body, and tail of the pancreas should first be identified (in both the longitudinal and transverse plains). Next, evaluate the shape, contour, and lie of the organ. Compare the texture to that of the liver. Identify the following structures that are located in and around the pancreas:

- The superior-mesenteric artery, gastroduodenal artery, and the aorta.
- The superior-mesenteric vein, portal vein, splenic vein, left-renal vein, and the inferior-vena-cava.
- The common-bile-duct, duodenal-bulb, back wall of the stomach, and the pancreatic duct.

The left lobe of the liver, stomach and colon can be used as windows to visualize the pancreas. To achieve this, the patient needs to ingest substances (such as water, glucagon, a fatty meal, or methylcellulose) that help the ultrasound waves "pass through the window" and "see" the pancreas.

SYMPTOMS, CLINICAL CORRELATION, AND ASSOCIATED COMPLICATIONS FOR DISEASES OF THE PANCREAS

The two most common symptomatic diseases of the pancreas are pancreatitis (inflammation of the pancreas) and pancreatic cancer.

Following are the most common symptoms of pancreatitis:

- Nausea and/or vomiting.
- A feeling of a fast pulse or sustained heart rate increase.
- A general feeling of illness.
- The presence of a fever.
- The presence of swelling in the upper abdomen.
- A build-up of fluid in the abdominal cavity (ascites).
- Low (or dropping) blood pressure readings.
- In acute pancreatitis there is usually moderate to severe pain in the upper abdomen.

Following are the most common symptoms of pancreatic cancer:

- Sustained pain in the upper abdomen.
- A loss of appetite.
- A rapid loss of weight.
- The presence of jaundice (yellowing of the skin and eyes).

- Chronic indigestion.
- Nausea and/or vomiting.

PHLEGMONOUS PANCREATITIS

Phlegmonous pancreaitis is a condition where the intense inflammation caused by exposure to the pancreatic juices causes the pancreatic tissue to become damaged or die. The affected areas of the pancreas become hardened and thickened.

The following ultrasound features are present:

- The hardened and thickened areas appear hypoechoic with good through transmission.
- There is no observation of collected pancreatic fluid.

LIQUEFACTIVE NECROSIS

Liquefactive necrosis (also called colliquative necrosis) is a condition where a lesion forms in an area of the pancreas that was digested by enzymes released by the pancreas during an episode of pancreatitis.

The following ultrasound features are present:

- A cystic structure is observed (without the presence of a pseudocyst).
- The cystic structure is hypoechoic.

CHRONIC PANCREATITIS

Chronic pancreatitis consists of repeated bouts of acute pancreatitis. This results in a sustained damage and scarring of the pancreatic tissue. The healthy tissue is replaced with an atrophied, calcified and thickened fibrous tissue. Inflammation and pseudocysts are frequently present. Patients with chronic pancreatitis have attacks of abdominal pain and digestive problems. The symptoms may become more frequent as the condition worsens. The condition is usually caused by alcohol abuse; however, chronic blockage of the pancreatic duct (typically due to a narrowing of the sphincter of Oddi) is also linked to chronic pancreatitis.

The following ultrasound features are present:

- There is an increase in echogenicity.
- Calcification, dilation of the pancreatic ducts, and an irregular outline are present.
- There is an enlargement of the pancreas.
- The presence of calcified stones.
- Shadowing may be present.

ACUTE PANCREATITIS

Patients with acute pancreatitis may have the following symptoms:

- Moderate to severe pain in the upper abdomen (usually after a meal or heavy drinking).
- The presence of fever.

They show an increase in white cell blood count (leukocytosis) and their serum amylase and serum lipase levels rise within one to two weeks of the onset of symptoms. In adults, acute pancreatitis is typically caused by biliary tract disease or alcoholism. Up to sixty percent of patients have gallstones. Problems occur when the pancreatic juices are not allowed to flow properly due to obstructions. The pancreatic juices cause the inflammation and destruction of pancreatic tissue when they back up and migrate to the surfaces of the organ. Ultimately, equilibrium occurs as the pocketed pancreatic juices are absorbed and replenished within the pancreas. Once proper flow is restored, the acute episode of pancreatitis ends. In children, trauma, drugs, infection, or congenital anomalies typically cause acute pancreatitis.

HEMORRHAGIC PANCREATITIS

Patients with hemorrhagic pancreatitis may have the following symptoms:

- A decrease in hematocrit and serum calcium levels.
- Low blood pressure (hypotension) even when the patient is infused with additional blood.
- The presence of metabolic acidosis.
- The presence of adult respiratory distress syndrome.

In hemorrhagic pancreatitis, there is a sudden escape of active pancreatic enzymes that attack the pancreatic tissue (parenchyma). These enzymes break down the fat protecting the pancreas, which in turn leads to rupture of pancreatic blood vessels and bleeding. In about half of these cases the condition occurs after eating an excessively large meal or a period of very heavy drinking.

The following ultrasound features are present:

- The fresh hemorrhage appears as a well-defined single mass.
- If the hemorrhage is more than one to two weeks old it takes on cystic features.

ANEURYSMS SECONDARY TO PANCREATITIS

Pancreatitis can cause aneurysms of the arteries that serve the pancreas. They are mostly found on the splenic artery. They can also be found on the pancreaticoduodenal arcades including the dorsal and transverse pancreatic arteries.

ABSCESS OF THE PANCREAS

An abscess of the pancreas is a collection of pus that results from pancreatic tissue death and infection. It is usually the result of pancreatitis. Its severity is related to the amount of tissue that is destroyed. It occurs in about five percent of patients that suffer from pancreatitis. There is a high probability of an abscess (in up to forty percent of patients) that suffer a bout of pancreatitis after an operation.

The following ultrasound features are present:

- A hypoechoic mass with smooth walls.
- The presence of small internal echoes.

ISLET CELL TUMORS

Islet cell tumors are derived from neuroendocrine cells. They tend to be slow growing tumors that are treatable even after they have metastasized. Islet cell tumors can produce dramatic symptoms since up to half of these tumors secrete excess hormones.

There are two types of islet cell tumors. They are:

- Non-functioning islet cell tumors (ninety two percent are malignant) account for one third of all islet cell tumors. Patients with non-functioning tumors do not have any symptoms from excess hormone secretion since the tumor does not release any hormones into the blood.

- Functional islet cell tumors produce dramatic symptoms because of excess release of hormones into the blood. There are two major types of these tumors, insulinoma (a tumor that produces excessive amounts of insulin) and gastrinoma (a tumor that produces excessive amounts of gastrin).

The tumors are located mostly in the body and tail of the pancreas.

PANCREATIC PSEUDOCYSTS

A pancreatic pseudocyst is a collection of pancreatic juice around the pancreas. A pseudocyst usually occurs after a bout of acute or chronic pancreatitis. The condition may appear directly (or take weeks to develop) after the patient recovers from pancreatitis. The most common location for the formation of a pseudocyst is towards the front of the pancreas at the back of the stomach. The typical symptoms may include pain in the abdomen and bloating (including digestive problems). Some complications of pseudocysts are pancreatic abscess, bleeding and blockage of the small intestine.

The following ultrasound features are present:

- The presence of sharply defined smooth walls.
- Pseudocysts show usual acoustic enhancement and internal echoes.
- There may be multiple septations.
- Pseudocysts may show similarities to cystadenoma or cystadenocarcioma.

A fluid-filled stomach, a dilated pancreatic duct, or the left renal vein varix may be mistaken for a pseudocyst.

MACROCYSTIC AND MICROCYSTIC ADENOMA

Actual pancreatic cysts (as opposed to pseudocysts) are lined by a layer of mucous and may be congenital or develop on their own. They are uncommon, accounting for less than two percent of all pancreatic tumors. Macrocystic adenoma is a slow growing, benign tumor. It usually appears as a large homogeneous cyst. It is more common in women than men. It occurs mostly on the head of the pancreas. Microcystic adenoma is a benign lesion. It consists of many small cysts lined by cells containing glycogen with little to no mucous. It is more common in women than men. It occurs mostly in the body and tail of the pancreas.

The following ultrasound feature is present:

- Actual pancreatic cysts are similar in appearance to pseudocysts.

CARCINOMA OF THE HEAD OF THE PANCREAS

The term "carcinoma of the head of the pancreas" encompasses carcinoma of the sphincter-of-Oddi, the lower part of the bile duct, and the functional cells of the pancreas. It typically affects men over fifty years old. The symptoms are often weight loss followed by a progressively worsening jaundice. Back pain and overall itching (pruritus) are common. The gallbladder may be enlarged along with thrombophlebitis (inflammation with the formation of blood clots) of the splenic vein causing congestive enlargement of the spleen (splenomegaly).

The following ultrasound features are present:

- A hypoechoic mass in the pancreas.
- The superior mesenteric vessels are displaced forward.
- The presence of multiple hypoechoic nodes along the pancreas, duodenum (first part of the small intestine), and porta/superior mesenteric vessels.

ULTRASOUND FINDINGS OF ACUTE AND CHRONIC PANCREATITIS

Pancreatitis is inflammation of the pancreas and may be characterized as acute (sudden onset) or chronic (long term). Ultrasound is often ordered if a patient presents with epigastric or abdominal pain in the presence of elevated pancreatic enzymes. Overlying bowel gas may make it difficult to visualize the entire pancreas, but every effort should be made to see the pancreas in its entirety especially when jaundice is one of the patient's symptoms because a tumor may be the cause of obstruction. The ultrasound appearance of acute pancreatitis may demonstrate an enlarged pancreas that appears hypoechoic. Due to the inflammation, the splenic vein may not be visualized well. Chronic pancreatitis may show an enlarged gland that is more echogenic than normal. The normal pancreatic duct is less than 3 mm and is larger in the pancreatic head.

ADENOCARCINOMA OF THE PANCREAS

The majority of pancreatic cancers are adenocarcinomas. These fatal tumors occur in the pancreatic head more often than in the body or tail of the pancreas, and they affect males more often than females. These masses can be the cause of obstruction and may create symptoms such as jaundice, abdominal or back pain, and nausea and vomiting with associated weight loss. Typical ultrasound findings of an adenocarcinoma include a hypoechoic mass with irregular walls. This mass may cause enlargement of the pancreas and dilation of the pancreatic duct. Depending on the location, the adjacent vessels may be displaced either anteriorly or posteriorly, and compression of the vessels is often noted. Gray-scale and color Doppler ultrasound should be used to determine the size and vascularity of these tumors. A follow-up computed tomography or magnetic resonance imaging test will be performed if the pancreatic duct or bile ducts are dilated without sonographic visualization of a stone or mass.

ANATOMY OF THE LIVER

The liver is the largest solid organ of the body. It is also the largest gland. It weighs about three pounds in an adult and is located below the diaphragm on the right side of the abdomen. The liver is made up of four **lobes**: right, left, quadrate, and caudate lobes. The liver is secured to the diaphragm and abdominal walls by five **ligaments**. They are called the falciform (which forms a membrane-like barrier between the right and left lobes), coronary, right triangular, left triangular, and round ligaments.

The liver processes blood once it has received nutrients from the intestines via the **hepatic portal vein**. The **hepatic artery** supplies oxygen-rich blood from the abdominal aorta so that the organ can function. Blood leaves the liver through the **hepatic veins**. The liver's functional units are called **lobules** (made up of layers of liver cells). Blood enters the lobules through branches of the portal vein and hepatic artery. The blood then flows through small channels called **sinusoids**.

FISSURES OF THE LIVER

The main lobar fissure definitively divides the liver into the right and left lobes. It is located along a line connecting the inferior vena cava and the gallbladder fossa. The middle hepatic vein runs within this fissure. The right segmental fissure divides the front and back parts of the right lobe of the liver. The front and back segments of the right portal vein run to the middle of each of these parts. The right hepatic vein also runs within this fissure. The left segmental fissure divides the middle and sides of the left lobe of the liver. The left intersegmental fissure delineates the top, middle, and bottom divisions of the left lobe of the liver. The ligamentum teres runs along the outer edge of the falciform ligament. The middle-third-of-left-intersegmental fissure runs along the front side of the caudate lobe.

CONGENITAL ABNORMALITIES OF THE LIVER

Congenital abnormalities of the liver are very rare and account for less than five percent of structural abnormalities. The possibility of a congenital abnormality should be kept in mind when an unexplained mass is encountered. One of the most well known (of these types of abnormalities) is called Riedel's lobe. This is a triangular-shaped projection (with the base of the triangle attached to the right lobe of the liver). It is usually located towards the front of the right lobe of the liver and is more common in women than men. Other types of congenital abnormalities of the liver include:

- Absence of one or more of its lobes
- Deformed lobes
- Decreased size of the lobes (In a normal liver, the right lobe is much larger then the left)
- Transposition of the gallbladder

FOUR FOSSAE OF THE LIVER

The left sagittal fossa is a deep groove that extends from the notch on the front of the liver to the upper border of the back. It forms a separation between the right and left lobes. The fossa for the umbilical vein provides space for the umbilical vein in the fetus. In the adult, it takes the form of the ligamentum teres (or round ligament) and is positioned between the quadrate lobe and the left lobe of the liver. The fossa for the gallbladder is a shallow "deflated balloon" shaped groove that provides space under right lobe of the liver for the gallbladder and the cystic duct. The fossa for the inferior vena cava is a short, deep cylindrical-shaped cut out that provides space for the vena cava. It extends upward and is located between the caudate lobe and the bare area of the liver.

FUNCTIONS OF THE LIVER

The liver is responsible for performing many vital functions in the body including:

- Production of bile
- Production of certain blood plasma proteins
- Production of cholesterol (and certain proteins needed to carry fats)
- Storage of excess glucose in the form of glycogen (that can be converted back to glucose when needed)
- Regulation of amino acids
- Processing of hemoglobin (to store iron)
- Conversion of ammonia (that is poisonous to the body) to urea (a waste product excreted in urine)
- Purification of the blood (clears out drugs and other toxins)
- Regulation of blood clotting
- Controlling infections by boosting immune factors and removing bacteria

The liver processes all of the blood that passes through the digestive system. The nutrients (and drugs) that pass through the liver are converted into forms that are appropriate for the body to use.

BILIARY ATRESIA

Biliary atresia is a congenital blockage of the bile ducts that affects infants less than a few months old. It occurs due to the failure of the bile ducts to form normally as a fetus. Bile flow from the liver (through the biliary tree and gallbladder) is reduced or completely blocked. This can lead to liver damage (including cirrhosis of the liver) and is eventually fatal to the infant.

CHOLEDOCHAL CYSTS

Choledochal cysts are congenital anomalies of the biliary tree. The common bile duct is structurally affected (the duct walls are widened and weakened), allowing bile to accumulate in the duct. The bile then forms a cyst that presses against the walls of the duct. This creates a condition in which bile may be prevented from reaching the small intestine. The bile then backs up towards the liver. The patient may experience jaundice, fever and abdominal pain (especially if the accumulated bile becomes infected).

LIVER FUNCTION TESTS

These diagnostic blood tests are used as a first course to determine the cause of potential liver-related problems in the patient. Some usual symptoms include; jaundice, dark urine, light or black colored feces, nausea/vomiting (including blood), swelling/pain in the abdomen, and unusual weight change. Higher elevations of AST and ALT can be signs of the death and damage of liver cells. This may be the result of acute and chronic diseases of the liver such as hepatitis and cirrhosis. Higher elevations of Alk Phos and bilirubin can indicate blockage of the bile ducts. This may be the result of gallstones or a structural tissue injury within the liver. Lower levels of albumin in the blood (and a longer PT time) are indicative of a severe problem with the liver's metabolic ability.

AST TEST

Aspartate aminotransferase (AST) (also called Serum glutamic oxaloacetic transaminase (SGOT)) is an enzyme primarily associated with liver and heart cells. Its level in the blood rises in direct proportion to the number of dead or damaged cells in these organs. Liver diseases such as acute hepatitis and cirrhosis cause sustained elevations of this enzyme in the blood.

ALT TEST

Alanine aminotransferase (ALT) is an enzyme (more sensitive to liver cells than AST) that is released into the blood when these cells die or are damaged. The level is in proportion to the number of dead or damaged cells (primarily in the liver). The AST and ALT tests may be performed at the same time to gain additional information. The ratio of AST to ALT may be used as an indicator as to whether the liver (or another organ) has been mostly affected.

PROTHROMBIN TIME

Prothrombin time (PT) is a test designed to measure the length of time it takes for blood to clot. It is typically used to determine bleeding problems. Prothrombin (factor II) is one of the clotting factors produced by the liver. The ability for the liver to produce prothrombin is determined by the availability of vitamin K. An increase in PT indicates damage to the liver cells (typically caused by disease).

ALBUMIN AND GLOBULINS

The blood levels of albumin and globulins are measured to determine liver function. Solely produced by the liver, albumin is the major blood protein used by the body (the remainder are globulins). Many drugs, fats, hormones and toxins are bound to albumin in the bloodstream and carried to the liver for processing to water-soluble forms. A low blood level of albumin indicates a significant impairment of the liver (usually caused by cirrhosis).

LDH Test

The presence of elevated levels of lactic acid dehydrogenase (LDH) results from the death or damage of cells in various tissues of the body (such as the heart, kidneys, or liver). The role of LDH is to convert lactic acid (produced by muscle tissue during stress) into pyruvic acid (that is necessary to produce energy within the cells). LDH isoenzymes can be used to isolate the specific tissue that has been affected.

Alk Phos Test

The presence of highly elevated alkaline phosphatase (Alk Phos or ALP) levels indicates a blockage of the bile ducts. Levels of ALP are also high in patients with liver or bone cancer. ALP isoenzymes can also be used to isolate their source (such as the liver or bones).

Indirect Bilirubin, Direct Bilirubin, and Total Bilirubin

Bilirubin is the major bile pigment that is produced when hemoglobin is broken down in the blood. The resulting indirect (or unconjugated) bilirubin is carried to the liver (by albumin) to be processed. Indirect bilirubin is fat-soluble and must be converted (by the liver) to a water-soluble form (called direct or conjugated bilirubin) in order to be eliminated from the body. Normally, only a low level of bilirubin exists in the blood. When the liver is damaged or unable to properly process indirect bilirubin, the total bilirubin level (indirect bilirubin plus direct bilirubin) increases in the bloodstream. When the total bilirubin builds to a high level, a yellowing of the skin and eyes (called jaundice) is typically observable in the patient. In adults, high blood levels of bilirubin are typically due to gallstones or liver diseases (such as cirrhosis or hepatitis).

Transjugular Intrahepatic Portosystemic Shunt

A transjugular intrahepatic portosystemic shunt is placed between the hepatic and portal veins to alleviate the pressure in the portal system that may be causing ascites or variceal bleeding. In patients that have severe portal hypertension, the flow of blood within the portal venous system tends to be in a hepatofugal direction (flowing away from the liver) instead of hepatopetal (flowing toward the liver). After the stent is placed, a baseline ultrasound should be performed to check the shunt with B-mode and color Doppler. When color Doppler is applied, the entire stent should demonstrate complete color filling. If the ultrasound operator does not see color flow, then one can assume that there is a blockage. If spectral waveforms demonstrate velocities that are extremely high or low when compared to the baseline exam, one may assume that there is a stenosis. Other indicators that the stent is no longer working correctly are a shift in directional flow within the portal vein, ascites that has increased, or the presence of collateral channels visualized with ultrasound.

Examining the Liver with Ultrasound

It is advisable to use the highest frequency abdominal transducer for obtaining the best image and for getting the proper penetration and depth. It is important to get the proper focal zone and depth placement for proper imaging. Take a systematic plan to view and document the liver in the transverse and longitudinal planes making sure to get the entire organ on record. Measure the longitudinal and anteroposterior diameter of the liver. Note the common hepatic duct as well as the bile duct. Color Doppler is used to identify the vasculature and record. Look for intrahepatic or extrahepatic bile ducts. Document and measure any abnormal findings including cysts, fluid in spaces, or masses.

Diseases of the Liver

Liver disease may originate in a number of areas. Hepatitis (liver inflammation) is usually caused by viral infection, exposure to toxins (including alcohol and drugs), or autoimmune factors. Portal hypertension and metabolic diseases also cause many liver problems. The liver can be injured by benign and malignant tumors (including cysts). The liver may also become involved in a number of systemic conditions, including autoimmune disorders, infections, and heart failure. Liver disease usually shows similar clinical manifestations. Initially, symptoms are typically mild. This sturdy and resilient organ can compensate for a surprising amount of damage. Eventually evidence of liver failure occurs; this is characterized by a marked decline in liver functions and the development of swelling (due to fluid retention) and portal hypertension.

Additional signs of liver disease include:

- Jaundice (hyperbilirubinemia)
- Cirrhosis (irreversible fibrosis and scarring)
- Hepatocellular carcinoma (primary malignant cancer of the liver)
- Hepatic failure (severe decline in all liver functions)

HEPATOCELLULAR DISEASE

Hepatocellular disease involves the hepatocytes (the main functional units of the liver). Since liver-function is affected by the death of liver cells, the serum liver enzyme levels will become elevated. The whole battery of liver-function-tests typically indicates the extent of disease.

BILE FLOW OBSTRUCTION DISEASE

Bile flow obstruction disease (cholestatis) refers to the stagnation or reduction of normal bile flow through the liver. This causes an elevation in alkaline phosphate and direct bilirubin levels in the blood. The blockage of bile can also cause problems in the livers ability to synthesize protein. This results in decreased blood albumen levels and clotting factors (PT time). The principle causes of this disease in adults are medications, cirrhosis, and a transient form that appears during pregnancy.

ACUTE AND CHRONIC HEPATITIS

Hepatitis (liver inflammation) is characterized by the injury/death of liver cells and the presence of inflammatory cells in the liver tissue. Acute hepatitis generally last less than six months. Acute hepatitis can be caused by viral infections (such as mononucleosis and hepatitis virus A, B, C, D, and E), bacterial infections, amoebic infections, certain medicines, and alcohol/fungal toxins. Acute infectious viral hepatitis usually improves without any intervention. Less than 0.3 percent of patients develop liver failure in the future. Chronic hepatitis generally lasts more than six months. Chronic hepatitis can be caused by contagious viral hepatitis (such as hepatitis B, C, D), certain medicines, toxins (such as alcohol), autoimmune disease, metabolic disorders (such as Wilson's disease (retention of too much copper) and haemochromatosis (retention of too much iron). About one in five of patients with chronic hepatitis B and C are at risk of developing cirrhosis or cancer of the liver in the future.

HEPATOCELLULAR CARCINOMA

Hepatocellular Carcinoma (HCC) is a cancer that involves the normal liver cells (hepatocytes). It is somewhat rare in the United States accounting for five percent of patients with existing cirrhosis. About eighty percent of cases involving HCC occur in patients with cirrhosis of the liver. Hepatitis (B and C) infections and exposure to aflatoxins (from contaminated food) also increase a patient's risk of HCC. HCC is usually discovered during an ultrasound (or CAT) examination of the liver. Elevated blood alpha-fetoprotein (AFP) levels are also present in about seventy percent of patients with HHC. The tumor itself can be a solitary mass, have multiple nodules, or infiltrate the liver in a

115

diffuse manner. It can affect the hepatic and portal veins, and sometimes the biliary tree. The liver usually becomes enlarged and the patient suffers from a mild fever and signs of cirrhosis.

SONOGRAPHIC FEATURES OF CIRRHOSIS OF THE LIVER

Cirrhosis is defined as the irreversible scarring of the liver. Scar tissue replaces healthy tissue due to the liver damage caused by toxins, viruses, and other disorders. Cirrhosis is a chronic condition that results in liver function failure and portal hypertension in its end stage. In America, cirrhosis of the liver kills about 26.000 people each year. The ability to determine the presence of cirrhosis may be difficult using ultrasound. The following features may be present:

- A coarsening of the normal liver tissue near the scarred area.
- Increased attenuation.
- Hepatosplenomegaly (an enlargement of the liver and spleen)
- Nodules on the liver's edge
- The fissures of the liver may be more visible.
- Portal hypertension
- Hepatoma tumors

CLASSIFICATION GRADES OF LIVER TEXTURE FOR FATTY LIVER

Echogenicity increases with the amount of fatty infiltration of the liver. There is typically an enlargement of the lobe of the liver affected. The portal vein structures may be obscured because of the increased attenuation. The three grades of liver texture used to classify the degree of fatty liver are:

1. Slight increase in the fine echoes of the liver tissue with a clear, normal view of the diaphragm and blood vessel borders.
2. Moderate increase in the fine echoes of the liver tissue with a slightly blurry view of the diaphragm and blood vessel borders.
3. Heavy increase in the fine echoes of the liver tissue with poor to no ability to view the diaphragm and blood vessel borders.

LIVER CELL ADENOMA

Liver Cell Adenoma is a benign tumor made up of normal liver cells (or hepatocytes). The tumor may grow as large as twelve inches in length. This tumor occurs most commonly in young women. It is associated with oral contraceptives containing hormones. The tumor should be recognized because it can clinically mimic a hepatocellular carcinoma. The tumor may also be present in the setting of glycogen storage disorders. Since the tumor grows in the presence of hormones, it has a tendency to rupture, especially during pregnancy.

During an ultrasound examination of the tumor, the following features are present:

- A solitary mass or a hyperechoic solid lesion.
- The mass shows an increase in size and appears heterogeneous in the presence of tissue damage or bleeding.

FATTY LIVER DISEASE

Non-alcoholic fatty liver (called steatosis) is a disease in which lipids accumulate to abnormally high levels in the hepatocytes. It is caused either by a physical injury to the liver or a systemic problem with the liver's ability to metabolize fat. In its milder form there is usually no damage to the liver. In its more severe form (called steatohepatitis) there is usually inflammation of the liver along with the formation of fibrous tissue. This can eventually lead to cirrhosis or liver cancer. Women are more likely to be diagnosed with fatty liver. It is found in all age groups although it is more common in middle-aged overweight/obese individuals. Contributing conditions are diabetes, high cholesterol, and high triglycerides (hyperlipidemia). The true prevalence of fatty liver is not known. The current estimate is that up to one third of American adults are affected by this disease.

CAVERNOUS HEMANGIOMA

Cavernous hemangioma is small tumor (about one inch). It is the most common benign liver tumor with an occurrence of 0.4 to 7.3 percent in the general population. Cavernous hemangioma typically occurs on the right lobe of the liver and originates with the endothelial cells that line the blood vessels. Walls made of collagen support its structure and the lesion itself consists of multiple, large vascular channels lined by a single layer of endothelial cells. In most cases, these tumors are without symptoms and discovered upon imaging, surgery, or autopsy. They can occur at any age and are more common in women (by about a five to one margin). When symptoms do occur, they are most likely caused by the compression of adjacent structures, rupture, or acute thrombosis.

FOCAL NODULAR HYPERPLASIA

Focal nodular hyperplasia is a rare benign tumor of the liver that takes the form of a nodule. It is composed of central scar tissue with masses of surrounding normal liver cells. The size of the nodule can vary in size and is located near the bottom edge of the liver. Typically, focal nodular hyperplasia does not cause symptoms and is normally discovered when the patient's abdomen is imaged (or during surgery). The tumor can sometimes cause pain, especially in situations where bleeding is present. The cause of focal nodular hyperplasia is uncertain. It may be caused by the abnormal development of blood vessels within the liver. Since this tumor is common in women under forty, there is a theory that this tumor is caused by hormones. Evidence shows that the nodules enlarge in women who are on contraceptive drugs containing hormones.

LIVER ABSCESS

Abscesses of the liver are very rare (about ten cases per one hundred thousand hospitalized patients). Symptoms may include abdominal pain, diarrhea, and low fever. Typically, the white blood cell count is also elevated (called leukocytosis).

There are three major forms of liver abscess. They are:

1. Pyogenic abscess (often polymicrobial in nature). Appendicitis can cause of this type of abscess. Pyogenic abscess accounts for eighty percent of all liver abscesses.
2. Amebic abscess caused by a parasitic amoeba (entamoeba histolytica). A person contracts the parasite through the ingestion of contaminated food and water. The infection is usually confined to the colon but can spread to the liver through the portal vein.
3. Fungal abscess (most often caused by the candida species).

The following sonographic features may be present:

- The abscess may be round or oval-shaped.
- The abscess will be hyperechoic compared to the surrounding liver tissue.

PATTERNS OF METASTASES SEEN IN THE LIVER BY ULTRASOUND

Bull's eye is one type of pattern. It has an echogenic center and areas around will be a darker echopenic image. Echopenic spots appear as dark spots in the liver. Echogenic areas appear different than the surrounding liver and will appear lighter, possibly due to calcification within a mass. Cystic spots are rare and difficult to impossible to determine by ultrasound from benign cysts. Diffuse refers to numerous lesions seen throughout the liver and will raise the question of lymphoma infiltration, an immunodeficiency disease, or multi-focal hepatoma. Necrotic areas are the last pattern seen with metastases by ultrasound and these areas appear as fluid-filled centers with irregular edges. It is useful to use color and pulsed Doppler to determine where the blood flow is and if there is an obstruction or flow interruptions within the liver. It is important to remember that lower-velocity shifts noted when scanning the liver tend to indicate hemangiomas, and high-velocity shifts may be more likely to show a malignant lesion.

LIVER HEMATOMAS

Liver hematomas typically occur when there is trauma to the liver. A hemotoma occurs when there is bleeding outside of a blood vessel, but the bleeding is contained within the surrounding tissue. It commonly appears as a pooling of blood (usually clotted), which is confined between the capsule (surrounding the liver and known as Glisson's capsule) and the surface of the liver. However, it is possible for a hemotoma to occur anywhere there are blood vessels within the liver. Hemotomas usually resolve themselves with time and do not require any intervention. In very rare circumstances, a liver hemotoma can become very large and rupture into the peritoneal cavity creating a very serious condition for the patient.

METASTASIS OF THE LIVER

Metastasis is the process by which cancer is spread from its originating site to other areas of the body (such as the liver). Cancer cells can migrate from a primary tumor and travel (via the lymphatic and blood vessels) to affect normal, healthy tissues elsewhere in the body. The liver is a prime site for metastatic disease due the large amount of blood that travels to and through the organ. The portal vein delivers blood from the digestive tract and provides a path for colon, stomach, pancreas, biliary-tree, and intestinal cancers to spread to the liver. More than half (54%) of all liver metastases are due to colon cancer. Breast and lung cancers also frequently pass to the liver. Liver metastases usually involve an enlarged and tender liver accompanied by elevated Alk Phos, ALT and AST levels (due to the damage done to the healthy liver cells.).

SIMPLE AND COMPLEX LIVER CYSTS

Simple liver cysts are also known as benign cysts, non-parasitic cysts, or solitary cysts. They occur in two to four percent of patients and are most often without any symptoms. They are typically discovered during ultrasound (or CAT) examinations of the liver. The lesion is round or oval shaped and varies in size from less than an inch to nearly eight inches. If simple cysts become symptomatic it is typically due to rupture (or bleeding) of the cyst, jaundice (due to bile obstruction), and portal hypertension.

Complex liver cysts can be caused by:

- Parasites such as echinococcus granulosus. This parasite is common among sheepherding peoples and appears as a simple oval-shaped cyst or a complex mass on a sonograph. Septations are also present.
- Hamartoma
- Hepatic cystadenoma and cystadenocarcinoma
- Cystic metastases

Other larger cysts may be due to infection caused by bacteria or infestations.

NECROTIZING FASCIITIS

Necrotizing fasciitis (NF) is a bacterial infection of the soft tissues that will affect the superficial and deep portions of the fascial planes. NF is rare, but it can be fatal if not treated. Often, patients that contract NF already have a chronic disease such as diabetes. A quick diagnosis can be difficult because in the early stage it may appear similar to cellulitis, but when collections of fluid are located within the deep fascia, NF is suspected. Cellulitis is a more superficial finding, and if NF is diagnosed early, the skin and muscles may not be affected. NF requires an emergent diagnosis, and ultrasound operators should look for "STAFF," which stands for demonstration of subcutaneous thickening, air, in addition to fascial fluid. Air can be seen when certain bacteria tend to form gas within the tissue that is affected. A high-frequency transducer should be used to better image the fascial plane and gas bubbles that often demonstrate posterior shadowing.

IMAGING THE APPENDIX

The five (or seven and a half) megahertz linear array probe should be applied with gradual and uniform pressure over the right lower quadrant. The linear array has a flat surface that makes it easier to perform compression maneuvers. The diameter of the appendix should be no larger than six millimeters. It should also be able to be compressed. A non-compressible appendix is a sign of appendicitis. If appendicitis is suspected, a five-megahertz linear array with a short focus should be utilized. If a hyperechoic focus with posterior shadowing is observed, it is a sign of an appendicolith (a calcification within the appendix).

ULTRASOUND TECHNIQUES TO DIAGNOSE PELVIC PAIN IN NONPREGNANT WOMEN

Ultrasound on a nonpregnant woman with pelvic pain is done most successfully with the endovaginal probe. It is a safe method and essential in diagnosing the cause of pelvic pain. Ultrasound can image a torted ovary or cyst, acute pelvic inflammatory disease, and an ectopic pregnancy. The pitfalls of ultrasound for pelvic pain are that some things can still be missed, for example an abdominal pregnancy or pelvic adhesions when the uterus is impregnated. A cervical pregnancy can look like an impending abortion or a uterine fibroid can mask a pregnancy. The endovaginal transducer should be used as with other types of vaginal exams, warming the medium gel, protecting the patient's privacy, and providing patient safety while doing the scan. The patient is most often preoperatively fasting or fasting until an acute surgical condition is ruled out.

SUPERFICIAL STRUCTURES AND ASSOCIATED PATHOLOGY ASSESSED WITH ULTRASOUND

Advancements in high-frequency transducers have enabled ultrasound users to assess superficial structures that could not be properly visualized in the past. Subcutaneous tissue is fat that is located just under the skin that will have different thicknesses depending on the amount of adipose tissue that the patient has. Lipomas are common masses found in the subcutaneous layer that often appear as elliptical, are compressible, and are typically isoechoic or hyperechoic when compared to the surrounding tissue. When scanning the thyroid, it is important that users are aware of the possibility of a third lobe called the pyramidal lobe. This should not be mistaken for a mass, and it will appear as normal thyroid tissue arising superiorly from the isthmus. Cutaneous hemangiomas are superficial masses that can be evaluated with ultrasound. They will appear as hyperemic masses with borders that are well defined.

ROLE OF ULTRASOUND IN CASES OF CRYPTORCHIDISM

Cryptorchidism can be defined as the failure of one or both testes to descend into the scrotum. If a clinician suspects an undescended testis and cannot palpate it within the inguinal canal, an ultrasound exam will often be ordered because it does not use ionizing radiation. When an ultrasound exam is ordered, it is important to perform a full scrotal ultrasound to confirm that the scrotum does not contain one or both testes. The gray-scale images should include a side-by-side comparison so that the radiologist can clearly see the missing testis. Once the measurements, color, and spectral Doppler images have been documented, the sonographer should scan the inguinal canal on the side of the missing testis. If located, measurements and color Doppler images should be provided. If the testis is not found in the inguinal canal, it is important to remember that testes form in the abdomen and may be found as superiorly as the kidneys. If it cannot be located, it may be beneficial to have a clinician present during the scan.

INFANTILE HEMANGIOENDOTHELIOMA AND LYMPHOMA

Infantile hemangioendothelioma is a benign tumor of the liver. There are usually multiple lesions present. The lesions are up to one inch in size and are round, smooth (with lobes) and have well defined edges. Each lesion is composed of vascular channels lined by endothelial cells. This tumor mostly affects patients who are six months of age or younger. The patients are predominantly females (by a two to one ratio). Accompanying symptoms can include gastrointestinal/internal bleeding, anemia, and jaundice. The tumor grows rapidly and then slowly regresses. The resulting liver damage may be fatal to the young patient.

A lymphoma is a rare benign slow-growing tumor made up of fatty tissue. Lymphomas are usually without any symptoms. They are typically small, but can grow up to two inches long.

RENAL LYMPHOMA

Renal lymphoma is often discovered in patients with known lymphoma. These tumors are often difficult to detect because their infiltrative growth results in preservation of the renal tissue (parenchymal structures) and renal shape. As these tumors enlarge, the surrounding renal parenchyma is compressed and destroyed. Eventually, the renal masses will extend beyond the renal contour and resemble primary renal tumors (neoplasms). Renal involvement occurs more commonly in non–Hodgkin lymphoma than in Hodgkin lymphoma. Patients with renal lymphoma may not have any symptoms, however, the renal function panel occasionally reveals elevated blood urea nitrogen (BUN) and creatinine levels, which may indicate an obstruction. The tumor may obstruct urine flow, resulting in dilation of the branches and pelvic cavity of the kidney due to an accumulation of urine (hydronephrosis).

GASTRIC CARCINOMA AND LYMPHOMA OF THE STOMACH

Up to ninety five percent of malignant stomach tumors are carcinomas. It is the sixth leading cause of death in older males. The lesions may be fungating, ulcerated, diffuse, polypoid, or superficial. Ultrasound shows a target and may show gastric wall thickening.

Lymphoma may occur as a primary tumor of the GI tract. Up to three percent of all lymphomas are malignant stomach tumors. Symptoms may include nausea, vomiting, and weight loss. On ultrasound, the tumor appears as a large hypoechoic mass. There may be thickening of the gastric wall and a spoke-wheel pattern within the tumor.

LYMPHADENOPATHY

There are many lymph nodes (about six hundred) distributed throughout the human body. Palpable lymph nodes exist just under the chin (submandibular), in the arm pits (axillary) and in the groin area (inguinal). Ultrasound may be used to image lymph nodes in other areas of the body (such as the splenic-hilum, porta-hepatis, renal-hilum, and the para-aortic area). Lymphadenopathy refers to nodes that are abnormal in size (larger than one centimeter). Lymphadenopathy is categorized as "generalized" if lymph nodes are enlarged in two or more separate areas or "localized" if only one area is affected. In patients with unexplained lymphadenopathy, about three fourths of patients will present with localized lymphadenopathy and one fourth with generalized lymphadenopathy.

ADRENAL GLAND PATHOLOGY VISUALIZED WITH ULTRASOUND

Normal adrenal glands can be extremely difficult to identify in adults during an ultrasound exam. If they are visible, it is usually because they are enlarged due to a mass. Masses of the adrenal gland are often an incidental finding. An adenoma of the adrenal gland is the most likely diagnosis when a solid, hypoechoic mass is present. Metastatic disease of the adrenals is common, and this is the second most likely tumor found if a patient has a history of cancer. The normal adrenal glands may be visualized by ultrasound when performing an abdominal scan on infants, however. A neuroblastoma is a primary malignant tumor found in children that presents as a large, solid intra-abdominal mass. Adrenal hematomas may be present after trauma or vaginal delivery, and their ultrasound appearance varies with the age of the bleed. They may be anechoic early on, whereas older bleeds are more echogenic.

ADRENAL GLANDS

The adrenal gland is an endocrine gland that is located on the top of each kidney. It is triangular in shape and measures about one-half inch in height and three inches in length. The gland consists of a medulla (the center of the gland) and is surrounded by the cortex (the outer surface of the gland). The medulla is responsible for producing epinephrine and norepinephrine (adrenaline). The adrenal cortex produces other hormones necessary for fluid and electrolyte (salt) balance in the body (such as cortisone and aldosterone). The adrenal cortex also produces sex hormones. Using ultrasound, the adrenal gland is seen as a distinct hypoechoic structure.

PHEOCHROMOCYTOMA

Pheochromocytoma is a tumor of the adrenal gland. These tumors cause the production of excess adrenaline into the bloodstream. Pheochromocytomas are formed in the central portion of the adrenal gland (called the adrenal medulla). The adrenal medulla is responsible for the normal production of adrenaline (that maintains blood pressure and helps the body cope with stressful situations). Pheochromocytoma can become a deadly tumor because of the severe elevation in blood pressure it causes. Symptoms may include those tied to excess adrenaline production such as sweating, headache, and a feeling of high anxiety. A serum catecholamines test (sometimes over a twenty-four-hour period) may be used to measure the level of adrenaline compounds in the blood. An abnormally high result may indicate that the condition is present.

METASTASIS OF THE ADRENAL GLANDS

The adrenal gland is a common site for metastases from cancers originating in the breast, lung, and kidneys. Lung cancer (due to smoking) is the leading cause of this condition. Adrenal metastasis occurs in up to ten percent of patients diagnosed with lung cancer. Most cases involve solitary, unilateral, small asymptomatic lesions. They are usually discovered incidentally when scanning the abdomen. Bilateral adrenal metastases are observed in less than three percent of patients with lung cancer. Again, most cases involve small, asymptomatic lesions. Hemorrhage (bleeding) is a rare but serious complication of adrenal metastases.

ADENOCARCINOMA OF THE GASTROINTESTINAL TRACT

Adenocarcinoma is the most common malignant tumor of the gastrointestinal (GI) tract. As the tumor grows, it can invade the intestinal wall. This allows the cancer to spread into adjoining lymph nodes and metastasize to other areas in the body. Most of the time adenocarcinoma occurs in the large intestine. Symptoms may include abdominal pain accompanied by nausea, bloating and loss of appetite. In advanced cases, signs of intestinal bleeding (vomiting blood and anemia) and jaundice may be present. Less than thirty five percent of patients diagnosed with adenocarcinoma of the intestines live more than five years after the cancer is discovered. This cancer is more prevalent in patients that have pre-existing Crohn's or Celiac disease.

FEATURES OF AN ULTRASOUND WHEN ABDOMINAL PATHOLOGY IS SUSPECTED

An abdominal mass is usually noncompressible and does not move. With a pathological image, the bowel may show three layers giving a bull's eye appearance when cross-sectioned. Fat and connective tissue appear swollen and the texture shows an increase in echogenicity. Vasodilatations will show on color Doppler. There will be an increase in vascularity when pathology is present. Fluid, shadows, and perforations may be present on the image. In large patients a low-frequency curved linear transducer may show a clearer image and an attempt to use all techniques available must be considered to get the best image and an accurate diagnosis.

BILIARY DYSPEPSIA

Biliary dyspepsia is a disease in which the gastrointestinal organs, primarily the stomach and first part of the small intestine, function abnormally. It is a chronic disease in which the symptoms fluctuate in frequency and intensity. It may be caused by a lack of enough bile (to the small intestine) to process fats in the diet. The primary symptoms of dyspepsia are upper abdominal pain, belching, nausea, and abdominal bloating. The symptoms most often appear shortly after eating.

BILIARY DYSKINESIA

Biliary dyskinesia has symptoms of intermittent upper abdominal pain that may be accompanied by nausea and vomiting. Scarring or spasms of the sphincter of Oddi muscle may cause it. The sphincter of Oddi muscle is a small circular muscle approximately one-half inch in length. The function of this muscle is to keep the bile duct and pancreatic duct muscles closed to prevent reflux of intestinal contents into the bile duct and pancreas duct.

LAYERS LINING THE GUT

Following are the different layers lining the gut:

- The innermost layer is called is called the mucosa. It is the moist membranous lining of the gut. It is made up of squamous cells through the esophagus, and is smooth thereafter. Connective tissue and smooth muscle are also present.
- The second layer is called the submucosa. It is made up of soft connective tissue, blood vessels, nerves and lymphatics.
- The third layer is called the muscularis-propria. It is made up of a circular inner layer, accompanied by a longitudinal outer layer consisting of smooth muscle.
- The fourth layer is called the serosa. This is a single layer that provides fluid to the gut.
- The fifth layer is called the adventitia. This is the outside connective tissue surrounding the gut.

ANATOMY OF THE GASTROINTESTINAL TRACT

The gastrointestinal (GI) tract begins at the mouth and continues through the esophagus, stomach, small intestine, large intestine, and rectum. Food is chewed in the mouth and travels to the stomach through the esophagus. The food is then stored and broken down in the stomach (using gastric acid produced by the stomach). The food then gradually enters the duodenum (the first part of the small intestine). The small intestine consists of three parts (the duodenum, jejunum, and the ileum). As the food travels though the small intestine, nutrients are absorbed into the bloodstream. Bile (from the liver), digestive enzymes (from the pancreas), and liquid (from the intestines) are added to assist with this process. By the time the food reaches the large intestine, most of the usable liquids and nutrients have been absorbed into the body. The resulting waste products continue to travel to the colon where they are finally eliminated from the body (through the rectum).

ADENOCARCINOMA

Pancreatic adenocarcinoma is a fatal tumor. It is the second most common cause of death from all gastrointestinal cancers. In fact, adenocarcinoma accounts for ninety five percent of all malignant tumors originating in the pancreas. It usually affects persons sixty to eighty years old (especially males). The tumor appears in the head of the pancreas sixty to seventy percent of the time. The tumor is seldom diagnosed at an early stage. The symptoms may include jaundice, weight loss, abdominal pain, nausea/vomiting, and a general feeling of poor health/weakness.

The following ultrasound features are present:

- The lesions show a different echodensity compared to the rest of the pancreas.
- The echopattern is hypoechoic.
- The borders are irregular.
- There may be an enlargement of the pancreas.
- Dilation of the pancreatic ducts is present.
- The spleen may be enlarged.
- Compression of components of the pancreatic vascular system may be caused by the tumor.

ROLE OF ULTRASOUND WHEN A HERNIA IS SUSPECTED

Not all abdominal hernias can be diagnosed clinically because physicians may not always be able to feel a palpable mass. Ultrasound provides low-cost, nonionizing, real-time imaging capabilities. Ultrasound can provide clinicians with information regarding whether or not a hernia is present; its contents (fat containing or bowel), size, and location; and if the hernia can be reduced. Ultrasound systems today combined with a picture archiving and communication system will allow end users to save an ultrasound clip that demonstrates the hernia during the Valsalva maneuver or while the hernia is being reduced. Combined, these tools offer increased diagnostic confidence, especially for radiologists who are not present during the ultrasound exam. Sonographers should note that sometimes hernias may reduce when the patient is in the supine position during the ultrasound exam. It is important to use the Valsalva maneuver and to have the patient upright during the ultrasound, especially in cases that appear negative when the patient is lying down.

ACUTE APPENDICITIS

Appendicitis is inflammation of the appendix. When the inflammation occurs suddenly, the condition is called acute appendicitis. The appendix is a small, tubular extension attached to the large intestine at the cecum. It occurs when feces, a swallowed foreign object, or a tumor obstructs the appendix. Symptoms may include a reduced appetite, nausea, vomiting, and fever. Usually, abdominal pain (located to the right of the navel) develops and becomes more severe as the condition progresses. A complication is that the appendix may rupture and cause a life-threatening infection (called infected peritonitis).

The following ultrasound features are present:

- A target lesion in the lower right quadrant.
- Thickening of the bowel wall.
- An echogenic core due to necrosis.
- The diameter of the appendix exceeds six millimeters.

CROHN'S DISEASE

Crohn's disease causes inflammation of the gastrointestinal (GI) tract. Its exact cause is unknown; however, it may be related to an abnormal immune response by the body. It may occur in any part of the GI tract. It occurs most often in the lower part (terminal ileum) of the small intestine or colon. The inflammation and swelling can be severe enough to cause pain and repeated bouts of diarrhea. Crohn's disease is unique in that it affects all layers of the intestine. Other inflammatory intestinal diseases such as irritable bowel syndrome and ulcerative colitis only affect the top layer. Crohn's disease is also known as ileitis or enteritis.

The following sonographic features may be present:

- Gut wall thickening (greater than three to five centimeters)
- Strictures
- Creeping fat (a mass effect adjacent to the bowel)
- Increasing vascularity

POLYPS AND LEIOMYOMAS OF THE STOMACH

Polyps are benign tumors usually observed when the stomach is imaged full of water. The patient should be asked to drink water (immediately before the examination) to distend the stomach wall. They appear as solid masses adhering to the stomach wall. The polyps show variable echogenicity.

A leiomyoma is the most common benign tumor of the stomach. It appears as a small mass (similar to a carcinoma). It is associated with other conditions such as cholelithiasis, peptic ulcer disease, adenocarcinoma, and leiomyosarcoma. On ultrasound, it appears as a hypoechoic mass attached to the muscular layer of the stomach.

PROSTATE

The prostate is a gland of the male reproductive system. It is located in front of the rectum and just below the bladder. It is about one inch in diameter (similar to the size of a walnut) and has a cone-like shape. It is made up of two lobes called the base (located directly against the bladder) and the apex (located downward and is in contact with the superior (upper) fascia of the urogenital diaphragm). The primary purpose of the prostate is to produce fluid for semen, which then transports sperm through the urethra during the male orgasm. Blood is supplied to the prostate from the prostaticovesical arteries that branch from the internal iliac.

PROSTATE'S CAPSULE AND ZONES

The prostate is enclosed in a fibromuscular layer (stroma) that is known as the prostatic capsule. This layer is most prominent along the base of the prostate gland.

Following are the zones of the prostate gland:

- Anterior Zone. The anterior zone is located in the front of the prostate gland. It is composed mostly of muscular tissue.
- Transition Zone. The transition zone is the innermost part of the prostate gland and surrounds the urethra where it passes through the organ.
- Central Zone. The central zone surrounds the transition zone.
- Peripheral Zone. The peripheral zone of the prostate gland is located in the back of the prostate gland (closest to the rectum). Prostate cancer forms in this zone eighty percent of the time.

PSA Lab Test

The PSA test measures the blood level of prostate specific antigen (PSA). PSA is a reproductive enzyme produced by the prostate that helps sperm move through the female's cervix. Generally, PSA levels less than 4 ng/ml (nanograms per milliliter) are viewed as normal for men less than fifty years of age. The PSA level tends to rise naturally with age, and some labs raise the level considered normal accordingly. In any case, PSA levels higher than ten may be associated with prostate cancer. Other causes of abnormally high PSA levels are benign prostatic hyperplasia (BPH) and infection of the prostate (prostatitis).

Ejaculatory Duct Cysts and Abscess of the Prostate

Ejaculatory duct cysts are typically small. The cysts cause dilation of the ejaculatory duct and are most likely caused by an obstruction of the duct itself. These cysts are associated with lowered sperm counts in affected men causing infertility.

An abscess should be suspected in cases where patients with acute prostatitis do not respond to treatment. Using ultrasound, abscesses of the prostate appear as an anechoic mass with or without internal echoes. Coliform bacteria (especially E-coli) cause more than seventy percent of prostatic abscesses. Surgical intervention is necessary (to drain the abscess) along with the administration of antibiotics.

BPH

Benign prostatic hyperplasia (BPH) is an enlargement of the prostate gland as a man ages. The prostate gland typically goes through two phases of growth. The first occurs during puberty, when the prostate typically doubles in size. Near age twenty-five, the gland begins to grow again. This second growth phase often results in BPH in older men (after age forty). More than half of men in their sixties and as many as ninety percent of men older than seventy have some symptoms of BPH. Typical symptoms include urination and bladder control problems (called prostatism) due to the enlarged prostate pressing against the urethra. The following ultrasound feature is present: An enlarged prostate that may be diffuse or focal.

Malignant Tumors of the Prostate

A malignant tumor of the prostate is classified as an adenocarcinoma (or glandular cancer). It occurs when the normal semen-producing prostate cells mutate into cancer cells. It is found most often in the peripheral zone of the prostate. Eventually, the tumor may grow large enough to spread to nearby organs such as the seminal vesicles or the rectum. The tumor cells may also metastasize (via the bloodstream and lymph nodes) to the bones and bladder. Malignant tumors of the prostate occur most often in men over fifty years old.

The following ultrasound features are present:

- The presence of a distinct hypoechoic lesion.
- An enlargement of the prostate.
- An irregular area of the prostate that distorts the normal hyperechoic pattern.

Prostatitis

Prostatitis is the term used to describe inflammation of the prostate gland. In most cases prostatitis is caused by a bacterial infection, but it can have other causes. Symptoms include painful urination and ejaculation. Prostatitis is the most common urological disorder in men over the age of fifty however, it may occur at any age. The four major types of prostatitis are:

- Acute bacterial prostatitis is inflammation of the prostate gland caused by bacteria. Severe complications may develop if not promptly treated. This condition can be fatal if the bacterial infection is left untreated and spreads to the bloodstream.
- Chronic bacterial prostatitis is a recurrent infection and inflammation of the prostate and urinary tract. Symptoms are less severe than those associated with acute bacterial prostatitis.
- Non-bacterial prostatitis is the presence of an inflamed prostate without bacterial infection.
- Prostatodynia is the occurrence of prostatitis symptoms, without any inflammation or bacterial infection.

ABNORMALITIES THAT MAY BE VISUALIZED IN THE URINARY SYSTEM AFTER A TRAUMATIC EVENT

In patients that are seen in the emergency department (ED) for trauma-related injuries, ultrasound is a relatively quick and easy method to determine the presence of free fluid within the abdomen and pelvis. An ultrasound can be performed in the ED so that an unstable patient does not have to be moved. Blunt trauma is more often the cause of injury when compared to penetrating forces involving the urinary system. Sonographers should be aware that if injuries are diagnosed in the kidneys due to trauma, the majority of cases will also include other organs. Computed tomography (CT) is often ordered when the patient presents with symptoms causes by trauma to the urinary system because ultrasound cannot diagnose all injuries, especially parenchymal involvement. Ureters are not often visualized due to bowel gas, but ultrasound operators should evaluate the urinary bladder. Rupture of the urinary bladder is better diagnosed with CT, but ultrasound may provide useful information pertaining to free fluid within the abdominopelvic cavity. Ureteral jets may be visualized with color Doppler if a distended urinary bladder is present to rule out the presence of an obstructed ureter.

EVALUATING PERFUSION OF VESSELS OF THE RETROPERITONEUM

The retroperitoneum consists of the abdominal aorta, inferior vena cava (IVC), and kidneys. These structures and their associated blood vessels or branches can be assessed with gray-scale, color or power Doppler, and spectral Doppler. When evaluating the aorta, longitudinal and transverse images and measurements should be taken in the proximal (at the level of the celiac artery), mid (close to where the renal arteries branch off the aorta), and distal (proximal to the bifurcation of the iliac arteries) portions. Vessel patency may be demonstrated with the use of color and spectral Doppler as well as demonstrating any pathology including an abdominal aortic aneurysm (AAA), any atherosclerotic changes, or to observe any leaks of a postsurgical endoluminal graft. In cases of an AAA in the distal aorta, it is important to demonstrate the position of the aneurysm to the renal arteries to determine if they are also affected. The IVC can also be evaluated for the presence of a clot with gray-scale and color Doppler. The renal arteries may be evaluated for any indication of stenosis.

DIAGNOSIS OF ABDOMINAL MASS

First, if a mass is palpated by a physician, the ultrasound is ordered to help determine the depth of the mass and whether it is superficial or deep in the abdominal cavity. The peritoneal fascial line will be universally used as a focal point for diagnosis. The transducer used during the scan can be used to compress the area and displace gas or bowel for a clear image of the mass. The mass can then be clearly marked on the scan with identifying surrounding structures, which allows the physician to look for sonographic characteristics. This can help lead to the identification of cysts, solids, irregular borders, movement of air or fluid, size (by using three-dimensional imaging), and vascularity (by using color and pulsed Doppler).

SPACES OF THE RETROPERITONEUM

The following are spaces of the retroperitoneum:

- Posterior-pararenal: The posterior pararenal space and iliac fossa are located between the posterior renal fascia and the transversalis fascia. The iliac fossa is known as the "false pelvis". It contains the ureter and major branches of distal great vessels (including their lymphatics). The space merges at the bottom of the anterior pararenal space. The psoas muscle makes up the medial border. There are no organs in this space however; blood and lymph nodes (embedded in fat) are present.
- Perirenal: The perirenal space is surrounded by the anterior and posterior layers of the renal fascia (Gerota's fascia). This space contains the adrenal glands, kidneys, and ureters.
- Retrofascial: The retrofascial space contains no organs and includes the posterior-abdominal-wall, muscles, nerves, lymphatics, and areolar tissue located behind the tranversalis fascia. It is divided into three compartments (psoas, lumbar and iliac).
- Anterior-pararenal: The anterior-pararenal space is bound in the front by posterior parietal peritoneum and in the back by the anterior renal fascia. The lateroconal fascia (the fusion of the front and back leaves of the renal fascia) forms the sides. The pancreas, duodenal sweep, ascending colon, and transverse colon lie in this space. This space merges with the bare area of the liver by the coronary ligament.

ANATOMY OF THE RETROPERITONEUM

The retroperitoneum is simply the anatomical space behind the abdominal cavity. The following are considered retroperitoneal structures/organs:

- Kidneys
- Suprarenal Glands
- Bladder
- Ureter
- Inferior vena cava (IVC)
- Rectum
- Part of the esophagus

The following are considered secondarily retroperitoneal structures/organs:

- Part of the pancreas.
- The second, third and fourth portions of the duodenum.
- The ascending and descending portions of the colon.

The borders of the retroperitoneum include the following:

- The posterior peritoneum (front)
- The transversalis facia (back)
- The lateral borders of the quadratus lumborum muscles and the peritoneal leaves of the mesentery. (sides)
- From the diaphragm to the pelvic brim (partitioned into the lumbar and iliac fossae). (top to bottom)

CONGENITAL ANOMALIES OF VESSELS THAT MAY BE DISCOVERED DURING ABDOMINAL ULTRASOUND

Congenital anomalies of the blood vessels located in the retroperitoneum are typically an incidental finding during an ultrasound exam. It is important to document any variants of the inferior vena cava, aorta, and their branches because critical injuries may occur during abdominal or pelvic surgeries. Although most patients may not have any associated issues with these variants, a diagnosis of congenital anomalies may explain symptoms for those patients that experience hematuria, display a left-sided varicocele, or have pain in the left flank region. These symptoms could be explained if the left renal vein is located posterior to the aorta. A retroaortic left renal vein may prevent adequate drainage of the blood from the left kidney because this vessel is being compressed between the aorta and spine. Another variant is the duplication of renal arteries and veins.

PSOAS MUSCLES

The psoas muscles are located in the lower back. There are a total of four muscles (two psoas muscles located on each side of the spine). The larger of the two is called the psoas major. The smaller one is called the psoas minor. The psoas major originates at the spine (near the bottom of the rib cage). It then continues to the thigh bone. The psoas major functions to flex the hip. The psoas minor originates in the same area as the psoas major but continues down to the bony pelvis. It functions to flex the lower spine or lumbar area. When using ultrasound to image the retroperitoneum, the psoas muscle appears as a striated structure located in back and towards the middle of the kidney.

RECTUS SHEATH HEMATOMA

The rectus sheath is made up of the rectus abdominis muscle (a paired muscle running vertically on each side of the front wall of the abdomen), a surrounding facial sheath, and the blood supply from the epigastric arteries and veins. When the rectus abdominis muscle contracts, the attached artery must move with the muscle to avoid tearing. During strong contractions of the rectus abdominis muscles (such as those during rigorous exercise), the artery may tear resulting in a hematoma. External trauma to the abdominal wall may also cause the condition. Abdominal pain in the region of the affected rectus abdominis muscle is usually present.

RETROPERITONEAL FIBROSIS

Retroperitoneal fibrosis is a condition in which a large, fibrous tumor grows within the retroperitoneum. Peak incidence occurs in people aged forty to sixty, and men are affected twice as often as women. The tumor usually originates near the aorta and iliac arteries. As the tumor increases in size, it pushes against the organs that lie within the retroperitoneum. The most commonly affected organs are the kidneys and ureters. The tumor may obstruct (or even cut off) the flow of urine from the ureters to the bladder. The affected patient may complain of moderate to severe pain in the lower back (usually in the abdominal or flank areas) and difficult urination. There may also be edema (swelling) in one or both legs (due to fluid retention). Serum blood urea nitrogen (BUN) and creatinine levels may show elevation.

Obstetrical and Gynecological Procedures

TRANSLABIAL ULTRASOUND

A translabial (also referred to as transperineal) ultrasound exam can be performed with a 4–8 MHz transducer (curved array) or by using the endovaginal transducer if penetration of the ultrasound beam is not required. A protective cover is placed over the probe face. Gel is applied in the cover as well as on the external surface in order to conduct the sound waves. The patient should be in the lithotomy position on an exam table used for pelvic scans, or a cushion should be used to elevate the hips. The operator should start in a sagittal orientation to identify the cervix and use the bladder as a landmark. The vagina will be positioned between the urinary bladder and the rectum. The probe may need to be rotated to help get rid of gas or to avoid shadowing from the pubic bone.

PREFERENCE FOR ENDOCAVITY TRANSDUCERS DURING PELVIC EXAMS

Endocavity transducers offer better spatial resolution because of the close proximity to the female organs. During a transvaginal (TV) or endovaginal (EV) ultrasound, the transducer is placed inside the vagina allowing excellent image quality. The transducers that are used during a transvaginal ultrasound are high frequency compared to the lower frequency transducers used during a transabdominal (TA) exam. This not only allows for better image quality when looking at the various pelvic organs and regions, but it is easier for operators to obtain Doppler measurements. The bladder is emptied during a TV study, which offers patients much relief because scanning TA while the patient's bladder is full is extremely uncomfortable. TV scanning may also be used in first-trimester OB scans because structures are better visualized, again, due to the close proximity to the transducer. For pelvic exams, clinicians may prefer a transabdominal and a transvaginal approach for a complete workup.

HARMONICS

Harmonic imaging is offered by modern ultrasound systems to improve the diagnostic capabilities, especially during exams that are technically difficult. When the harmonics application is in use, the fundamental (transmitted) frequency offers improved diagnostic quality because the beam is altered less. The ultrasound harmonics are produced within the anatomical tissue of the patient. Tissue and contrast are two common types of harmonics used. Harmonics are useful during exams to help eliminate reflectors seen inside of cysts and side-lobe artifacts. Harmonic tissue applications used during OB ultrasounds are especially useful in the second trimester to provide improved visualization of organs and other anatomy, especially when the patient is obese. The use of tissue harmonics has especially increased the resolution of the heart or when the user would like to rid the image of any associated noise.

INCREASING AND DECREASING THE SCAN LINE DENSITY AND IMAGING DEPTH

If a sonographer decreases the scan line density and imaging depth, these adjustments will have a positive effect on the temporal resolution. Recall that an increase in frame rate will improve the temporal resolution because it more accurately portrays the location of signals in time. Both of the aforementioned adjustments will improve this frame rate. If a user decreases the line density, fewer pulse sequences are required to produce each image. Decreasing the line density will, however, degrade the lateral resolution. Decreasing the imaging depth also increases the frame rate because less go-return time is required because the reflectors are located at a shallow depth.

M-Mode

Motion mode (M-mode) is used mainly during cardiac imaging, and it displays the depth of echoes in regards to time represented by an x axis and a y axis. The x axis relates to time and is the horizontal plane. The y axis is a vertical axis that displays the depth of the anatomy. As the tracing moves from left to right across the screen, if the line rises up it indicates that the structure is closer to the transducer. A line that drops down is moving away from the probe, and a horizontal line means that the anatomy is not moving. M-mode offers excellent temporal resolution because data are gathered from only one ultrasound signal that is sent and received by the transducer. Even structures that are moving extremely fast can be accurately measured with M-mode. The location of the line can quickly be changed by the ultrasound operator, but care should be taken because more accurate measurements are calculated when the line is perpendicular to the structure. In addition to adult and pediatric echocardiography, M-mode is the preferred method of obtaining a fetal heart rate because less power is required, and it is also used during fetal echocardiograms.

Importance of Correlating Findings from Previous Ultrasound Exams

Often, pelvic and OB ultrasound exams are performed in order to follow up on pathology or to track the well-being and progression of the fetus. If a follow-up scan of an ovarian cyst or uterine fibroid is requested, it is important that the sonographer examines the prior ultrasound and report in order to know the number, size, and location of these structures. Today's ultrasound systems allow the sonographer to import parameters from previous OB studies in order to track interval growth of a fetus. Graphs can be used by the clinicians to serve as a visual aid in understanding the growth that has taken place. It is also important to compare previous studies because clinicians should not redact the estimated date of delivery if an exam was performed correctly earlier in the pregnancy. Follow-up scans for interval growth should not be performed weekly because the measurements may be incorrectly evaluated because a margin of error can exist. It is typically suggested that these follow-up exams are performed over a span that ranges from two to four weeks.

Translabial Method

Sometimes, the more conventional methods of performing an ultrasound are contraindicated or additional views are required to provide clinicians with a correct diagnosis. The translabial technique may be beneficial during a pelvic, OB, or bladder ultrasound. A translabial (also referred to as transperineal) approach can be performed when an endovaginal ultrasound exam cannot be performed or if it is too painful for the patient. A translabial approach is a useful method to measure the cervix or assess the placenta and lower genitourinary structures in cases of placenta previa. This is the ultrasound method of choice in cases of uterine prolapse or incontinence. The translabial method can add value because imaging with this technique can also be done in multiple planes. The ultrasound user should always be familiar with anatomy when performing additional views.

4D Ultrasound Applications

The 2D imaging mode is still used to obtain various measurements of the fetus during obstetrical (OB) exams, but 3D and 4D technology have offered even more applications for OB patients. The 3D imaging mode offers one more dimension to the 2D study. The 4D study is real-time 3D, and it offers not only a 3D image, but one that shows the movements of the fetus. The 3D and 4D imaging modes offer family members a more realistic portrayal of the fetus than 2D imaging. The 4D mode imaging is more than just a lifelike picture of the fetus. Many 4D applications offer improved diagnostic confidence during an OB ultrasound: Echocardiograms, looking at the fetal face for cleft lip/cleft palate deformities, watching the fetus swallow, viewing the fetal spine, checking for skeletal dysplasia, measuring lung volumes, and diagnosing diaphragmatic hernias are just a few examples of what can be studied in greater detail with 4D imaging.

General Uses of Sonography in Obstetrical Practice

Sonography may be used in obstetrical practice to assist in diagnosis of pregnancy. Ultrasound can detect the gestational sac at about 5 weeks or when corresponding beta-hCG levels are 5000 mIU/ml. Ultrasound serves as the most accurate determination of gestational age, this is often done in the late first trimester to early second trimester. Doppler devices are used to monitor fetal heart activity throughout pregnancy. Ultrasound is also the most accurate tool in assessing fetal growth and activity. It may also be used to assess fetal abnormalities. Sonography can indirectly help assess fetal maturity, but this is not the most accurate or first-line test for fetal maturity assessment.

Pelvic Preparation for Pelvic Sonography

As with any patient encounter, a brief introduction and a thorough history it imperative. Do not rely solely on the sonography order, as this may contain human error or if handwritten, penmanship may be difficult to read. Question the patient about their symptoms and their location, allergies, past surgeries, and what exam they are having done. Not only does this support the order for the imaging study, but gives you a clue as to the patients experience with such a procedure. Determining if previous imaging studies have been done on the pelvis/abdomen, as well as dates and location is helpful for comparison and interpretation. The procedure should be explained and questions and concerns answered. Equipment should be properly cleaned, and protocols followed. It is often recommended that the transducer sheath or condom be placed over the transducer while the patient is observing, further reassuring the patient of infectious disease control.

AIUM Guidelines for Equipment and Documentation of Ultrasound Evaluation

Female Pelvis

Guidelines for use and maintenance of sonographic equipment used to evaluate the pelvis should be known and reviewed periodically by all personal. AIUM as well as individual manufacturer guidelines should be followed. Appropriate infectious disease protocols should be recognized and applied as well. Real-time equipment with sufficient transducer frequency should be used. Transducer frequency should be adjusted to the level that allows for the least ultrasound exposure, yet yields adequate and useful results. Transducer frequency is chosen based on the unit used, the approach (transabdominal versus transvaginal), and body habitus. Thorough interpretation and documentation is necessary for quality of care and legal record-keeping purposes.

Antepartum Examination

The AIUM guidelines for equipment and documentation for antepartum sonographic evaluation are much like those of any ultrasound evaluation. They include use of real-time equipment and use of appropriate transducer, using the lowest exposure required to gain the most accurate information. Testing should be done only in situations that are medically necessary or as per protocol screening guidelines. Appropriate infectious disease control and sterile measures must be followed. Detailed documentation of all findings, measurements and tests should accompany the patient's medical record. All images should be clearly labeled with the minimum patient identifiers (name and date of birth), exam date and image details.

First Trimester Sonography

American Institute of Ultrasound in Medicine guidelines for sonography in the first trimester includes use of real-time equipment. The minimum necessary approach should be performed. If transabdominal approach gathers accurate and appropriate information, then transvaginal approach need not be completed and vice versa. Both approaches may be needed. Presence, location, and content of gestational sac should be noted. If applicable, crown rump measurements should be included versus gestational sac measurements; these allow for more accurate gestational age determinations. An embryo or yolk sac must be present before noting the presence of a gestational sac. Note cardiac motion if crown rump is at least 5 mm. Determination of fetal number can only be based on embryo number, not on multiple sac-like structures. Document evaluation and appearance of all surrounding structures including adnexa and cul-de-sacs.

APPROPRIATE TIMING OF THE FIRST OBSTETRICAL SONOGRAM

The optimal timing of the obstetric sonograph is dependent on the purpose that is hopes to achieve. If it is strictly gestational age that is sought, the earlier the sonograph can be performed and the measurements taken, the better. Gestational age determination is most accurate in the first trimester. If fetal monitoring, development, and screening for anomalies are the goal of sonography, then early second trimester sonography is preferred. Most fetal images can be viewed with great detail, and anomalies detected by 18 weeks of gestation. If only one ultrasound can be performed, selecting a time in between these two ideals is suggested. A single ultrasound between the 12th and 16th weeks is acceptable and widely used.

DETECTION OF SOLID PELVIC MASSES

In the presence of a sonographic finding of a solid mass during obstetrical sonography, it is important to determine whether this mass arises from the ovary or the uterus. In the presence of the sonographic "claw sign" (uterine distortion around the solid mass), the solid mass arises from the uterus. In the absence of uterine distortion, the solid mass likely originates from the ovary. Masses associated with pregnancy include: leiomyomas, uterine fibroids, solid ovarian masses, and focal myometrial contraction. Leiomyomas are the most common and sonographically appear with a well-defined border and usually hyperechoic; in some instances they may contain central cysts. Documentation of mass location and growth is important in prenatal planning and monitoring, as solid masses can affect placental implantation and delivery.

OBTAINING FETAL HEART RATE DURING 11-WEEK OBSTETRICAL ULTRASOUND

The best method of obtaining the fetal heart rate with ultrasound during the first trimester is with M-mode (motion mode). Using M-mode allows ultrasound users to follow the as low as reasonably achievable (ALARA) principle because the intensity of M-mode is less than what is obtained during pulsed-wave Doppler interrogation. M-mode should be the first choice to attain the fetal heart rate because the energy is distributed along the entire wave that is sent into the patient. In contrast, a spectral display should not be used because the energy is only located within the sample gate, which can lead to tissue heating. M-mode doesn't allow the patient to hear the heartbeat, but the user can explain that it is a safer choice for early pregnancies.

USE OF M-MODE TO OBTAIN FETAL HEART WITH REGARD TO TIME

Regarding A-mode (amplification), B-mode (brightness), or M-mode (motion), the only one that offers information pertaining to time is M-mode. M-mode is illustrated by bumpy lines that tend to roll across the monitor from left to right. M-mode is used predominantly in echocardiography or to obtain a heart rate during an obstetrical exam. M-mode is advantageous because it allows greater temporal resolution, so even structures that are moving rapidly can be accurately measured and recorded. The data are obtained from a single line of sight, which allows the user to change the location if necessary. Sometimes this can create erroneous measurements if the single line is not perpendicular to a structure.

OB ULTRASOUND BETWEEN 10 AND 14 WEEKS OF GESTATION

An ultrasound performed between 10 and 14 weeks of gestation should include the presence (and number) of a fetus; sonographers should also check for movement of the fetus. Cardiac activity should also be documented by using a video clip in addition to calculating the heart rate. Today's ultrasound systems provide excellent resolution compared with machines used in the past, and many anatomical structures can be visualized and measured to provide an estimated due date. Many labs still use the crown-rump length (CRL) measurement during this time to provide an accurate estimate of gestational age, especially between 10 and 13 weeks. CRL is a measurement of the embryo or fetus from the top of the head to the bottom of the buttocks. This measurement does not include the lower extremities, and it is the most accurate for dates as long as the measurement is performed correctly. If a CRL measurement is provided in the first trimester of pregnancy, the due date should not be changed later on.

USE OF CROWN-RUMP LENGTH IN ESTABLISHING THE GESTATIONAL AGE

Once the embryo can be visualized with ultrasound, the crown-rump length measurement becomes the most accurate and preferred method of gestational age determination. In this situation, the gestational sac diameter measurements are no longer useful for gestational age determination. The embryo can me visualized when it is as small as 2 mm; this often correlates with a gestational age of about 6 weeks. The most accurate crown-rump length, and thus most accurate gestational age, should be taken from the average of three good measurements at maximal length. Although the embryo can be imaged earlier, a clearer sonographic image is established after week seven.

GENERAL PARAMETERS OF DETERMINING GESTATIONAL AGE

Since there are limitations to obtaining accurate gestational or menstrual age from the patient (irregular menstrual cycles and inaccurate recall), sonography has become the mainstay and most accurate determinant of gestational age. In the first trimester, the most accurate sonographic gestational age determinants are crown-rump length and biparietal diameter. These can be used individually or in combination. The crown-rump length may be easier to determine initially. The head circumference, femur length, and abdominal circumference may also support sonographic gestational age determinations. If sonography is performed after the first trimester, its accuracy for determining gestational age declines. In this case, all of the above measurements plus last menstrual period should be used to determine the most likely gestational age.

COLOR FLOW IMAGING DURING PELVIC AND OB EXAMS

Color Doppler can be used during pelvic ultrasound exams to determine ovarian torsion or to provide more diagnostic information in cases in which a uterine, ovarian, or adnexal mass is identified. Color Doppler can also provide important clues as to whether a mass portrays benign or malignant color flow characteristics. Benign masses tend to demonstrate peripheral flow, whereas malignant masses tend to display feeding vessels that are more centrally located. Often, malignant tumors may show hypervascularity, because malignant tumors require a fair amount of blood flow in order to proliferate. Color Doppler is also helpful in identifying an ectopic pregnancy or corpus luteal cyst. Sonographers should remember, especially during OB exams, that color Doppler requires an increase in output power, but it can be used in conjunction with spectral analysis to sample various vessels or the umbilical cord when necessary.

PELVIC MASSES AND CORPUS LUTEUM CYSTS

A corpus luteum cyst is the most common occurring ovarian mass seen in pregnancy. They are generally small, but can reach a size greater than 5 cm. Regardless of the size, a large percentage of corpus luteum cysts resolve by the 18th gestational week. In the case of a corpus luteum cyst that is greater than 5 cm and symptomatic (pelvic or abdominal pain), surgical intervention may be considered due to the increased risk of bleeding into itself and twisting on itself (torsion). Higher incidences of these cysts are seen in females that have used fertility drugs such as Clomid.

DYSGERMINOMA AND YOLK SAC TUMORS

Dysgerminomas are germ cell tumors, commonly unilateral, malignant, affects those under 30 years of age and are often diagnosed in pregnancy. They are the most common germ cell tumor seen in patients with gonadal dysgenesis. Sonographically monitoring will result in observation of rapid growth and a multilobular textured, solid mass. Yolk sac tumors are germ cell tumors also known as endodermal sinus tumors. They are malignant, affect patients at an average age of 20 years, and are unilateral. Sonographic appearance is usually a solid mass that is encapsulated and has varying shape and size.

HUMAN DEVELOPMENT FROM FERTILIZATION TO EMBRYO

Fertilization occurs when a female oocyte unites with a male sperm cell. Together, these form a zygote that implants itself into the female endometrium. Implantation of the zygote is the official beginning of pregnancy. The zygote goes through mitotic divisions and forms the placenta, umbilical cord, and eventually the embryo. The embryonic phase starts at about week 3 and continues through week 8. Early in the embryonic phase, the growth centers around what will be the spine and spinal cord. By week 6, the embryo produces chemicals to cease the menstrual cycle. Brain activity can be noted at this time and the heart beat starts. Organogenesis begins, limb buds form and the head is over half of the mass of the embryo. By week 8 of embryogenesis, the embryo is capable or movement, eyes are forming and blood type develops. At the end of the 8th week, the embryo state is complete and moves into the fetal stage.

DOUBLE BLEB SIGN AND THE EMBRYO IN EARLY INTRAUTERINE PREGNANCY

The double bleb sign is a sonographic finding seen from about 5.5 weeks up to 7 weeks gestation. Two adjacent, circular shapes with echogenic outer borders mark this sign. These represent the yolk sac and the amniotic sac. Lying in between these "blebs" is a small echogenic embryo. This follows that the embryo may first be visualized by ultrasound at about 5 weeks. If imaging this early, the transvaginal approach is recommended and may be the only means of viewing the 1-2 mm embryo at this stage. Embryo heart movements may be seen as early as 5 weeks, but is best recorded when the embryo itself is at least 5 mm and the gestational sac 16 mm.

PROSENCEPHALON AND MESENCEPHALON

The prosencephalon is also known as the forebrain and is therefore the most anterior located portion of the brain. When it divides, during embryonic development, it forms the diencephalons and the telencephalon. When the prosencephalon fails to divide in the developing fetus, holoprosencephaly (often times with facial anomalies) occurs. The prosencephalon is responsible for directing impulses to our senses, personality, and intelligence. The mesencephalon is also known as the midbrain and made of the tectum and tegmentum. The mesencephalon helps process visual and auditory cues.

ZYGOSITY AND CHORIONICITY

Zygosity refers to the number of fertilized ova that a multiple birth fetus develops from. Monozygotic refers to multiple fetuses developing from a single ova. Trizygotic refers to multiple fetuses developing from three separate eggs. Monozygotic twins are also known as "identical twins" because they arise from same fertilized egg and share similar genetic material. Dizygotic, and higher, are also known as "fraternal" and do not have the same genetic structure. For example, when delivering dizygotes one may be male, one female, one with brown hair, and the other with blonde hair. Chorionicity basically refers to the number of placentas present in a pregnancy. A dichorionic pregnancy will have two placentas; a trichorionic pregnancy will have three placentas and etc. Both descriptors are necessary to determine pregnancy management and identify possible complications. A monochorionic pregnancy, of any zygosity, increases the likelihood of twin-to-twin transfusion syndrome and other complications.

SONOGRAPHIC IDENTIFICATION OF TWINS OR HIGHER ORDER MULTIPLES

First trimester sonography is preferred for the most accurate assessment of chorionicity and amnionicity. Chorionicity can be determined slightly earlier at five weeks gestation. Sonographic determination of amnionicity is optimal after the 8th gestational week. Both chorionicity and amnionicity determinations are optimal prior to ten weeks of gestation. Identification of chorionicity and amnionicity requires diligent sonographic assessment of the number of gestational sacs/yolk sacs and the number of amniotic sacs. Furthermore, determination of the number of embryonic heartbeats within each gestational sac will correlate directly with each other.

GESTATIONAL AGES TO DISCERN VARIOUS BONES OF EXTREMITIES

When an ultrasound is performed around the 8th week in utero, the sonographer may see tiny limbs extending from the body of the embryo. Movement of the limbs will be seen after 11 weeks because the long bones of the skeleton are easily seen by this stage because ossification has taken place. After 13 weeks, the sonographer may use various biometric measurements instead of the CRL to determine the gestational age. One such bone that is often used in fetal measurements is the femur length. The femur (thigh bone) can often be visualized after 9 weeks, and it is one parameter used to estimate fetal age by 14 weeks. The humerus (upper arm bone) can be visualized after 9 weeks, and it may also be used to determine gestational age. The bones of the forearm (radius and ulna) are seen around 10 weeks, with the phalanges more readily seen after 11 weeks. The bones of the lower leg (tibia and fibula) are also visualized well after 10 weeks with the digits of the foot seen after 11 weeks.

ASSIGNMENT OF GESTATIONAL DATES USING VISUALIZATION OF THE CHORIONIC SAC AND ITS CONTENTS

Gestational dates can be estimated with a great degree of accuracy based on sonographic visualization of the gestational or chorionic sac. This is true regardless of the actual gestational sac measurements and is secondary to the fact that there is very little size variability in the first 8 gestational weeks. Sonographic viewing of only the gestational sac suggests a gestational age of 5 weeks. Sonographic visualization of the gestational sac plus yolk sac suggests a gestational age of 5 weeks and 5 days. Sonographic imaging of the chorionic sac plus yolk sac plus a small embryo suggests a gestational age of 6 weeks.

GESTATIONAL AGE

The gestational age refers to the time since conception. Conception refers to the event and time at which the blastocyte implants itself into the endometrium. The gestational age is usually two weeks later than the first day of the last menstrual period. The term gestational age is often used interchangeably with menstrual age, even though the two terms or definitions technically differ by two weeks. Menstrual age is the time from the first day of the last menstrual period. This is the more commonly used age determinant, although inaccurate patient reporting limits this method.

ACCURACY OF GESTATIONAL AGE ESTIMATION IN THE FIRST TRIMESTER

Sonographic first trimester gestational age determination is the most accurate and widely used. Even if second and third trimester sonographic measurements of crown-rump, biparietal, head circumference, and femur length suggest a different gestational age; the earliest sonographic measurements will be deferred to for gestational age determinants. The gestational age is either determined by chorionic sac diameter when this is between 2 mm and 14 mm, or by the earliest crown-rump measurement. Although first trimester measurements are preferable is gestational age determination, accuracy can still be maintained up to 20 weeks.

GESTATIONAL SAC IN EARLY INTRAUTERINE PREGNANCY

Gestational sac is synonymous with chorionic sac. The earliest sonographically visualized gestational sac is about 4.5 weeks gestation. It is viewed as a small, well-defined echogenic ring with a hypoechoic center. The horizontal line below the gestational sac is the endometrial cavity; the appearance of this is called the intradecidual sign. This must be present to identify a true intrauterine gestational sac. The gestational sac may be visualized at 2 mm diameter with transvaginal technique. With transabdominal technique, the gestational sac may not be apparent until it is at least 5 mm diameter. The gestational sac should be visualized near the fundus of the uterus. Measurements of the gestational sac (length, width and depth) are highly correlated with hCG levels and gestational age up to 8 weeks.

GESTATIONAL SAC AND YOLK SAC IN EARLY DETERMINATION OF PREGNANCY

The gestational sac can be viewed with sonography as early as 4 weeks. This is the first sonographic evidence of pregnancy. Gestational sac diameter may be measured and correlated with gestational age initially, but after 8 gestational weeks, this is no longer used. The diameter of the gestational sac at 5 weeks is usually about 5 mm. The yolk sac can be viewed at about 5 weeks with sonography. The presence of the yolk sac on sonogram is the first sign of embryonic structure or formation. It is located between the chorion and the amnion and its measurements are recorded along with those of the gestational sac.

DECIDUAL THICKENING AND YOLK SAC IN EARLY INTRAUTERINE PREGNANCY

Decidual thickening is literally a thickening of the endometrium at the site of implantation. This has an echogenic appearance on sonography and may actually be the earliest sonographic sign of pregnancy. However, it is rare to define pregnancy solely on this finding. The yolk sac may be identified within the gestational sac as early as 5 weeks, via transvaginal imaging. The presence of a yolk sac is the truest determination of an valid gestational sac. The yolk sac is echogenic and sphere shaped. The yolk sac is usually positioned at a border of the gestational sac.

DECIDUA BASALIS, DECIDUA CAPSULARIS, DECIDUA VERA, AND DECIDUA PARIETALIS

The decidua basalis is the term used to describe the maternal endometrium that is located directly inferior to the fetal placenta. This is the site in the inner uterine wall, where implantation occurs. Decidua basalis is synonymous with decidua serotina. Decidua capsularis may also be known as decidua reflexa. The decidua capsularis is a thin portion of endometrium that has direct contact with the chorionic villi. The decidua vera and decidua parietalis are used interchangeably and describe all other areas of the endometrial lining that is not in contact with the chorion.

AMNIONICITY

Amnionicity describes the number of amniotic sacs in multiple gestations. However, amnionicity is not an independent description and is used alongside zygosity and chorionicity. The importance of these descriptors becomes especially important in identifying possible multiple gestational complications. For example, a monochorionic-monoamniotic twin pregnancy is one in which two fetuses are within the same amniotic cavity and share a single placenta. This situation increases the likelihood of umbilical cord entanglement, increasing the risk for fetal mortality. Amnionicity is highly correlated in a one to one ratio with the number of yolk sacs present.

MEASURING THE YOLK SAC

The yolk sac is often the first structure visualized within the gestational sac during an early pregnancy because it can be identified even earlier than the embryonic pole. When an extremely early intrauterine pregnancy is identified sonographically, the yolk sac may be the only structure visible (other than the gestational sac). The yolk sac can be measured to provide clinicians with information about the pregnancy or when the yolk sac appears abnormal (shape, size, solidity, or calcification). Measurements should be taken from the inner leading edge to the opposite inner leading edge. Yolk sacs that measure greater than 6 mm without the presence of a fetal pole suggest fetal demise, and this should be followed up accordingly. Ultrasound users should be aware that the number of yolk sacs will be the same as the number of amniotic sacs as long as the embryos are alive.

LENGTH OF THE EMBRYONIC POLE BY THE END OF THE 10TH WEEK

During human development, weeks 6 through 10 are considered to be the embryonic period. In this stage, the proportions and the shape of the embryo are considerably altered. At the beginning of this stage, the head is disproportionate, and it consumes nearly half of the entire embryonic pole. By the end of the embryonic period, the head becomes more proportionate with the rest of the crown-rump length (CRL). The CRL will measure about 30 mm near the end of this period. With the exception of the heart, the other organ systems are present, but they are not yet fully functional by the end of the 10th week. It is important to note that the gastrointestinal organs develop quickly, and the intestines are temporarily displaced within the umbilical cord. This makes the GI tract a common site for anomalies to occur.

EMBRYONIC CARDIAC ACTIVITY

Cardiac activity correlates highly with embryo/fetal well-being. This correlation exists because it is a marker of adequate fetal oxygenation. In the early embryonic stage, transvaginal sonograph may be the best way to determine cardiac rate. In the fetal stage, better methods of fetal heart monitoring exist. In the first 6 gestational weeks, embryonic heart rate is at its lowest at 100 – 120 beats per minute. The normal embryonic heart rate peaks to about 140 beats per minute between gestational weeks 8 and 10. If embryonic cardiac rate remains less than 100 bpm in the first 6 weeks; the rate of miscarriage increases. Likewise, miscarriage is more likely with cardiac rates less than 120 bpm between 6- and 8-weeks gestation.

NORMAL FETAL STRUCTURES THAT CAN BE MISTAKEN FOR FETAL ANOMALIES IN EARLY PREGNANCY

Along with nuchal translucency measurements, a few other normal fetal structures can be mistaken for abnormalities. Defective brain or bony cranial vault development cannot be determined or diagnosed with first trimester sonography. Sonography of anencephaly (or lack-thereof) in the first trimester is not predictive of actual development later. Diagnosis of herniation has been made mistakenly; it is normal for bowel to herniated into the umbilical cord base between 8-13 weeks. This regresses by week 14. Between weeks 7 and 9, a posterior fossa cystic mass may be misdiagnosed. This is a normal finding as the fourth ventricle develops (rhombencephalon).

NUCHAL TRANSLUCENCY

Nuchal translucency measurements deserve much attention. Accurate sonographic measurement is highly technique and position dependent. Misinterpretation or measurement can result in a misinformed patient and mismanaged pregnancy. The nuchal translucency test measures the hypoechoic space between the back of the fetal neck and the skin overlying this area. However, it is an "inside to inside" measurement that should only measure the translucent portions and not the skin or soft tissue. It is best measured with the fetus neck flexed. If possible, observe fetal movement away from the amniotic sac periphery, so that unfused amnion is not mistaken with fetal skin for accurate measurement end points. It is first visible on sonograph at 10 weeks. At about 14 weeks, nuchal translucency measurements are maximal up to 2.8 mm, then thins through the rest of the pregnancy. Both transabdominal and endovaginal measurements are recommended.

ULTRASOUND INDICATORS OF ABNORMAL YOLK SAC

An early intrauterine pregnancy will be demonstrated on an ultrasound exam as an anechoic sac that correlates with the gestational sac. The next structure that will be identified within the gestational sac with ultrasound is the yolk sac. During an endovaginal ultrasound, the yolk sac is visualized during the fifth week. The ultrasound operator should examine not only the size of the yolk sac, but also how it is displayed sonographically. Yolk sacs that have an unusually large diameter (greater than 6 mm) may be associated with fetal demise. Yolk sacs should not be calcified, echogenic (except for the rim), asymmetrical, or absent if the mean sac diameter exceeds 8 mm. If any abnormality of a yolk sac is demonstrated, serial ultrasound exams should be performed because a full-term pregnancy could still be possible.

FETAL BLADDER OUTLET OBSTRUCTION

Fetal bladder obstruction can be detected as early as 12 weeks gestation by ultrasound. Sonographic and diagnostic findings include insufficient amniotic fluid, hydronephrosis, echogenic kidneys, pelvic diameter greater than 4mm, and an enlarged fetal urinary bladder. The most common cause of lower urinary tract obstruction in a fetus is the presence of posterior urethral valves. This is seen in as many as 1 in 5000 male fetuses, with a mortality rate as high as 63%. With these occurrence and mortality rates, the search for definitive treatments and urinary bladder decompression methods has been sought. Several in utero procedures have been attempted, usually during the second trimester and usually involving some sort of catheter placement or various shunting methods. Many fetal bladder decompression techniques have been limited by device dislodgement, short functional life, and obstruction.

INTRADECIDUAL SIGN AND DOUBLE DECIDUAL SIGN

The main value of the sonographic appearance of the intradecidual sign is to exclude the possibility of an ectopic pregnancy. The intradecidual sign is defined as the presence of a fluid collection surrounded by a echogenic border that is located directly adjacent to the central endometrial cavity. This is the earliest sonographic sign of pregnancy and should be differentiated from a similar described finding located *within* the central endometrial cavity that would indicate a pseudogestational sac or ectopic pregnancy. The double decidual sign may first be observed at 5.5 weeks of a normal intrauterine pregnancy. It is comprised of the decidua vera and decidua capsularis that form an echogenic ring. This will not be present in an ectopic pregnancy.

EVALUATING THE MIDDLE CEREBRAL ARTERY IN THE MANAGEMENT OF FETAL ANEMIA

Evaluation of the middle cerebral artery peak systolic velocity (MCA-PSV) is a technique used with increasing frequency to manage fetal anemia. This technique has proven to be very accurate and noninvasive and carries less risk than amniocentesis and cordocentesis in fetal anemia management. When obtaining the MCA-PSV study, the fetal middle cerebral artery closest to the mother's skin should be used. The angle of blood flow to the ultrasound beam should be as close to zero degrees as possible. The middle cerebral artery should be measured as close as possible to its origin in the internal carotid artery. Record the highest peak systolic velocity and generate a curve with the MCA-PSV as a function of gestational age. These measurements are accurate up to 35 weeks gestation. The more severe the fetal anemia, the more accurate the MCA-PSV technique is. However, at a fetal hemoglobin of < 1-3 gm/dl, the MCA-PSV no longer increases.

HETEROTOPIC MULTIFETAL PREGNANCY

A heterotopic multifetal pregnancy is a dangerous diagnosis in which an extrauterine pregnancy occurs simultaneously with an intrauterine pregnancy. This is a difficult clinical diagnosis, and like all ectopic pregnancies, if not correctly diagnosed it can be life-threatening. Transvaginal sonography is an important method to aid in this diagnosis. Sonographers must be aware of this phenomenon, especially with the prevalence of assisted reproductive methods that so many patients undergo. More cases of heterotopic multifetal pregnancies occur with those that have sought the assistance of fertility specialists or have had prior pelvic surgeries, but it may also take place in natural pregnancies. It is important that sonographers check for an ectopic pregnancy when an adnexal mass is seen or when free fluid is present. If the adnexal mass proves to be hyperemic and demonstrates a reduced resistive index, then a heterotopic pregnancy should be considered even when a normal intrauterine pregnancy has been identified.

CLASSIC HYDATIDIFORM MOLE

Classic hydatidiform mole, also known as complete hydatidiform or complete mole, is a condition only seen in pregnancy. It is caused when either a single haploid sperm or a 2 normal sperm fertilize an egg that does not contain a nucleus. This results in edema of the chorionic villi and an increased number of trophoblastic cells. The incidence of hydatidiform mole (type unspecified) in the US is about 1 in 1000 pregnancies. It is also an incidental finding in as many as 1 in 600 abortions. The incidence in Asian countries is 15 times that of the US for reasons unknown. Approximately 15% of those with complete mole have uterine involvement and about 4% develop metastasis. Risk of developing complete hydatidiform mole is highest with teenage pregnancy and 7-fold with pregnancy greater than age 40.

SUBCHORIONIC HEMORRHAGE IN EARLY PREGNANCY

Subchorionic hemorrhage in early pregnancy is an abnormal sonographic finding. A subchorionic hemorrhage is basically blood or a blood clot found collected between the uterine wall and the outside of the chorionic membrane. This blood may then leak through the cervical canal, thus causing the gravid female to complain of vaginal bleeding and often prompting an ultrasound. In the embryonic stage, a subchorionic hemorrhage is the most common sonographic finding. Prognosis depends on three factors: clot size, gestational age, and maternal age. Miscarriage is more likely the larger the subchorionic hemorrhage, the older the mom, and the later the finding (late first trimester, early second trimester).

ECTOPIC PREGNANCY

An ectopic pregnancy is one that results in the fertilized egg and sperm unit implanting anywhere outside of the uterine cavity. Some causes of ectopic pregnancy include: previous ectopic pregnancy, PID, abortion, adhesions, endometriosis, pelvic tumors, and use of oral contraceptives (in some cases). Ectopic pregnancy is not compatible with fetal development, and if undetected places the mother at risk. Some studies report incidence as great as one ectopic pregnancy for every 66 intrauterine pregnancies. This is thought to be due to increasing incidence of PID. Despite increasing rates of ectopic pregnancy, maternal mortality rates have been significantly reduced due to earlier diagnostic capabilities. Clinically, ectopic may present as bleeding, pain, a palpable pelvic mass, fever, tenesmus, referred pains to the shoulders, and syncope. Maintain a high index of suspicion, as these symptoms are shared by many other disorders.

CORRELATION OF SERUM BETA-HCG AND SONOGRAM IN DIAGNOSIS

Quantitative beta-hCG serum level monitoring is often the first clue that a pregnancy is not progressing normally and also may raise the first suspicion for the diagnosis of ectopic pregnancy.

This is true because the physical signs and symptoms may not always be apparent early on or may be mild in their presentation. In normal pregnancy, serum beta-hCG levels should increase by about 66% every 48 hours. If beta-hCG levels are not increasing as expected, ectopic pregnancy should be suspected. To further the diagnosis, sonography is primarily used to "rule-out" intrauterine pregnancy. Sonography does not always image extrauterine pregnancy, but may image findings that increase the possibility. By the time the serum beta-hCG levels reach 1500 mIU/ml, transvaginal ultrasound should be able to identify an intrauterine pregnancy. For transabdominal technique to view an intrauterine pregnancy, serum beta-hCG levels need to be at least 5000 mIU/ml.

SONOGRAPHIC FINDINGS

Sonographic findings for ectopic pregnancy are largely nonspecific or exclusionary. In fact, about one quarter of patients with ectopic pregnancy will have a normal pelvic and transvaginal sonogram. Probably the most definitive sonographic finding of ectopic pregnancy would be visualization of an adnexal ring and yolk sac with cardiac activity anywhere outside of the intrauterine cavity. Any patient with a positive serum beta-hCG, no sonographic evidence of intrauterine pregnancy, sonographic evidence of fluid in the pelvis, or adnexal mass need to be followed closely. Monitoring should at least include repeat beta-hCG levels and sonography every 48 hours.

SITES IMPLICATED

Sonography may be helpful in identifying the location of the ectopic pregnancy, however, Laparoscopy remains the gold standard. The highest percentages of ectopic pregnancies occur in the fallopian tube. This is why one will often hear the terms ectopic and tubal pregnancy used interchangeably, although this is not entirely accurate. About 5% of ectopic pregnancies occur in the fimbria (the very distal, finger-like projections of the fallopian tubes). Approximately 1-2% of ectopic pregnancies may occur at an abdominal source. Less than 1 % occur in the cervix and ovary. Of the approximated 95% of ectopic pregnancies occurring in the fallopian tube, 78% of those occur in the distal most portion or ampullary.

DIFFERENTIATING BETWEEN EARLY INTRAUTERINE PREGNANCY AND ECTOPIC PREGNANCY

The sonographic appearance of a cystic sac viewed within the endometrium may in fact represent a pseudogestational sac of ectopic pregnancy. However, this small cystic endometrial sac may also represent a decidual cyst or a very early but normal intrauterine pregnancy/gestational sac. The double sac sign is helpful in diagnosing an early pregnancy, but does not absolutely eliminate the possibility of ectopic pregnancy. Even with the appearance of an intrauterine yolk sac and embryo, it is important to evaluate the adnexa. A heterotopic pregnancy may exist in which a normal intrauterine gestation and an abnormal extrauterine gestation coexist. It is often recommended to start with the transabdominal sonograph, as this often allows for better viewing of adnexa and extrauterine structures. Follow this technique with transvaginal technique for better uterine and endometrium viewing.

DIAGNOSING FETAL DEMISE

Fetal demise is primarily diagnosed by inability to obtain a fetal heartbeat. Whether that be through sonographic monitoring or fetal stress testing, lack of fetal heart tones is equivalent to fetal death. Other sonographic findings may include a cystic and degenerating placenta, edematous findings (almost anywhere), poorly defined abdominal organs, and a positive Spaulding sign, which is a finding of overlapping skull bones. Fetal demise is diagnosed before the fetus and conceptus are extracted from the mother. If fetal death occurs prior to 20 gestational weeks, it is considered early. Intermediate fetal demise is diagnosed if the criteria are met between gestational weeks 21 and 28. If fetal death occurs after 28 gestational weeks it is termed late fetal demise.

ANEMBRYONIC PREGNANCY

An anembryonic pregnancy (referenced in the past as a blighted ovum) suggests an early failed pregnancy. In this situation, the embryo failed to grow, or death occurred before it could even be seen with ultrasound technology. In either case, the ultrasound will exhibit a gestational sac without a yolk sac or embryo. An embryo with cardiac activity should be seen during a transvaginal exam when the mean sac diameter (MSD) is greater than 16 mm. A yolk sac should be visible when the MSD is 8 mm or greater when using the same technique. Transabdominally, an embryo with positive fetal heart tones should be visualized when the MSD is 25 mm or greater. If an empty gestational sac is visualized and the measurements are less than the aforementioned parameters, then a follow-up ultrasound should be performed, and serial beta human chorionic gonadotropin levels should be measured. These serial exams will help clinicians determine if the empty gestational sac is due to an extremely early intrauterine pregnancy or an ectopic pregnancy with an associated false gestational sac.

ABNORMAL GESTATION SAC

Early pregnancy abnormalities or complications may first be suspected when a gravid female complains of vaginal bleeding, pain or fever. This usually prompts evaluation with sonography. Gestational sacs that are anywhere other than the intrauterine position, are abnormal. If gestational sac size or visualization does not correlate with beta-hCG levels, consider an abnormality. If a gestational sac is at least 8 mm with no yolk sac or at least 16 mm without sonographic visualization of an embryo, the pregnancy is not developing normally. Furthermore, if a 5 mm or greater embryo is visualized but without cardiac activity, this is abnormal. Many of the above findings warrant correlation with beta-hCG and repeat sonography evaluation in a few days to support and confirm diagnosis. The exception to repeat sonography would be extrauterine implantation and ectopic pregnancy findings, which would warrant immediate action.

NEURAL TUBE DEFECT

Neural tube defect describes a broad category of developmental birth defects involving the brain and/or spinal cord. Disruption in embryologic closure and formation of the spinal cord and fetal nervous system is responsible for neural tube defects. Neural tube defects are classified according to the type and location of the failed neural tube closure. Neural tube defects develop in the first four gestational weeks, often times before a female is aware of pregnancy. It is thought that at least 400 micrograms of folic acid daily, prior to and during pregnancy can reduce the occurrence of neural tube defects.

LITHOPEDION, INFARCTION, AND EXOPHTHALMOS

Lithopedion, also known as 'stone baby', describes a rare condition in which fetal tissue becomes calcified and too large to be reabsorbed by the maternal body. This is more likely to be seen after an ectopic pregnancy.

Infarction describes any condition or location in which there is a sudden (or prolonged) disruption of blood flow (arterial or venous) to a tissue or organ structure. Infarction then results in cell, tissue, or organ death of the structure to which blood supply is compromised.

Exophthalmos describes a congenital or acquired condition in which there is a unilateral or bilateral increased protuberance of the eyeball(s).

3D IMAGING

The majority of measurements during an OB ultrasound are still obtained during a 2D B-mode exam, but 3D and 4D technologies offer improved diagnostic confidence because more detail is provided than ever before. Contrast resolution is greatly improved when using 2D array transducers because they offer a thin slice thickness of the ultrasound beam. When the beam is not any wider than the anatomy being examined, it improves the contrast resolution. The use of 3D and 4D imaging during an OB exam includes imaging the fetal heart, spine, diaphragmatic hernias, extremities, lungs, and fetal face as just some of the anatomical structures that are better visualized. The 3D ultrasound offers yet another dimension to the traditional 2D exam, and 4D ultrasound is real-time 3D. Along with the diagnostic importance of 3D and 4D studies, these applications can offer parents and family a chance to bond with their baby because they can offer a more lifelike picture.

IMAGING BARRIERS AND RECOMMENDATIONS FOR SECOND OR THIRD TRIMESTER FETUS

Advanced technology and techniques have made accurate sonographic images a reality over the past several decades. However, even technology has not quite overcome maternal obesity. Furthermore, fetal movement and position cannot be controlled for, thus limiting visualization of certain anatomy. Sonographic image quality may be compromised depending on the amount of amniotic fluid. Optimal sonography, requires the operator to first assess fetal positioning. From there, the best plane and axis by which to view a particular fetal anatomy may be established. Use of real-time equipment is optimal as well as appropriate transducers and parameters.

MEASURING CIRCUMFERENCE DURING AN OBSTETRICAL ULTRASOUND

After the first trimester, the sonographer may use the ellipse feature to measure the perimeter of the fetal head and abdomen. The user is trying to obtain a circumference measurement when evaluating the fetus. Circumference can be thought of as the perimeter or distance around a circle. Most fetal heads are not circular in shape, but the circumference measurement is used along with other anatomical measurements in order to determine the fetal weight, estimated age of gestation, and the due date. The head circumference can give the clinician important information pertaining to not only the weight of the fetus when combined with other parameters such as the biparietal diameter, femur length, and abdominal circumference, but also information pertaining to brain development.

SONOGRAPHIC BIPARIETAL DIAMETER MEASUREMENTS

Sonographic biparietal diameter measurements are best obtained at about week 14. To obtain the most accurate measurements, the following three anatomical structures must be clearly identifiable: the midline falx, symmetrical thalmi, and the cavum septum pellucidum. A high degree of accuracy can still be obtained with measurements through any plane that crosses through the thalami and ventricle. This forms an oval shape and measurements should be recorded from leading edges at greatest width of the oval. The transducer must remain perpendicular to the parietal bones during measurements. Limitations for accurate sonographic biparietal diameter measurements include later gestational age, increased transducer pressure on the abdomen, abnormal fetal position, and a fetus with a "flat head". In these instances, use measurements in conjunction with head circumference, cephalic index and femur length to determine the most accurate gestational age.

ANATOMICAL STRUCTURES VISUALIZED WHEN CORRECT LEVEL FOR BPD MEASUREMENT IS LOCATED

The biparietal diameter (BPD) is one of the main measurements used to determine fetal weight and gestational age. This measurement is typically performed in the second trimester; the CRL is often used in the first trimester. The BPD can be measured at the widest level that includes the third ventricle, thalami, and cavum septum pellucidum. The first cursor should be placed on the outer edge of the skull closest to the transducer with the second set at the inner edge of the skull that is farthest away from the probe. One main disadvantage of using the BPD is that it is affected by the shape of the skull. When BPD shape correction is used, the BPD will be the same as the head circumference (HC). The accuracy of the HC is not affected by the shape of the head. The following formula can be used for the shape-corrected BPD:

$$\text{shape corrected BPD} \ = \ \text{BPD} \times \frac{\text{OFD}}{1.265},$$

where OFD is the occipitofrontal diameter.

APPROPRIATE PLANE FOR FETAL HEAD CIRCUMFERENCE MEASUREMENT

Fetal head circumference measurements should be taken with the transducer positioned correctly from three planes. Optimal fetal head circumference measurements will be obtained when the plane is parallel to that of the skull base. This arranges the plane in the anterior portion of the cranium. This plane may also be known as the transverse axial plane. A measurement perpendicular to the above aforementioned plane should also be taken, from outer edge to outer edge; this is known as the occipitofrontal or anterior/posterior diameter measurement.

MEASURING THE HEAD CIRCUMFERENCE

Measurement of fetal head circumference is useful in determining fetal age and making fetal weight determinations. Fetal head circumference measurements are essentially an average of two measurements: the biparietal diameter and the anterior/posterior diameter. Therefore, many of the landmarks used to measure biparietal diameter, need also be located for head circumference measurements. Measurements should be taken through the third ventricle and thalamus. The posterior brain should contain visualization of the tentorial hiatus and the anterior brain should show the cavum septum pellucidi. Sonographic measurement arrows should be placed on the outer calvarial wall edges opposite each other, but should not contain the outer skin edge.

CEPHALIC INDEX

The cephalic index is useful to obtain accurate sonographic measurements despite variants in fetal head shape. Some head shape variants can be greater, especially in circumstances of breech fetal position, ruptured membranes and multiple gestations. The cephalic index is an equation that divides occipitofrontal measurements into biparietal diameter measurements and multiplies this by 100. It should be noted that a true biparietal diameter is not used in this equation, rather the maximal width, perpendicular to the maximal anterior/posterior length, is used. Expected values are between 74 and 83. A second equation may be used based on an "ideal" cephalic index of 78. This equation takes the total of the multiplied biparietal and occipitofrontal diameters and multiplies it by 1.265. The result is the "shape-corrected biparietal diameter".

NUCHAL FOLD, FEMUR, AND RENAL PELVIS IN EVALUATING A FETUS FOR POSSIBLE DOWN SYNDROME

Measurements of the nuchal fold, femur and renal pelvis should be standard and performed whether one is looking for Down syndrome, other anomalies, or evaluating a normal fetus. The nuchal fold is best measured with the fetal head in the transverse plane. Measurement is taken from outer occipital bone to inner skin margin and should be less than 7 mm. Nuchal thickening may resolve later in pregnancy. After obtaining sonographic fetal femur measurements, the following equation should be utilized: 0.9028 x biparietal diameter – 9.3105 = expected femur length. If there is approximately a 10% reduction in actual and expected femur measurements, suspect Down syndrome. Down syndrome may also be suspected if fetal anteroposterior diameter measurements of the renal pelvis are greater than 3 mm.

MEASUREMENTS OF THE ORBITS

During an evaluation of the fetal face, the sonographer must also look at the orbits. Typically, an evaluation of the orbits does not require any measurements, unless the ultrasound operator believes that the orbits are too close together (hypotelorism), too far apart (hypertelorism), or appear smaller than expected (microphthalmia). Evaluating the orbits is subjective, but a good rule of thumb to follow is that the bony orbits should be the same size and the space between the two orbits should be the same width as one orbit. If the width between the orbits is concerning to the sonographer, then it is possible to provide measurements because they can be compared to standardized recorded normal values. Sonographers should be aware that holoprosencephaly may be present when hypotelorism is suspected. In exams that suggest hypertelorism, the sonographer should look for a number of chromosomal malformations or median cleft face syndrome.

The orbits are not routinely measured during an OB ultrasound, but in certain cases these measurements may provide insight on various fetal abnormalities. During ultrasounds performed later in the pregnancy, the internal structures of the orbits may be identified, such as the lens and optic nerve. If a fetus is diagnosed with hypertelorism (a greater amount of space separating the orbits), the sonographer should interrogate further to rule out median cleft face syndrome. If hypotelorism is present, the space between the eyes is reduced. Orbital measurements can be taken at a level that runs parallel (but below) the biparietal diameter and head circumference in a transverse axial cut. There should be two orbits that are symmetrical in size with the space between them being about the diameter of an orbit. The inner orbital measurement is taken from the inside of an eye socket to the inside of the contralateral eye socket (also known as the interocular distance). The outer orbital diameter is measured at the outside edges of each eye socket; it is also referred to as the binocular distance. These measurements vary with gestational age, so it is important to have a good reference for comparison.

FETAL ABDOMINAL CIRCUMFERENCE MEASUREMENT

For optimal abdominal circumference measurements, location of abdominal landmarks and positioning in the correct plane is necessary. Locate the lower ribs, as these are symmetric and usually readily identifiable. Locate the liver (the largest fetal abdominal organ) and the point at which its length is greatest from end to end. The greatest 'diameter' of the liver is usually found where the left and right portal veins become continuous with each other. The optimal plane for this is the cephalocaudal plane. In this plane, be sure the umbilical segment of the left portal vein is at its shortest. Measurements are from skin edge to skin edge; do not mistake these for the rib edges. Add the transverse diameter plus the anteroposterior diameter and multiply by 1.57 to obtain abdominal circumference.

INHERENT DIFFICULTIES

Measurement of fetal abdominal circumference via sonography is the least accurate method of gestational age determination. The decreased accuracy of abdominal circumference measurements is due to several different factors. First, it is difficult in a technical sense, because the abdomen is not symmetrical. Second, landmarks are difficult to locate consistently. Third, the margins are not as clearly defined and visualized on sonography like those of the calvarium of the head. Fourth, excessive transducer pressure can distort the abdominal shape and thus the abdominal circumference measurements. Finally, the abdominal cavity is highly affected by fetal abnormalities and therefore measurements may be quite variable in this circumstance.

ROUND RULE

The "round rule" may be utilized with sonographic measurements of abdominal circumference when less than optimal circumstances present themselves. The most common of these situations would be difficulty locating the fetal landmarks required for abdominal circumference measurements. If this is the case, measure the anteroposterior diameter and transverse diameter where they are thought to be approximately equal. Abdominal circumference measurement results when using the "round rule" will not be highly accurate but they will be acceptable as long as care is taken to not apply too great of transducer pressure.

MEASURING THE LENGTH OF THE HUMERUS

When an OB ultrasound is performed between 18 and 22 weeks, most of the bones of the extremities will be able to be identified. The humerus length (HL) is a common long bone measurement that is used in addition to the femur length to estimate gestational age and weight. It is important to note that when measuring the HL, the operator should make every attempt to make sure that it is laid out in a horizontal orientation on the monitor with the more superficial limb being measured. This will enable the sonographer to visualize the entire diaphysis of the bone and reduce any possible errors associated with foreshortening. The calipers should be placed at the areas that are the most reflective at the proximal and distal ends of the humerus, taking care not to include the epiphyseal end of the bone. If the humerus tends to be shorter, several measurements should be taken, and skeletal dysplasia should be considered.

AIUM GUIDELINES FOR PERFORMANCE OF SECOND AND THIRD TRIMESTER SONOGRAPHY

AIUM guidelines for ultrasound in the second and third trimester include real-time imaging with evaluation and documentation of fetal number, position, amniotic fluid measurements and fetal activity (including heart rate). If sonographic gestational age has not already been determined in the first trimester, second trimester measurements are the last chance for the most accurate findings. Gestational age can be determined with head circumference and/or femur measurements. Fetal weight estimates can be determined by measurements of abdominal circumference. Do not overlook the importance of routine examination and documentation of cervix and adnexal structures. If readily visualized, include any other organ findings and measurements including brain and heart details.

FETAL FEMUR LENGTH MEASUREMENT IN THE SECOND AND THIRD TRIMESTER

Sonographic measurement of the fetal femur length is less important as a gestational age determinant than it is to determine fetal skeletal growth and exclude anomalies such as dwarfism. Sonographic technique should begin with the transducer positioned at abdominal circumference. The transducer should then be moved in the inferior direction, transecting the bladder. At this position, the transducer should be rotated about 30 degrees for optimal femur viewing. If the angle is greater than 30 degrees to the horizontal, femur length measurements will not be accurate. Furthermore, measurements are only accurate if taken from two blunted ends. The femoral head and greater trochanter are not included in the measurement. Do not mistake the tibia for the femur and remember the femur is straight on the lateral side and curved on the medial side.

OTHER BONES MEASURED DURING AN OB ULTRASOUND

It may be necessary to measure the long bones of the forearm and lower leg to provide additional information pertaining to abnormalities of the appendicular skeleton. As with the femur and humerus, only the ossified portion of the bone should be measured when the bone is in a horizontal orientation on the screen. The bones of the forearm include the radius (positioned on the thumb side) and ulna (located on the side of the fifth digit). The ulna is longer than the radius because it articulates with the humerus in the elbow joint. If the hand is pronated, the sonographer should be aware that the two bones will appear to be situated on top of one another. In the lower leg, the operator should demonstrate two bones of almost equal length with the tibia being the bone positioned medially and the fibula laterally. The operator should take a picture of the foot positioned perpendicular to the lower leg.

LENGTH OF CERVIX AS FACTOR IN PRETERM DELIVERY

Sonographic measurement of the endocervical canal, by transvaginal approach, to determine cervical dilation and length is the most accurate method of determining preterm labor risks. Cervical length is measured as the distance from internal cervical os to external cervical os, including funnel length. In assessing risk, it also determines cervical competency. If first trimester sonographic findings include a vertical cervical measurement of less than 3 cm, dilation or a funneled cervical canal appearance, the likelihood of miscarriage is high. These findings in the second trimester, without concurrent ruptured membranes or uterine contractions, indicate an incompetent cervix. Sonographic evaluation of a cervix dilation >5 mm and length < 3 cm in the third trimester increases the risk of preterm labor and delivery.

APPEARANCE OF ABDOMEN AND PELVIS IN SCAN DONE BETWEEN 10 AND 14 WEEKS OF GESTATION

The fetal stomach will be visualized by 13 weeks of gestation as a sonolucent "bubble" in the left upper quadrant. Sonographers should remember that the midgut extends into the umbilical cord and returns between 10 and 12 weeks. Fetuses scanned after 12 weeks may not display any of the aforementioned herniation because the midgut has likely already returned to the abdomen. Organs of the urinary system may be seen at 12 weeks. The kidneys are often visualized in a transverse plane located on both sides of the spine. The echogenicity of the kidneys tends to increase as the pregnancy progresses due to the amount of perinephric fat. The renal pyramids may be visualized as anechoic areas within the middle portion of the kidneys. The urinary bladder can often be visualized as a small anechoic structure that will change in size as the bladder fills. If the ultrasound user does not see the bladder at the beginning of the scan, it should be reevaluated at the end, especially in the second trimester to help determine renal function. The umbilical cord insertion may be visualized as well, especially during TVUS by 11 weeks.

STRUCTURES OF THE BRAIN VISUALIZED WITH ULTRASOUND BETWEEN 10 AND 14 WEEKS OF GESTATION

The sonographer should be able to see the fetal head by 12 weeks of gestation, and with the resolution of today's machines, many structures of the central nervous system should be seen by the end of the 14th week. A measurement of the nuchal translucency (NT) is often performed between weeks 10 and 14, and it is taken in the posterior portion of the fetal neck to help determine the possibility of chromosomal abnormalities. The sonographer must make sure that the NT is evaluated when the neck of the fetus is in a neutral position and that the calipers are placed correctly on the inside portions. A measurement greater than or equal to 3 mm is considered abnormal. The cerebral hemispheres, cerebellum, ventricles, thalami, and brain stem are visible by 12 weeks. The fetal face can be seen, with the facial profile by 13 weeks. Sonographers should check for the presence of these intracranial structures so that anencephaly can be ruled out. In this condition, the majority of the brain and skull are missing, but usually the fetus has orbits and facial structures.

DIENCEPHALONS AND RHOMBENCEPHALON

Diencephalon refers to the midline portion of the human brain, superior to the brainstem. The diencephalon contains the forebrain structures such as the hypothalamus, thalamus, prethalamus, epithalamus, pretectum, and a portion of the pituitary gland. The diencephalon is responsible for much of the autonomic and visceral functions in the human body. The rhombencephalon is also known as the hindbrain. The rhombencephalon is comprised of the cerebellum, pons, and medulla oblongata. These structures contain many of the cranial nerves. It is often further broken down into the metencephalon and myelencephalon. The rhombencephalon is responsible for: complex muscle movements, simple learning, autonomic function, attention, and sleep.

DEVELOPMENT OF THE FETAL FACE

Facial structures develop in the fetus as early as 6 weeks gestation. At this stage the orbits are seen on the sides of the face. The nasal and palate structures also start out high and on the sides of the face at this stage. It is at about this time that a cleft palate may develop if these structures do not migrate normally to their midline position. As early as gestational week 8, the above aforementioned structures will turn to bone, and by about the 11th gestational week, sonographic examination of these structures becomes feasible. Of particular sonographic interest at this stage is orbital measurements. Maximal orbital diameter should be about equal and the distance between the orbits should be about that of the orbital diameter itself.

IMAGING THE FETAL HEAD AND FACE

Sonographic evaluation of the fetal facial features is becoming increasingly routine, especially if other fetal anomalies are suspected. For optimal sonographic viewing and facial descriptions, it is necessary to view the fetal face and head in multiple planes. Some fetal features are viewed more optimally through these planes. For example, the axial view probably provides the most detailed examination of the most superficial features: forehead, orbits, nose, cheek and jaw bones, lips and tongue, and neck. The mid and hard palate, tongue, mandible, neck soft-tissue structures, and more detailed view of the lips and nose can be obtained from the frontal plane. Three-dimensional imaging allows for a better profile view of the fetal head and face, and often allow for better imaging of the ears and neck structures.

NORMAL ANATOMY OF THE FETAL PELVIS AS VIEWED SONOGRAPHICALLY

Sonography of the fetal pelvis includes the skeletal structures such as the iliac bones, pubic symphysis, and sacrum. The fetal pelvis also contains the urinary bladder, colon, rectum and pelvic vessels, which can be identified readily during the second and third trimester ultrasound. Imaging of the fetal pelvic vessels helps confirm the 3-vessel composition of the umbilical cord. The posterior fetal rectum and anterior fetal bladder are equally echogenic. If the fetal bladder is without fluid, it may be missed or confused with colonic and rectal structures.

NORMAL ANATOMY OF THE FETAL SPINE AS VIEWED SONOGRAPHICALLY

The fetal spine serves an important landmark for sonographic studies, as well as an important anatomical structure to evaluate and record to determine normal development. Determination of the continuity of the spinal column and the skin above it should be first determined in an overview in the transverse plane. Each vertebral body should be evaluated, along with the right and left posterior elements. These should be viewed in at least two different planes. By the second and third trimester, the spinal cord can be visualized under optimal sonographic conditions and fetal positioning. The spinal cord has bright margins and a central and is hypoechoic.

NORMAL ANATOMY OF THE FETAL EXTREMITIES AS VIEWED SONOGRAPHICALLY

Sonographic evaluation of the extremities is important to monitor growth and screen for any abnormalities. The limbs (arms and legs) can usually be readily evaluated with ultrasound, and good images can be obtained in many planes. The hands, feet, fingers and toes must all be evaluated. Sonographs of the fetus may detect limb absence, abnormal number of digits, clubfoot, and fetal length. Normal fetal leg bones include a longer fibula distally. Proximally, the tibia and fibula are level. In the normal fetal forearm, a similar situation exists. The ulna is the longer bone. The ulna and radius are equal at the distal end, but the ulna extends beyond the radius proximally.

147

Sonographs done later in the third trimester may show ossification centers, this is a sign of a mature fetus. Ossifications develop a few weeks earlier in the female fetus, and may be demonstrated as early as 32 weeks.

EVALUATION OF FETAL HANDS AND FINGERS

Sonographic exams of the fetus will include a survey of both fetal hands. This should include the position of the thumb and fingers compared to the hands and wrists and the number of digits. Typically, the hands will demonstrate fingers that are slightly bent. The operator should try to capture images as the fetus opens and extends the fingers, and ideally it should be noted that the fetus opened the hand at least once during the exam. A fetus that does not open the hands completely during the course of the exam may be at a higher risk of trisomy 18. Also, any abnormalities concerning the fetal hands such as polydactyly (too many digits) should facilitate further investigation because they are often connected to aneuploidy. Whether abnormalities of the fingers (and toes) are an isolated incident or are an associated abnormality, parents can be better prepared for the situation once the baby is born.

DETERMINATION OF AMNIONICITY AND CHORIONICITY IN THE SECOND AND THIRD TRIMESTER

The sonographic criteria for amnionicity and chorionicity become more difficult in the second and third trimester; furthermore, the criteria are different than the same determinations in the first trimester. Fetal gender should be determined at this stage. The number of placenta indicates the chorionicity; however, fused and single placentas are difficult to evaluate. The interfetal membrane should be sonographically documented with the presence of a 'Lambda' or 'twin peak' sign. The interfetal membrane should be further described in terms of number of layers and thickness. Thick membranes are between 1 and 2 mm and a thin membrane is less than 1 mm. However, the membrane naturally decreases in thickness with pregnancy progression so measurements of membrane thickness are only useful before 26 weeks of gestation.

DETERMINING FETAL LIE

Fetal lie is the comparison of the long axis of the fetus to the maternal long axis with the most common being a longitudinal lie. Fetal lie must be determined while performing an OB ultrasound so that the sonographer can ascertain the normal anatomy. Fetal lie is not a parameter that can be controlled by the sonographer (nor can the amount of amniotic fluid or maternal body habitus), which all may limit an exam. Some anatomical structures are more readily visualized with the fetus in a certain position. Starting in a longitudinal scan at the cervix, determine the general position of the fetus (breech, cephalic, transverse, or oblique). Next, determine the position of the spine. If the fetus is in a transverse or oblique orientation, then manipulation of the transducer will be necessary to find the long axis. During first- and second-trimester exams, the fetus will often move, so it is important to be aware of the body plane when trying to find the best window for an anatomical survey.

IMPORTANCE OF ESTABLISHING FETAL PRESENTATION

Fetal presentation is the body part of the fetus that is leading into the birth canal. Fetal lie and presentation are often established at the beginning of an OB exam so that the sonographer can determine if the anatomical structures are in the correct places. The most common fetal lie and presentation are longitudinal and cephalic. This indicates that the long axis of the fetus is parallel to the long axis of the mother with the head closest to the cervix. A fetus that is breech is also parallel to the long axis of the mother, but, instead, the buttocks (frank breech) or at least one of the feet (footling breech) are the body parts that are closest to the cervix. In cases of a transverse lie, the fetal shoulder, arm, or back could be the presenting part. There is a greater risk of mortality with breech presentations, so it is important to provide this information to the doctors because they may opt to turn the fetus prior to birth or may perform a cesarean section.

SONOGRAPHIC VISUALIZATION OF THE FETAL FACE DURING THE SECOND AND THIRD TRIMESTERS

Accurate imaging of facial features, particularly the nose and lips, is important medically for the diagnosis of cleft lip deformities. These deformities can be best viewed in the coronal plane, along with the maxilla, anterior jawbone and the orbits. Many fetal facial structures can be identified even when positioning is not optimal. Optimal viewing of facial bones, nasal bones, jawbone, and soft tissue of the face are obtained with a fetal profile angle. Imaging the fetal face in the axial plane allows for optimal images of the anterior palate, oropharynx, tongue, and the same structures viewed in the coronal plane. The ears, eyebrows, eyelids and cheeks are often viewed with good clarity. By about 20 weeks, tooth buds along the gingival ridge can be seen. By the late second trimester and early third trimester it is not unusual to view intraorbital contents with great clarity.

BINOCULAR MEASUREMENT AND TRANSCEREBELLAR MEASUREMENT

Sonographic binocular measurements and transcerebellar measurements are rarely used in obstetrics to determine gestational age, especially with all of the other options and measurements available and their high degree of accuracy. However, in rare circumstances, binocular and transcerebellar measurements may be used to determine gestational age if fetal head and femur measurements cannot be obtained. Binocular measurements can be obtained with the fetal head in the occipital posterior position. In this position, measure the diameter of the outer orbits to estimate gestational age. With transcerebellar diameter measurements in the transverse direction, then measurement in millimeters should equal that of the gestational week.

OBSTETRICAL IMPORTANCE OF DETERMINING AN ACCURATE GESTATIONAL AGE

Determining an accurate gestational age is important for obstetrical management and planning. It is also imperative for monitoring fetal development and normalcy. If an anomaly is found, it is important to know if this is a "normal variant" or a true concern based on gestational age. Accurate gestational age determination is important for scheduling and interpreting routine obstetrical tests. If the need for invasive obstetrical testing arises, such as amniocentesis and chorionic villus sampling, correct timing and appropriate windows are imperative. Gestational age determination allows for more accurate estimation of delivery, whether that be spontaneous or a planned cesarean delivery. If a serious abnormality is discovered, accurate gestational age is important in helping the mother determine her options for management.

ACCURATE ASSESSMENT OF GESTATIONAL AGE AND WEIGHT IN SECOND AND THIRD TRIMESTER

If possible, it is important to first determine the estimated gestational age by using the first day of the last menstrual period. This allows for a baseline gestational age estimate, by which to proceed with obstetrical management, scheduling of routine obstetrical tests and determination of most appropriate time to perform an obstetrical ultrasound to gain the most amount of information possible. A gravid female may only get one chance at ultrasound due to cost, availability and insurance coverage. If there is a single best time to perform obstetric sonography, it should be about the 15th week for all-purpose evaluation, earlier for most accurate gestational age determination. Sonographic gestational age determination is determined by crown rump length (first trimester only). In the second trimester, biparietal diameter measurements are the gold standard. These may be used in combination with the head circumference and femur measurements. Less frequently, abdominal circumference and cephalic index are used.

GESTATIONAL DATING USING ULTRASOUND IN THE SECOND AND THIRD TRIMESTER

Sonographic gestational age determination in the second or third trimester is most accurate with biparietal diameter measurements. Measurements of fetal head circumference and femur length may be supportive to the biparietal diameter measurements. Measurements from poor or suboptimal images should not be included. If the fetal age estimate is already known, it should not come into play when obtaining sonographic images and measurements. This recommendation arises from the tendency of a sonographer to alter measurement technique, repeat measurements, and second guess good measurements if they do not fit with the known gestational age. It is recommended that the sonographer remain unbiased to gestational age.

ESTIMATION OF AMNIOTIC FLUID VOLUME

Several methods exist for the estimation of amniotic fluid volume. Amniotic fluid volume estimation is primarily attempted through sonographic routes and many methods are qualitative in nature, which limits their use and consistency. If a qualitative method is being used, the subjective findings are ranked on a scale of 1 to 5. One represents no amniotic fluid and five represent severe excess of amniotic fluid. The AFI (amniotic fluid index) attempts to quantify the amount of amniotic fluid. The AFI is determined by adding the depth of the largest vertical pockets from four areas of the uterus. An AFI of < 5 cm indicates insufficient amniotic fluid and > 20 cm indicates excessive amniotic fluid.

AMNIOTIC FLUID

Amniotic fluid surrounds a fetus throughout pregnancy and is constantly recirculated by the fetus "inhaling" and swallowing it and returning it by "exhalation" and urination. The amount of amniotic fluid increases to a peak volume of 800 mL at 34 weeks gestation, then decreases slightly. By delivery, about 600 mL still remains, surrounding the fetus. Amniotic fluid functions to protect and cushion the fetus from outside trauma. Amniotic fluid also maintains a consistent temperature for the fetus, to prevent against heat loss. Fetal movement is made possible by the amniotic fluid, which allows for fetal musculoskeletal development. Amniotic fluid is also largely responsible for fetal lung development.

UMBILICAL CORD

Anatomically, the umbilical cord is comprised of two arteries that transport deoxygenated blood from fetus to placenta. The umbilical cord also contains one vein that transports oxygen-rich blood from the placenta to the maternal liver. Wharton's jelly surrounds these vessels within the umbilical cord, acting as a connective tissue and protectant. Sonographically, the umbilical cord can be viewed as early as 8 weeks. It will about the same length as the crown-rump length and appears thick and straight, maintaining a diameter of less than 2 cm throughout pregnancy. Thorough sonographic evaluation of the umbilical cord is important in identifying a number of possible fetal abnormalities and pregnancy complications.

ASSESSMENT WITH DOPPLER

A normal umbilical cord transports oxygenated blood from the placenta to the fetus. The umbilical cord comprises two umbilical arteries and one vein. The arteries return deoxygenated fetal blood to the placenta to become the iliac arteries. Two umbilical arteries may be confirmed with color Doppler interrogation in the region around the fetal bladder because paired umbilical arteries will be demonstrated on both sides of the bladder. The umbilical vein conveys oxygenated blood to the fetal liver from the placenta. Doppler performed on the umbilical cord may provide pertinent information, especially when the patient experiences preeclampsia or in cases of suspected intrauterine growth restriction. The appearance of the Doppler waveform will vary depending on where the gate is placed, but measurements of impedance should be lower at the placental end of the cord and greater when measured closer to the fetus. The direction and velocity of blood flow can be measured as well as the quantity of blood flow. Doppler of the umbilical vein may provide clues related to heart failure or hypoxia.

EVALUATION OF DV

The ductus venosus (DV) is an anatomical fetal structure that enables oxygen-rich blood to pass from the placenta to the inferior vena cava. After birth, the DV will close and eventually become the ligamentum venosum. During the first trimester, it is useful to image the DV in order to assist in the diagnosis of an abnormal number of chromosomes. The assessment of the DV may provide additional information regarding anemia, possible defects in the heart, or intrauterine growth restriction in the second trimester. The DV should be examined in the superior portion of the abdomen using an oblique scan plane or midsagittal plane with the focus (and magnify) on the area where the DV unites with the umbilical vein. Doppler and spectral ultrasound should be used to determine if a normal forward flow is seen. Ultrasound operators should expect variations of blood flow within the DV during the activity of the fetus, so this is best evaluated while the fetus is inactive.

SIGNIFICANCE OF PLACENTAL SIZE AND APPEARANCE

The normal placenta is flat and circular and weighs approximately one pound. The thickness in millimeters usually correlates with the gestational age in weeks; therefore, the placenta should not exceed 40 mm thickness. Suboptimal viewing planes, contractions, and increased or decreased amounts of amniotic fluid may hamper accurate placental thickness measurements. Abnormal placental thickness may be seen in diabetes, hemorrhage, infection, maternal anemia, incompatible blood groups, and chromosomal abnormalities. Decreased amniotic fluid and contraction may make the placenta appear falsely thickened. Decreased placental thickness may indicate hypertension, diabetes, toxemia or infection, chromosomal abnormalities, and growth restrictions. Increased amniotic fluid may give the placenta a falsely thin appearance.

ROLE OF THE PLACENTA AND ITS SONOGRAPHIC EVALUATION IN NORMAL PREGNANCY

The placenta is the fetal lifeline. It allows for fetal survival, growth, development, nutrition, oxygen and carbon dioxide exchange, waste removal, hormone production, and protection from toxins and infections. This is all done through the placental connection to the uterus and umbilical cord, these allow for connection to the mother's blood supply. Due to the dependent nature of the fetal survival on the health of the placenta, routine monitoring with ultrasound is necessary. With sonographic exam of the placental, a number of points should be noted, including: placental size, shape, weight, position, and attachments.

PLACENTAL GRADING

Placental grading is all but an obsolete practice in modern medicine. Its remaining and rare usage is in describing the appearance of a Grade III or mature placenta too early in pregnancy. This may signal fetal abnormalities. Initially, placental grading was formulated to determine lung maturity of the fetus based on sonographic appearance of the placenta. Increased technology and testing parameters have determined that fetal lung maturity and placental appearance do not correlate well. Grades are given 0 through III. Grade 0 represents a uniform placenta with a smooth chorionic plate. Each successive grade describes increasing echogenic calcifications, densities and cysts.

EVALUATING THE FETAL HEART

On routine fetal sonography, the heart should be evaluated in as much detail as the fetal positioning will allow. At minimum, a cross-sectional four-chamber view should be obtained. Chambers should be symmetrical, valves should be documented, and often times the foramen ovale may be seen. A short-axis view through the sagittal plane (with rotation and depending on the level) allows for more detailed evaluation of the left ventricle, ventricular septum, aortic arch, and the mitral valve. Viewing of the outflow tracts is difficult with routine screening, and may be better obtained with off-axis views, segmental views, and/or Doppler studies.

SONOGRAPHIC APPEARANCE

With routine fetal heart sonography, the fetal heart should consume one-third of the thorax in the cross-sectional plane. The atria should be of about equal size and appearance. The ventricles should be of equal size. The foramen ovale should be slightly bowed towards the left atria. The internal left ventricle is smooth and the right internal ventricle is rough appearing. Two papillary muscles should be visualized within the left ventricle. The outflow tracts will demonstrate the crossing of the great arteries. Furthermore, the pulmonary artery should show division into its right and left branches.

MEASURING THE CEREBELLUM

The cerebellum is a dumbbell-shaped structure in the posterior fossa that is situated just anterior to the cisterna magna. Abnormal measurements of these posterior fossa structures can provide clinicians with clues about Dandy–Walker malformation. One such example that a sonographer should look for is the simultaneous visualization of an enlarged cisterna magna and a malformation of the cerebellar vermis that provides a pathway between the cisterna magna and the fourth ventricle. To measure the cerebellum, the calipers should be placed on the outer margins of the cerebellum. The transcerebellar diameter distance has been found to correlate well with the gestational age in weeks (if you drop the period), and it may be useful because this measurement is not dependent on the shape of the head. The transcerebellar diameter measurement can also be helpful in providing another parameter to estimate the age for twins as well.

IMPORTANCE OF EVALUATING THE CEREBELLUM

The development of the cerebellum is quite extensive because it is one of the first areas to develop in the brain, but it is one of the last portions of the brain to be formed completely. The cerebellum is one of the main portions of the brain that is essential for motor function such as coordination, performing fine motor movements, and balance. The cerebellum is located in the posterior fossa, and it can be imaged when moving the probe to an inferior and posterior position from where the biparietal diameter and head circumference measurements are taken. The cerebellum will appear as a dumbbell-shaped structure, and transcerebellar diameter measurements can be provided. The cisterna magna will be located posterior to the cerebellum with the nuchal fold just posterior to the bone of the skull.

EVALUATION OF FETAL BRAIN AND CRANIUM DEVELOPMENT

Although the fetal nervous system development starts very early, the earliest sonographic evidence of this is at the 5th week of gestation. At this time, the fetal spine can be visualized and the neural tube is forming within this. At about 13 weeks, the brain ventricles can be visualized at about their maximal transverse diameter of about 7 mm. The rest of the fetal brain grows and develops progressively around the ventricles throughout the pregnancy. The choroid plexus will continue its growth from the anterior position moving posteriorly as gestation progresses, eventually dominating the posterior ventricular region. At about the time the ventricles can be viewed, the corpus callosum begins its development. Furthermore, sonography at 10-15 weeks should visualize the fetal calvarium. These developments can all be monitored as the corpus callosum continues to develop through the 20th gestational week. At this stage (18-20 weeks) the cavi septi pellucidi can be seen beneath the corpus callosum. The inferior cerebellar vermis can also be seen at the 18th week.

NORMAL ANATOMY OF THE FETAL CEREBELLUM AND EARS DURING THE SECOND AND THIRD TRIMESTERS

Sonographic viewing of the cerebellum during the second and third trimesters is best accomplished in the transverse plane. In this view, fluid is a normal finding between the hemispheres of the cerebellum and the occipital bone of the fetal skull. The sonographer will already be in this area when evaluating the nuchal translucency measurements. The transverse plane images the cerebellum with the cavum septum pellucidum anterior. The cavum septum pellucidum lies midline between the lateral ventricles, if filled with fluid, and is not evident at term. External ear structures can be sonographically imaged in great detail. Care must be taken to thoroughly describe the plane in which the ear image is being obtained as well as identifying adjacent landmarks, so as not to misdiagnose a normal fetal ear as an encephalocele.

ASSESSING THE FETAL DIAPHRAGM

The diaphragm is a muscle that is a necessary component of the respiratory system that differentiates the thoracic cavity from the abdominal cavity. Sonographically, the diaphragm should present as a hypoechoic, uninterrupted line separating the fetal heart and lungs from the abdominal organs such as the liver and the stomach. Congenital diaphragmatic hernias (CDHs) are one abnormality that are ruled out when evaluating the fetal chest; these are the most prevalent anomaly of the diaphragm. Although they are more common on the left side, CDHs may develop on the right side or could even be bilateral in some cases. If present, a sonographer often sees the stomach bubble or loops of bowel in the chest. It is important to diagnose CDHs during an OB ultrasound because there is a high mortality rate due to the associated pulmonary hypertension and hypoplasia. The diaphragm is an important structure to watch during a biophysical profile because the sonographer must see an episode of breathing for at least 30 seconds within a 30-minute exam window.

DURAL AND VENTRICULAR ANATOMY OF THE FETAL CRANIUM IN THE SECOND AND THIRD TRIMESTERS

The fetal head and brain are a commonly imaged entity due to gestational age determination imaging of the biparietal diameter and head circumference. Taking these measurements further, the sonographer evaluates the rest of the cranial contents from superior to inferior. The falx and tentorium are dural structures that should be noted, and are necessary landmarks for biparietal measurements anyway. These are usually best viewed in the axial plane. Transaxial views allow for optimal imaging of the ventricles. The atrial measurements remain relatively consistent throughout the second and third trimesters. The temporal and occipital horns of the lateral ventricles are readily viewed.

THORACIC DEVELOPMENT AND SONOGRAPHY OF THE NORMAL LUNG

The healthy fetal lung develops under the following conditions: sufficient thorax cavity, normal fetal breathing, fetal pulmonary fluid production, and normal amniotic fluid amounts. The first signs of fetal lung development occur as early as the 5th gestational week with the development of the lung buds. By the 20th week, all of the bronchi will have developed. The alveoli develop through the 24th week. However, it is not until the 35th gestational week that sufficient amounts of lung surfactant are present. Lung surfactant is crucial to the maintenance of breathing and air pressure. Sonographically, normal fetal lungs should be moderately homogeneous and more echogenic than the nearby liver. The lungs should occupy one third of the thoracic cavity with the right lung being slightly larger than the left lung, due to heart placement.

SECOND AND THIRD TRIMESTER THORAX EVALUATION

SONOGRAPHIC VISUALIZATION OF THE FETAL GREAT VESSELS, AORTIC ARCH VESSELS, AND ESOPHAGUS

Optimal viewing of the great vessels in a fetus can be obtained after imaging the four-chamber view of the fetal heart. From the fetal heart images, the transducer should be moved toward the fetal head. This places the transducer in a transverse axial plane. From here, images of the ascending and descending thoracic aorta, the pulmonary artery, the superior vena cava, and the ductus arteriosus can be obtained. The branching vessels from the aortic arch can be imaged best from the sagittal view. From the descending thoracic aorta, moving the transducer anterior from this landmark can sometimes allow for visualization of portions of the esophagus. However, the esophagus is much more difficult to view than the great vessels of the fetus.

SONOGRAPHIC VISUALIZATION OF THE FETAL LARYNX, TRACHEA, DIAPHRAGM, AND LUNGS

The second and third trimester sonograph allows for visualization of the larynx. This is most readily viewed as the constricted portion of the fluid column of the trachea superiorly. The fluid-filled hypopharynx allows for easy viewing of the larynx. If visible, the trachea will be filled with fluid as well. It may be optimal to trace the distal trachea from its location behind the aortic arch, and image it moving superiorly. The fetal diaphragm separates the lungs from the liver and ultimately the chest from the abdominal contents. Check for diaphragmatic herniation. Although the lungs and liver may be seen on ultrasound from early in the second trimester, the later in pregnancy they are imaged, the more they separate out to define themselves with increasing echogenicity of the lungs.

SONOGRAPHY OF THE FETAL LIVER, GALLBLADDER, SPLEEN, AND FETAL ASCITES

A sonographically normal appearing fetal liver should appear homogenous. Any hypoechoic areas signify an abnormal mass. Calcifications may be viewed as abnormal from vascular injury or infection. An enlarged fetal liver is abnormal and secondary to Rh disease, infection, and a number of syndromes. If the fetal gallbladder cannot be identified sonographically by 15 weeks, consider cystic fibrosis, or atresia somewhere in the surrounding GI tract. The normal fetal spleen is not always visualized sonographically; therefore, it is the presence of splenomegaly that would be an abnormal finding and suggest infection. The sonographic finding of fetal abdominal ascites is always an abnormal finding and can signify a number of conditions and therefore requires close evaluation of all other fetal structures.

NORMAL ANATOMY OF THE FETAL ABDOMEN AS VIEWED SONOGRAPHICALLY

Abdominal sonography is best performed in the transverse plane, and abdominal circumference is a common measurement. Fetal abdominal anatomy that may be visualized with ultrasound include: abdominal muscles, stomach, duodenum, colon, liver, umbilicus with cord insertion, kidneys and adrenal glands, ureters, bladder, abdominal aorta, and inferior vena cava. The muscular portion of the abdominal wall is hypoechoic and should not be confused with ascites. Fluid in the stomach, gallbladder and bladder are normal findings. Any other fluid-containing structure should be considered abnormal and further evaluated. The umbilical cord should contain three vessels identifiable via sonography.

SONOGRAPHIC FINDINGS OF THE DEVELOPING GASTROINTESTINAL TRACT

The fetal gastrointestinal system can be seen sonographically by the 14th gestational week. However, at this stage there is poor differentiation between large and small bowel, as it all appears echogenic. At 20 weeks gestation, the colon diameter measures up to 5 mm and steadily increases to about 18 mm by delivery. Sonographic differentiation is possible after 22 weeks by observing the meconium-filled colon. Normal sonographic position of the fetal stomach or foregut should be in the left upper quadrant, its position in relation to the heart apex (left side) is important to note.

FETAL DEVELOPMENT OF THE GASTROINTESTINAL SYSTEM

During embryologic development, the GI (gastrointestinal) tract is discussed in three categories: foregut, midgut, and hindgut. The foregut comprises the most superior abdominal structures such as the esophagus, stomach, anterior duodenum, pancreas and liver. The midgut forms the rest of the duodenum, small intestine, and the first portion of the colon. The hindgut will give rise to the more inferior abdominal cavity structures including the colon, rectum, and portions of the genitourinary tract. The 6th gestational week sees foregut dilation. By the 12th gestational week, the midgut herniates into the umbilical cord at its base, rotates, and descends back into the abdominal cavity by the 14th gestational week.

DEVELOPMENT OF THE FETAL SKELETON

The first sonographic signs of fetal bony development can be seen at 6 gestational weeks. Ossification of skeletal bone begins between gestational weeks 9 and 13, starting with the collarbone, skull, vertebrae, long bones, and pelvic girdle (usually in that order). Normally the change of fetal skeleton to bony material occurs earlier in the fetal female. Sonographic descriptors of abnormal fetal skeletal development may include: agenesis, duplication, abnormal differentiation, hypoplasia, hyperplasia, or constriction band presence. Furthermore, the individual descriptors above need to identify whether the abnormal skeletal condition affects a localized area or the entire fetal skeleton.

DEVELOPMENT OF THE FETAL GENITOURINARY SYSTEM

Development of the kidneys of the fetal genitourinary system can be seen sonographically as early as 7 weeks gestation. By the 11th gestational week, the kidneys have located to their permanent anatomical location in the fetal flank, adjacent to the thoracolumbar spine. By 17 weeks gestation, the fetal kidneys are responsible for almost 100% of amniotic fluid production via fetal urination. Fetal urination and complete bladder emptying occurs at least twice per hour. Normal fetal kidney circumference remains slightly less than 1/3 of the fetal abdominal circumference measurements throughout pregnancy. Sonographically, the fetal kidneys should be readily imaged by the 14th week as individual, hypoechoic, elliptical structures. Many fetal kidney anomalies may not be apparent via sonographic evaluation until the third trimester.

STRUCTURES ASSESSED IN THE FETAL NECK

The 3D and 4D ultrasounds have greatly improved the visualization of structures in the neck that can be assessed during an OB ultrasound. Gray-scale imaging in two planes is still very useful to determine any abnormalities of the shape of the neck. The first thing a sonographer may want to examine is the contour of the neck. Any interruption of the normal contour of the neck region may be the first clue of an abnormality. Next, it is important for the ultrasound technologist to inspect for any mass (cystic or solid) that is projecting from the neck. Normal anatomical structures that can be assessed in the neck region of a fetus include the esophagus, trachea, thyroid, carotid arteries, and lymphatic sacs of the jugular region. The nuchal fold can be measured in the posterior neck, and the cervical vertebrae are visualized as well.

SONOGRAPHIC SCORING SYSTEM FOR FETAL ANOMALIES ASSOCIATED WITH CHROMOSOMAL ABNORMALITY

A scoring system has been formulated based on the presence of a number of sonographic findings and their correlation with chromosomal disorders, with a slightly higher specificity for trisomy 21. The scoring system takes into account the presence of 7 sonographic findings: cardiac or duodenal defect, thickened nuchal fold, decreased femur length, dilated renal pelvis, choroid plexus cyst, and echogenic bowel. Each of these is given a score of one or two. If a fetus scores a ≥ 2, amniocentesis is recommended. The higher the score, the greater the likelihood for Down syndrome. Although many other chromosomal anomalies would score high using this method, it is likely that these other disorders would be accompanied by more extreme organ and structural defects.

CDH

Congenital diaphragmatic hernia occurs as frequently as 1 in every 2,500 live births. Diaphragmatic herniation occurs from failure of diaphragmatic structures to fuse normally be the 10th gestational week. CDH more frequently involves the left diaphragm. The prognosis is based on the area of herniation and the abdominal contents that have herniated. Sonographic evaluation of a diaphragmatic hernia will likely reveal fetal heart displacement to the right side of the thorax. Abdominal contents such as the bowel, stomach, and even the liver, may be seen in the thoracic cavity. The presence of a congenital diaphragmatic hernia is highly correlated with trisomy 18 and its associated anomalies.

POTTER'S TYPE I

Potter's Type I, better described as autosomal recessive polycystic kidney disease (ARPKD), is a rare and most often fatal form of renal cystic disease. ARPKD usually involves both fetal kidneys and there is usually an insufficient amount of amniotic fluid during pregnancy. Sonographically, the kidneys will be enlarged with multiple cysts. Centrally, the kidney is echogenic with hypoechoic borders. If a hypoechoic halo of cortical tissue borders the kidney, this finding is diagnostic. Often biliary duplication cysts and liver defects are associated with Potter's Type I kidney disease. Close sonographic evaluation of the entire fetal development is necessary, as several other conditions may have similar kidney findings, especially Meckel-Gruber syndrome and trisomy 13.

TRISOMY 18 AND TRISOMY 13

Trisomy 18, also termed Edward's syndrome, with an incidence of 1 in every 3,000 births. It is 3 times more common in females and holds a poor prognosis, with 90% not surviving beyond the first year of life. Sonographic evidence of trisomy 18 includes: multiple congenital heart and kidney defects, abnormally small placenta, excess amniotic fluid, low-set ears, clenched hands, micrognathia, and microcephaly. Trisomy 13, also called Patau syndrome, is another congenital and chromosomal defect with a poor prognosis. An estimated 80% of trisomy 13 babies do not survive beyond the first month of life. Incidence is about 1 in 5,000 births. Sonographic characteristics of trisomy 13 include: multiple cardiac defects, single umbilical artery, holoprosencephaly, cleft lip and palate, multiple eye and ear defects, polydactyly, and situs inversus.

TRISOMY 21

Trisomy 21, perhaps more commonly termed Down syndrome is the most common chromosomal and congenital syndrome. Estimated incidence is 1 in every 730 births. The incidence rises dramatically to 1 in 75 pregnancies with a maternal age greater than 40 years. A large number of cases are diagnosed at birth, as fetal sonographic findings are vague and sometimes nonspecific. The best chance for prenatal diagnosis is amniocentesis, AFP, and triple screen tests. If the aforementioned tests are positive, a number of sonographic findings may support the diagnosis of Down syndrome. The following sonographic findings may be associated with trisomy 21: shorter-than-expected-for gestational age femur and humerus, underdeveloped 5th middle phalanx, dilated renal pelvis, thick nuchal fold, disproportionate short head, echogenic bowel and left intraventricular region, underdeveloped nasal bones, absent duodenal opening, and multiple heart defects.

AUTOSOMAL RECESSIVE DISORDERS AND AUTOSOMAL DOMINANT DISORDERS

An autosomal recessive disorder is caused when each parent contributes an abnormal gene to one of the non-sex chromosomes of the child. In this case, the child will display the disorder. If only one parent contributes the abnormal gene to the chromosomal pair, the child will be a carrier of the defective gene but will not display symptoms of the disorder. If both parents carry the abnormal gene, the child has a 25% chance of displaying the disorder. An autosomal dominant disorder is present in a child when he or she receives a defective gene from one parent. Usually that parent also displays the disorder, since it is dominant. If one parent does not carry the defective gene, and the other parent has the chromosomal disorder (one defective gene and one normal gene), the child has a 50% chance of displaying the autosomal dominant disorder.

X-LINKED DISEASES IN THE FETUS

An X-linked recessive disorder, since it is contained on the X-chromosome only, will be seen in more males than females. If a mother carries one abnormal X-chromosome and the father does not have the disorder, the male child has a 50% chance of displaying the disorder and a female child of the same parents has a 50% chance of carrying the disorder. An X-linked dominant disorder is more likely seen in females. A male with an X-linked dominant disorder will pass the disease on to all of his daughters and none of his sons, regardless of the mother's status. A mother with an X-linked disorder, assuming an unaffected father, gives both a male fetus and a female fetus a 50% chance of displaying the disease.

IMPORTANCE OF MEASURING THE CISTERNA MAGNA

A thorough evaluation of the posterior fossa will include measurements of the cisterna magna. This anatomic structure receives cerebral spinal fluid from the fourth ventricle of the brain. Normal parameters for the cisterna magna during a 2D ultrasound exam fall between 2- and 10-mm. Mega cisterna magna is suspected for any measurement greater than 10 mm, and if it is determined that the cisterna magna is connected to the fourth ventricle, then Dandy–Walker malformation should be considered. Dandy–Walker malformation may aid in the diagnosis of any chromosomal abnormalities because it has been associated with trisomy 13, 18, and 21. It is important to diagnose these abnormalities as early as possible to help the family decide on the direction of the rest of the pregnancy. Trisomy 18 is a deadly disorder that typically causes spontaneous abortion or causes the baby to be stillborn, and those with trisomy 13 typically die shortly after they are born. Imaging in 3D can also be used to document and measure the cisterna magna.

CHOROID PLEXUS CYSTS IN THE FETAL BRAIN

Choroid plexus cysts describe fluid-filled sacs that develop in the choroid glomi, the portion of the brain that makes cerebrospinal fluid. The choroid glomi can be seen on ultrasound as early as five weeks gestation. The fetal brain essentially forms around these structures. Small choroid plexus cysts, in and of themselves, are generally not an ominous finding and they always resolve through the pregnancy. However, if the choroid plexus cysts are large enough to be seen on ultrasound, they are thought to be associated with an increased risk of fetal chromosomal disorders.

PROBABILITY RATIO OF DOWN SYNDROME FOR INDIVIDUAL MARKERS TYPICAL OF TRISOMY 21

Independent sonographic findings have been rated on their correlation-to and likelihood ratio for developing Down syndrome. These likelihood ratios are not based on "grouped" findings or their correlation with amniocentesis results, AFP testing, and triple screen results. If one of the sonographic findings is not present, the risk of the fetus developing Down syndrome by 50% or 40% of its pre-sonographic marker. The isolated sonographic finding of nuchal thickening increases

157

the odd of a fetus having Down syndrome by a factor of 11. Other independent ratios include: echogenic bowel increases likelihood by 6.7, decreased humeral length increases ratio by 5.1, decreased femoral length by 1.5, intracardiac echogenicity with a 1.8 ratio, and dilated renal pelvis has a likelihood ratio of 1.5.

MEASURING THE NASAL BONE

The nasal bone should be documented on an OB ultrasound because fetuses are at a higher risk for having trisomy 18 or 21 when they have an absent or hypoplastic (shortened) nasal bone. This absence or shortening of the nasal bone is apparent in more than half of the cases of fetuses with trisomy 18 or 21, but there is a higher association with trisomy 21. While imaging the fetal face, the nasal bone can be identified as parallel reflectors best visualized on a midsagittal plane. In the second trimester, the length of the nasal bone increases with increasing gestational age, but some ethnicities tend to demonstrate a shortened nasal bone in the absence of chromosomal anomalies. Both 2D and 3D ultrasound can be used to provide the best images of the nasal bone. Skeletal dysplasia may demonstrate a nose that appears to be flat as well as the appearance of micrognathia and a forward-protruding forehead.

MECKEL-GRUBER SYNDROME AND TRIPLOIDY

Meckel-Gruber syndrome is a rare genetic disorder linked to chromosome 17 abnormalities. Worldwide incidence has huge variability with the highest incidence (1 in 9,000) seen in the Finnish population. The multiple defects associated with Meckel-Gruber syndrome are not compatible with life. Common sonographic findings include: polycystic kidneys, occipital encephalocele, postaxial polydactyly, genital abnormalities, cleft lip and palate, multiple central nervous system defects, and a fibrotic liver. Triploidy is a lethal fetal diagnosis occurring in about 1% of all pregnancies. A large percentage of triploidy cases result in a miscarriage or termination. Sonographic findings in triploidy will always reveal severe intrauterine growth restriction and some degree of molar gestation. Sonographic defects in all major organ systems are likely.

OMPHALOCELE

An omphalocele is the herniation of fetal abdominal contents (usually intestine) through the umbilical cord opening, with the development of these contents outside of the fetal abdominal cavity. A thin membrane covers the ruptured abdominal contents. The incidence of omphalocele is similar to that of gastroschisis. Omphalocele has a high percentage of associated fetal and chromosomal anomalies. Common chromosomal anomalies associated with omphalocele are trisomy 18, 13, and 21. Common fetal anomalies associated with omphalocele are a number of cardiac defects. Diagnosis is with AFP testing and ultrasound findings. Prognosis for omphalocele is dependent of the extent of the secondary anomalies.

BECKWITH-WIEDEMANN SYNDROME

Beckwith-Wiedemann syndrome is a congenital disorder marked by larger-than-expected body and organ size. Often omphalocele and asymmetric fetal limbs are characteristic of Beckwith-Wiedemann syndrome. Up to 80% of cases involve a defect on chromosome number 11. The diagnosis of Beckwith-Wiedemann syndrome is usually made in infancy by a number of findings including: hypoglycemia, enlarged fontanelle, x-ray of long bones, abdominal CT scan, and testing for defects on chromosome 11. The prognosis for Beckwith-Wiedemann syndrome is variable. Individuals with this disorder are at increased risk for tumor development. If the survive infancy, prognosis is improved.

ECHOGENIC SMALL BOWEL

Echogenic small bowel, if present, is usually seen in the second trimester ultrasound. Sonographically, the bowel is hyperechogenic and brighter than the nearest fetal bone. Echogenic small bowel may be seen after amniocentesis if the fetus swallows bloody amniotic fluid. The presence of echogenic small bowel raises the possibility of a fetus with cystic fibrosis, as this finding is present in up to 80% of these fetuses. Echogenic small bowel is also highly correlated with several chromosomal anomalies. Echogenic small bowel may be the result of any number of congenital infections. There is increased likelihood of late pregnancy fetal demise in the presence of hyperechoic small bowel.

UPJ OBSTRUCTION, REFLUX AND UVJ OBSTRUCTION, AND PYELECTASIS

Ureteropelvic junction (UPJ) obstruction is a condition in which there is a blockage at the junction of the renal pelvis and the ureter. This obstruction is manifest by kidney enlargement. It is more common in the male fetus. Ureterovesical junction (UVJ) obstruction or reflux may be seen with sonography of the fetal kidney when both the renal pelvis and the ureter are enlarged. Sonography is unable to differentiate obstruction versus reflux at this site. This finding is more common in the female fetus. Pyelectasis refers to the mildest form of hydronephrosis or enlarged renal pelvis of the kidney. Pyelectasis is seen as an independent finding in about 1% of chromosomal anomalies and in 2% of normal fetuses. Pyelectasis is found in up to 25% of fetuses with trisomy 21.

CEPHALOCELES/ENCEPHALOCELE

When the contents of the cranium protrude through the skull via a defect at a particular region it is termed a cephalocele. Rarely is a cephaloceles an independent fetal defect finding, it is often seen in conjunction with Meckel-Gruber syndrome. Suspect this syndrome in the presence of an occipital cephaloceles, renal dysplasia and in the presence of greater than 5 digits on the hand(s) or foot. When the contents of a cephaloceles include brain tissue, it is termed an encephalocele. Bifid cranium, craniocele, and cranial meningoencephalocele are synonymous with encephalocele. The most common location for an encephalocele is the fronto-orbital and posterior skull region. An encephalocele in the posterior skull is often associated with severe intellectual disability; where as a fronto-orbital encephalocele is less likely to cause retardation.

JEUNE SYNDROME AND ELLIS-VAN CREVELD SYNDROME

Jeune syndrome is an autosomal recessive disorder occurring in 1 in every 100,000 births. It has a poor prognosis, usually secondary to respiratory and renal problems. It is marked by many of the characteristics of skeletal dysplasia with markedly short and horizontally placed ribs, giving the thorax a cloverleaf appearance on fetal ultrasound. Ellis-Van Creveld syndrome is a rare autosomal recessive skeletal dysplasia marked by sonographic findings of shortened distal limbs and polydactyly of the feet. There is an increased incidence in the Amish and prognosis depends on degree of associated defects of the heart and lungs. Postnatally, one will observe characteristic anomalies of the hairline, teeth spacing and nails.

POTTER'S TYPE III AND POTTER'S TYPE IV

Autosomal dominant polycystic kidney disease (Potter's Type III) is primarily an adult-onset disorder that usually affects both kidneys. In the rare cases that it would be seen on fetal ultrasound, multiple cysts formation will be noted in the kidneys as well as other organ structures such as the liver, pancreas and spleen. Potter's Type IV or obstructive renal dysplasia classification system is largely dependent on the underlying cause of the obstruction. In many cases it is secondary to obstruction at the ureteropelvic junction and posterior urethral valves. Sonographically, cysts will be apparent but the renal pyramid(s) will not be visualized.

ACHONDROGENESIS

Achondrogenesis is a rare skeletal dysplasia that is almost always fatal. The overall incidence is estimated at 1 in 40,000. Achondrogenesis is broken down into type I and type II, with type I being more severe and least compatible with life. Polyhydramnios, breech presentation and hydrops may be present with achondrogenesis. Sonographic characteristics of type I include: extreme micromelia, appendages are "flipper-like", short neck, short and barrel-shaped thorax, protuberant abdomen, cardiac defects, and an average birth weight of 1200 g. Type I is associated with multiple craniofacial anomalies including: microcephaly, soft skull, flat nasal bridge with horizontal groove, small nose with anteverted nostrils, sloping forehead, and overall convexity of facial plane. Type II sonographic findings include many of the same craniofacial, neck, and abdominal findings. Micromelia is present, but to a lesser degree in type II. Birth weight is slightly greater at 2100 g and the thorax is bell-shaped in type II achondrogenesis.

CAMPOMELIC DYSPLASIA, MILD OSTEOGENESIS IMPERFECTA, AND METATROPIC DYSPLASIA

Campomelic dysplasia is a rare congenital disorder secondary to a mutated gene on chromosome 17. Sonographically, campomelic dysplasia is marked by severe bilateral bowing of the long bones especially those of the femur and tibia. The curvature and angulation is so great that it may be mistaken for a fracture. Those with campomelic dysplasia often have clubfeet and prominent occiput and there is a moderate association with ambiguous genitalia. Osteogenesis imperfecta is a set of disorders in which the collagen is either deficient in quantity, quality or both. In its mildest form, osteogenesis imperfecta is conducive to survival. It may also be known as brittle bone syndrome. Mild forms of osteogenesis imperfecta may not be identifiable in utero. Metatropic dysplasia is extremely rare, but can be diagnosed prenatally via characteristic ultrasound findings. Characteristic findings of this short-limbed dysplastic disorder are dumbbell-shaped long bones and a coccygeal appendage or tail.

FETAL ASSESSMENT FOR SUSPECTED SHORT-LIMB SKELETAL DYSPLASIA

If short-limb skeletal dysplasia is suspected in the fetus, thorough sonographic examination, description and measurements in a number of areas are needed. When measuring the extremities and long bones (including hands and feet), it is important to differentiate whether shortening occurs in the proximal segment (rhizomelic), middle segment (mesomelic), distal segment (acromelic), middle and distal segments (acromesomelic), or all three segments (micromelia). This helps identify the type of short-limb dysplasia. Fetal skull measurement, shape, flexibility, density, and ossification need to be noted. Sonographic detail of the fetal skeletal thorax should be obtained including notes on circumference at various levels and symmetry. The fetal spine imaging should include detail on the ossification of the vertebrae. Finally, note any facial anomalies that may be present to help with the diagnosis of the type and extent of skeletal dysplasia present.

OSTEOGENESIS IMPERFECTA TYPE II

Osteogenesis imperfecta type II is the most severe form of the said class of skeletal dysplasia. Osteogenesis imperfecta type II is caused be a gene mutation that affects collagen formation. Sonographically, this disorder is characterized by crumpled, fragmented, and/or fractured skeletal bones in utero. The fetal thorax is narrow and small, thus affecting lung development. Extremities appear short and bowed. Skull bones are thin, soft, and flexible. Osteogenesis imperfecta type II is not compatible with life, and those with this disorder are either stillborn or succumb shortly after birth from respiratory failure.

SHORT-LIMB SKELETAL DYSPLASIA

Short-limb skeletal dysplasia, also known as dwarfism, refers to a group of disorders in which the fetus develops a disproportionate short skeletal stature and limbs. There are several sub-groups of skeletal dysplasia, many dependent on when in the gestational age that the skeletal development becomes abnormal. A short stature is generally defined as any height measurements that are greater than 3 standard deviations below those expected for age. The true incidence of skeletal dysplasia is difficult to determine because many diagnosis are made well into childhood, but incidence is estimated at 1 in every 4000 births. If marked sonographic evidence of skeletal dysplasia occurs before the 20th gestational week, the prognosis is poor and the fatality rate is high.

SHORT-RIB POLYDACTYLY SYNDROME AND LETHAL HYPOPHOSPHATASIA

Short-rib polydactyly syndrome is a rare and always fatal skeletal dysplasia. Diagnosis is usually made prenatally by the presence of key sonographic features. Key sonographic findings in short-rib polydactyly syndrome include: macrocephaly, poorly-formed and low-set ears, cleft palate and lip, atrophied or bifid tongue, severely reduced and bell-shaped thorax, thick umbilical cord (>3.5 cm), micromelia, and polydactyly usually in the toes. Lethal hypophosphatasia is a rare, inherited metabolic skeletal dysplasia with estimated occurrence at 1 in 100,000. Sonographic features may include: micromelia with metaphyses cupping, significant variability and alternating of bone ossification, short and fragmented ribs, and butterfly-shaped vertebral bodies.

THANATOPHORIC DWARFISM

Thanatophoric dwarfism is the most common lethal skeletal dysplasia. The prevalence is estimated at 1 in every 25,000 live births. Classic sonographic characteristics of thanatophoric dwarfism are marked micromelia in all limbs, megacephaly, and reduced thorax circumference but with a normal length. Thanatophoric dwarfism is further broken down into two types with many overlapping features; however, probably the most obvious differentiator is in type I the skull normally shaped and in type II the skull is a cloverleaf shape. Sonographic diagnosis is usually made in the late second or third trimester. Other sonographic possibilities (type undifferentiated) are: curved "telephone receiver" long bones, especially the femur; extremely short and straight proximal long bones; short ribs; protuberant abdomen; polyhydramnios; flat nasal bridge; proptotic eyes; hydrocephalus; and an average term length of < 40 cm. The presence of polydactyly suggests another type of skeletal dysplasia and is never seen in thanatophoric dwarfism.

TORCH INFECTIONS

TORCH infections are a group of five common intrauterine infections that physicians and sonographers should be aware of during the reproductive years of a woman's life. TORCH is an acronym for toxoplasmosis, other, rubella, cytomegalovirus, and herpes simplex virus (types 1 and 2). Providers can test for TORCH, but this may first be diagnosed during an abnormal OB ultrasound. When the fetus is affected, physicians can provide more thorough and effective prenatal and antenatal care for the fetus as well as provide better care in any subsequent pregnancies. Ultrasound indicators of TORCH include intrauterine growth restriction, microcephaly, hydrocephalus, calcifications within the brain, cataracts, cardiac malformations, and fetal hydrops. If mothers have not been tested for these infections, they may not be aware of the risk associated with passing these infections onto their babies. Not all babies with TORCH can be diagnosed sonographically because sometimes the infections cause intellectual disabilities and sensory issues.

CYSTIC HYGROMA

A cystic hygroma is created when the lymphatic system cannot effectively drain the lymphatic fluid, causing retention. Cystic hygromas will present as a cyst or multiple cysts on ultrasound. These fluid-filled structures are typically on the posterior or posterolateral portion of the fetal neck, but they can also be found in an anterior location. Often, these cysts contain thick septations that may give the appearance of a mass that is solid. These thick septations can have a similar appearance to a teratoma, but it is important to try to discern between the two. The prognosis for a teratoma can be more promising if they are small. However, a cystic hygroma may give insight to chromosomal malformations that are often present, such as Turner syndrome and trisomies 18 and 21, although these tend to contain more septations and are bigger in Turner syndrome.

HEMANGIOMA

Hemangiomas, otherwise known as birthmarks, are the most common type of lesion seen in newborns. They are yet another type of tumor that may be visualized during a scan of the fetal head and neck. If a hemangioma can be detected with ultrasound, they typically include bigger vessels that are within the deeper layers of the skin such as the hypodermis and dermis as well as the smaller channels in the epidermis. These will display hypervascularity when color Doppler is used, and they can become quite large. Exophytic hemangiomas may cover the entire neck and face and appear to be a solid mass with an echotexture that resembles the placenta. Follow-up ultrasounds may show an increase in size. Regardless of the type of mass present in the region of the fetal neck, they are important to note because the airway may be compromised at birth.

FETAL DIAPHRAGMATIC HERNIA REPAIR

In utero diaphragmatic hernia repair is indicated if a large fetal herniation is diagnosed on sonography. It is also indicated due to the high fetal mortality rate of an untreated diaphragmatic herniation. Diaphragmatic herniation occurs when fetal abdominal contents press through a hole in the diaphragm into the chest cavity. This usually occurs in the posterolateral left hemidiaphragm. This leads to fetal respiratory distress and atrophied fetal lung(s). Repair of this condition is done by laparoscopy. The fetal trachea is clamped, causing the fetal lung volume to gradually increase with fluid. This increased fetal lung volume, within the thorax, pushes any herniated abdominal contents back into the abdominal cavity.

GOITER

Most fetal thyroid conditions are the result of a maternal thyroid condition, but primary hypothyroidism can occur in a fetus. When mothers have thyroid conditions such as Hashimoto's thyroiditis or Graves' disease, these antibodies that are produced in the mother can be passed on to the fetus via the placenta. It is important to provide doctors with clinical and diagnostic information about thyroid dysfunction because, if untreated, these conditions may increase neonatal mortality rates. Goiters that are found on OB scans will demonstrate the soft tissues of the neck bulging anteriorly. The thyroid will be enlarged because of the presence of a homogeneous, bilateral mass in the anterior portion of the neck. If these are not a solitary finding, it is typically the result of hyperthyroidism, in which case the fetus may also demonstrate hydrops and a rapid heart rate.

STRUCTURES VISUALIZED SONOGRAPHICALLY IN AN ABNORMAL FETAL NECK

The fetal neck is important to evaluate thoroughly during an ultrasound exam to rule out cystic hygromas, goiters, teratomas, hemangiomas, and proximity of the umbilical cord. Diagnosing these anomalies may help improve the mortality rate after birth, and although some have a similar appearance, it is important to try to discern the type. Determining if a mass is cystic, solid, or complex is an advantage of the use of ultrasound during an OB exam. Sonographers should try to determine the size of the mass, where the mass originated from, and if there is an association with other fetal structures. Sometimes even in the presence of abnormalities of the neck, the skull or face may be involved. Color, power, and spectral Doppler are useful to determine the vascularity of these structures.

Invasive Hydatidiform Mole

Invasive hydatidiform mole or chorioadenoma destruens is a gestational disease of the trophoblastic cells. Invasive hydatidiform mole occurs when a partial or classic hydatidiform mole grows into the muscular uterine wall. Invasive hydatidiform may develop in up to 20% of complete hydatidiform mole pregnancies. About 15% of chorioadenoma destruens cases metastasize and require chemotherapy. Signs and symptoms of invasive hydatidiform mole include heavy or prolonged postpartum bleeding and increasing serum beta hCG levels in the postpartum period. Sonography is helpful to evaluate the location and extent of uterine wall invasion by molar tissue.

Complete Mole

With the increasing use and availability of obstetrical sonography, complete hydatidiform mole may be diagnosed early before severe maternal symptoms develop. Possible maternal symptoms of complete mole include: vaginal bleeding, hyperemesis, preeclampsia, and hyperthyroidism. Sonographically, uterine enlargement that is greater than expected for gestational age is a classic sign. The fetus is not visible in a complete mole. The echogenic placenta will appear enlarged and cystic. The sonographic term, "bunch of grapes" is often used to describe this finding. In almost half of the cases of complete mole, bilateral theca-lutein ovarian cysts are present. Both ovaries usually appear enlarged with septated cysts.

DES and Effects on the Fetus

Diethylstilbestrol (DES) is a medication that has a long and controversial history. Its original indications were for the treatment of gonorrhea, atrophic vaginitis, vasomotor symptoms of menopause and lactation suppression. It started being used "off label" to help prevent miscarriages (1940s) and this soon became one of its labeled indications. After several years of this use, DES was found to cause multiple severe risks to the mothers and their offspring. DES is thought to increase the risk of breast cancer in women taking it. Female offspring, of mothers treated with DES, have an increased risk of developing vaginal and/or cervical adenocarcinoma, genitourinary defects, infertility, autoimmune disorders, and pregnancy complications of their own. Male offspring (of mothers treated with DES during pregnancy) are at increased risk for the development of feminization, epididymal cysts, and autoimmune disorders. It is unclear if and how third generation offspring of DES will be affected. DES is no longer available in the US

Fetal Macrosomia

Macrosomia is a retrospective diagnosis, meaning it can only be diagnosed upon obtaining the birth weight of a newborn after delivery. Macrosomia refers to a birth weight of greater than 90% expected for gestational age or a birth weight between 8 lb 12 oz and 9 lb 15 oz. Several factors increase the risk for delivering a large-for-age baby including: gestational diabetes, maternal obesity, Hispanic race, excessive maternal weight gain, and male fetus. Cesarean delivery, neonatal and maternal birthing injuries, and neonatal morbidity are common complications associated with fetal macrosomia.

Relationship of Down Syndrome and Iliac Angle, Under-Ossified Nasal Bones, and Duodenal Atresia

There has been some correlation between sonographic findings of an increased angle between iliac bones and Down syndrome. However, this is a difficult measurement due to varying iliac angles that are dependent on varied sonographic planes. Sonographic plane and measurement parameters have not been established. Up to 70% of Down syndrome fetuses have been observed to have an underdeveloped nasal bridge. Proposed calculations based on nasal bone length and biparietal diameter have limitations with test specificity, sensitivity, and false-positive rates. A sonographic finding of duodenal atresia suggests a 30% risk of the fetus having Down syndrome. This finding is not available until at least the 22nd gestational week and therefore is not useful for pregnancy continuation or termination planning but may be used in conjunction with other findings to ready and educate the parents on having a child with Down syndrome.

PULMONARY HYPOPLASIA AND PLEURAL EFFUSIONS

Pulmonary hypoplasia may develop if optimal fetal lung development conditions are not present. Among the conditions that might impair the normal development are: inadequate thoracic space secondary to mass or effusion, abnormal fetal breathing, abnormal amniotic fluid volume, and deficient fetal production of lung fluid and surfactant. An insufficient thoracic space may be diagnosed if it is significantly smaller than the fetal abdominal circumference. Fetal pleural effusion can be a primary or secondary condition occurring in one or both fetal lungs. The prevalence of fetal pleural effusion is approximated at 1 in every 15,000 pregnancies.

VEIN OF GALEN ANEURYSM IN THE FETAL BRAIN

A vein of Galen aneurysm in the fetal brain is not an aneurysm at all; rather it is a vascular malformation. This arteriovenous malformation shunts blood into the dilated vein of Galen from the cerebral arteries. The malformation develops by the 11th gestational week, but is not likely to be detected before the 32nd gestational week and more often until after birth. The best chance for fetal detection is with Doppler ultrasound. In the delivered infant, often the first sign of vein of Galen aneurysm is congestive heart failure. Although rare in terms of overall vascular malformations, vein of Galen aneurysm accounts for up to 30% of all fetal and infant vascular malformations.

AGENESIS CORPUS CALLOSUM

Agenesis of the corpus callosum describes a condition in which the portion of the brain (corpus callosum) that connects the two brain hemispheres is either absent or poorly formed. This condition can be seen independently or with other congenital malformations such as Dandy-Walker and Arnold-Chiari. Sonographic evaluation can identify corpus callosum agenesis between weeks 12 and 18. Associated sonographic changes may include: absent cingulate gyrus, lateral ventricles are further from each other, ventricles appear slightly more vertically positioned when viewing in the coronal plane, and transverse diameter of posterior ventricle is greater than the anterior horn.

DANDY-WALKER MALFORMATION

Dandy-Walker malformation is a very rare congenital malformation with variable prognosis. It primarily involves the cerebellum and fourth ventricle of the brain. Dandy-Walker malformation is present when there is an absent or poorly developed cerebellar vermis, cystic fourth ventricle dilation, and posterior fossa enlargement. The diagnosis cannot be made until later in the second trimester. There have been several variants of Dandy-Walker malformation described but all are associated with other fetal defects. Dandy-Walker malformation should be sonographically differentiated from an arachnoid cyst of the posterior fossa. A posterior fossa arachnoid cyst will maintain the presence of the cerebellar vermis and will not be associated with any other fetal malformations.

HYDRANENCEPHALY AND PORENCEPHALY

Hydranencephaly is a rare condition in which the fetal cerebral hemispheres are completely absent and, in their place, reside cerebrospinal fluid-filled sacs. Sonographic evaluation will reveal an intact falx and meninges. The cerebral cortex is absent or with severe abnormal appearance. If the fetus is delivered, head size, reflexes and general examination may be within normal limits initially. Within the first few weeks of live, changes in muscle tone and development become increasingly apparent. Rarely does an infant born with hydranencephaly survive past the first year of life.

Porencephaly is also rare and involves a cystic sac filled with cerebrospinal fluid within the ventricle or subarachnoid space. The sac is lined with white matter. It involves a smaller area than hydranencephaly. Prognosis is dependent on the area of the brain involved and the size of the cyst.

MILD LATERAL CEREBRAL VENTRICULOMEGALY

Mild lateral cerebral ventriculomegaly may also be termed borderline lateral cerebral ventriculomegaly. By definition, this is a slight enlargement of the lateral brain ventricles to an atrial width between 10-15 mm. This condition can be unilateral or bilateral. The cause of this is unknown and its effects range from none to hydrocephalus and other fetal central nervous system defects. If this sonographic finding or diagnosis is present, a thorough search for other fetal defects and associated conditions should be undertaken. Fetal karyotyping should be offered and explained to the mother in this situation.

SCHIZENCEPHALY, MICROCEPHALY, AND INTRACRANIAL CALCIFICATIONS

Schizencephaly is a rare birth defect characterized by slits through the cerebral hemispheres. These abnormal slits can be unilateral or bilateral. Cortical brain matter lines the slits. Microcephaly is a condition in which the fetal head is smaller than expected for gestational age or relative to abdominal circumference and femoral length measurements. Microcephaly is often times associated with other conditions of abnormal brain development. Intracranial calcifications seen in the fetal head with sonography, usually later in pregnancy, may be the result of infection or conditions involving vascular abnormalities/thrombosis.

VENTRICULOMEGALY AND HYDROCEPHALY

Ventriculomegaly is defined as abnormally enlarged lateral ventricles (>15 mm atrial width) in the absence of other central nervous system anomalies on sonography. However, often times other sonographic findings will be associated with ventriculomegaly thus limiting the use of the formal definition. Ventriculomegaly is often seen with hydrocephaly or when the size of the choroid plexus pales next to the size of the ventricle. Hydrocephaly refers to excessive amounts of cerebrospinal fluid often resulting in excess accumulation and dilation of within the ventricles. The presence of hydrocephaly often increases intracranial pressure. However, ventricular enlargement can occur independent of increased intracranial pressure.

ANENCEPHALY

Anencephaly is a neural tube defect in which the cephalic portion of the neural tube fails to close during development. This stage of closing/development usually happens between the 23rd and 26th days of gestation. Lack of neural tube closure at this stage results in anencephaly, which is marked by absence of most of the fetal brain, skull, and scalp. The majority of cases of anencephaly are stillborn. Anencephaly is the most common open neural tube defect. If a live birth occurs, survival is not expected much beyond several hours. Although anencephaly develops within the first 4 weeks of gestation, sonographic diagnosis is difficult to make before 10 weeks gestation. Anencephaly is associated with several other fetal anomalies.

CLEFT LIP AND CLEFT PALATE

Cleft lip is a facial abnormality that results when the lateral and median nasal prominences fail to fuse during fetal development. Cleft palate describes a condition in which a fissure develops along the median and anterior palate, also affecting the normal fusion process in fetal development. These terms are often used synonymously, but the conditions can be seen independently or coexist. Cleft palate is further categorized to describe the severity and depth of involvement of the hard palate. The midline cleft may extend to involve the nostrils.

Facial Anomalies, Dorsal Cyst, and Holoprosencephaly

Holoprosencephaly can result in a number of facial defects and anomalies. Close-set eyes (hypotelorism), an abnormally small head (microcephaly), absent incisor teeth, cleft lip and or palate, flat and single nostril (cebocephaly), and multiple nasal deformities are commonly seen in an infant born with holoprosencephaly. Cyclopia (a single midline eye) is another possibility, but this is rare and usually accompanied by the most severe form usually associated with fetal mortality. A dorsal cyst may accompany the diagnosis of holoprosencephaly. This is a space-occupying cyst that often develops in the posterior region, displacing the posterior cerebral hemispheres into the frontal fossa. Holoprosencephaly must be sonographically differentiated from hydranencephaly and hydrocephaly. Both of these conditions maintain a central falx not seen in holoprosencephaly.

Types of Holoprosencephaly

Holoprosencephaly is a condition in which the fetal brain does not divide normally into two hemispheres. The term also describes a variety of fetal brain and facial defects. There are 4 main types of holoprosencephaly. First is alobar holoprosencephaly describes complete failure of hemispheric division and an absent third ventricle. Second is semilobar holoprosencephaly is partial hemispheric division in the posterior brain with a single ventricular cavity. The third type is lobar holoprosencephaly in which hemispheric division is complete but there is an interhemispheric fissure and some structures may remain fused. The fourth type is the middle interhemispheric variant in which the frontal, posterior and parietal portions of the middle brain are not divided. All forms are usually correlated with a small head and close-set eyes. The prognosis is variable from minimal facial defects and normal intelligence to severe deformity and intellectual disability.

Fetal Facial Anomaly of Hypotelorism

Hypotelorism is defined as abnormal eye spacing, in which the eyes are abnormally close-set. This condition is usually seen as a result of abnormal or premature fusion of the metopic skull suture. Hypotelorism is seen in conjunction with other brain and facial malformations under the term holoprosencephaly. Hypotelorism can be further divided into subgroups. Cyclopia is its most severe form in which the orbits have fused and there is only a single middle orbit ("cyclops"). Ethmocephaly is a facial formation with abnormally close-set eyes with a proboscis (nose-like protuberance) that starts high above the orbits. Cebocephaly is a form of hypotelorism in which the normally formed and place nasal bridge, but only one nostril is present. The three described forms of hypotelorism are usually associated with fetal mortality.

Micrognathia and Macroglossia

Micrognathia refers to an abnormally small jaw. This is a fetal anomaly often associated with many other fetal syndromes and defects although it can be seen independent of another condition. Micrognathia can correct itself with growth and development. Micrognathia may interfere with normal respiration and feeding early in life and teeth malalignment later on. Macroglossia refers to a condition in which the tongue is larger than normal. Macroglossia is associated with a number of other fetal abnormalities and syndromes. It may be seen on sonography later in gestation. If the fetal tongue repetitively extends beyond the fetal lips on sonographic evaluation, suspect the diagnosis.

Fetal Echocardiography and Fetal Cardiac Abnormalities

Congenital heart defects are present in up to 1 in every 100 births, thus necessitating advanced imaging techniques. Fetal echocardiography allows for a detailed assessment of the fetal heart structure and function. The use and application of fetal echocardiography is well documented. Fetal echoes are a relatively non-invasive and low to no-risk procedure, even so, they are not currently recommended for routine screening. Fetal echocardiography allows for early diagnosis of a wide variety of congenital heart defects; furthermore, early detection of defects allows for management plans in utero or during and after delivery.

SINGLE VENTRICLE AND PERSISTENT TRUNCUS ARTERIOSUS

Abnormal development or absence of the ventricular septum leads to a rare congenital heart defect of single ventricle. This condition may also be termed univentricular heart. In this condition, the two atria are normal and there may be one or two atrial ventricular valves. Common surgical repair procedures include: Fontan operation, Blalock-Taussig shunting, Glenn shunting, and banding the pulmonary artery. Without surgical intervention, a univentricular heart is not conducive to sustained life. Persistent truncus arteriosus is essentially a large ventricular septal defect often times with a large vessel anomaly in which there is only one ventricular artery. Prenatal diagnosis may be made with sonographic viewing along the long-axis of a large outflow tract and four-chamber view of a ventricular septal defect. These findings would necessitate further evaluation with Doppler studies and fetal echocardiography.

HYPOPLASTIC LEFT HEART SYNDROME AND COARCTATION OF THE AORTA

Hypoplastic left heart syndrome is a congenital heart defect in which the entire left side of the heart, including the aorta; aortic valve; left ventricle; and mitral valve are poorly developed. Atrial septal defects and large patent ductus arteriosus are often present with hypoplastic left heart syndrome. Hypoplastic left heart syndrome is responsible for about 8% of all congenital heart defects and is more common in boys. Prenatal diagnosis is more likely with fetal echocardiography. Coarctation of the aorta is a narrowing of the aorta. It is among the top 3 most common congenital birth defects. It may be an independent finding and condition, but more commonly is seen with other heart defects including: a bicuspid aortic valve, ventricular septal defect, stenosis of the aortic or mitral valve, and patent ductus arteriosus. Routine fetal ultrasound may not detect this condition.

CARDIOMYOPATHY AND AVC DEFECT IN FETAL HEART

If an enlarged fetal heart is seen on routine fetal sonography, further detail and measurements should be obtained, as this is a sign of fetal cardiomyopathy. The heart chambers themselves may be larger or the muscular septum and heart walls may be thickened causing the enlargement. Note must be made if this is diffuse thickening and enlargement or localized to a single heart chamber. Atrioventricular canal (AVC) defect is a condition in which the mitral and tricuspid valves do not form normally and individually and a single defect/hole/valve forms that communicates between the atrium and ventricles. This is usually readily seen in routine fetal heart sonography. Sonographically, AVC is seen as a gooseneck deformity with left ventricular outflow narrowing. Doppler studies are then needed to estimate the degree of defect.

ATRIAL VENTRICULAR SEPTAL DEFECTS AND EBSTEIN'S ANOMALY

Septal heart defects are further categorized into atrial or ventricular, thus describing the location in which the defect occurs. Essentially these are a hole in the muscular septal wall that divides the chambers. Ventricular septal defects are difficult to diagnose with routine fetal sonography, especially if the defect is small. Atrial septal defects are also difficult to detect because of the normal fetal blood flow that occurs through the foramen ovale. Ebstein's anomaly is a congenital heart defect with an abnormal tricuspid valve. This valve is displaced further into the right ventricle. As a result of this displacement, signs of an Ebstein's anomaly may include right ventricular enlargement and pulmonary artery narrowing. It is common for atrial septal defects to coexist with Ebstein's anomaly.

INDICATIONS FOR FETAL ECHOCARDIOGRAPHY

Since fetal echocardiography is not currently a standard screening procedure, guidelines have been established for those that should undergo it. Certainly, if there is a family history of congenital heart disease the fetal heart should be evaluated with echocardiography. Maternal conditions such as type I diabetes, early drug or chemical exposure (some seizure medications and illegal drugs), and infections should warrant a fetal echocardiogram. An abnormal amniocentesis, fetal arrhythmia, or abnormal fetal heart structure are indications for fetal echocardiography. If routine obstetrical sonography detects abnormal amniotic fluid amounts, fetal situs inversus, decreased fetal size, 2-vessel umbilical cord, or the absence of a fetal spleen echocardiography should be considered.

SITUS ABNORMALITIES, CARDIAC TUMORS AND FETAL HEART RATE AND RHYTHM ABNORMALITIES

Situs inversus, also called situs transverses, is a condition in which the abdominal and/or thoracic contents are reversed. If only the heart is involved (located on the right side) it is termed dextrocardia. Care must be taken in imaging these individuals, with special attention to landmarks, positioning, and labeling "left" and "right". Fetal cardiac tumors are an extremely rare finding. When they are present, about 90% of them are benign. The most common benign cardiac tumor is a rhabdomyoma. Fetal sonography may detect the mass, but cannot differentiate tumor-type. Evaluation of fetal heart rate is important, as up to 2% of all fetuses have an arrhythmia. Many of these resolve spontaneously. Normal fetal heart rates range from 120 – 180 beats per minute. If irregularities are sonographically detected, the duration, frequency and type of irregularity should be documented and followed.

TETRALOGY OF FALLOT AND DOUBLE-OUTLET RIGHT VENTRICLE

Tetralogy of Fallot is a congenital heart defect comprised of a ventricular septal defect, pulmonary stenosis, an abnormal or overriding aortic valve, and right ventricular hypertrophy. Tetralogy of Fallot is present in up to 6 in 10,000 births. Tetralogy of Fallot may initially be seen as an overriding aorta in the long-axis view on routine fetal heart sonography. Double-outlet right ventricle is a congenital heart defect in which both the aortic and pulmonic arteries arise from the right ventricle. In the presence of a double-outlet right ventricle is a ventricular septal defect. Short-axis view on routine fetal cardiac sonographic evaluation may best demonstrate this defect initially.

TRANSPOSITION OF THE GREAT ARTERIES IN THE FETAL HEART

Transposition of the great arteries is a congenital heart defect in which the aortic artery is connected to the right ventricle (instead of the left ventricle) and the pulmonary artery is connected to the left ventricle (instead of the right ventricle). This transposition compromises the circulation of oxygenated and deoxygenated blood to and from the body. The "D" in D-transposition refers to dextro-transposition of the great arteries and describes the position of the aortic artery to be anterior and to the right of the pulmonary artery. L-transposition of the great arteries refers to the location of the aortic artery anterior and to the left of the pulmonary artery.

FETAL CARDIAC ANOMALIES VISIBLE IN THE FOUR-CHAMBER VIEW

The four-chamber view allows for visualization of many structures and since it is usually the easiest and most standardized view to obtain, it allows for detection of a number of anomalies. Among the ventricular anomalies that may be detected with four-chamber viewing are: single ventricle (absence of ventricular septum), atrioventricular canal, poorly developed ventricles, or enlarged ventricles. Four-chamber imaging of the fetal heart may also reveal valvular anomalies such as: absent mitral valve, absent tricuspid valve, and a displaced tricuspid valve (Ebstein's anomaly).

EVALUATING ABDOMINAL WALL DEFECTS

In obstetrical sonography, evaluation of fetal abdominal wall defects is important to identify independent anomalies as well as defects that are correlated with additional fetal anomalous conditions. The first sonographic protocol is to establish abdominal landmarks, specifically in relation to the umbilical cord. Second, sonography needs to establish if a membranous material covers the defect, and this needs to be thoroughly described. Third, identify the fetal organ structures that are involved in the defect and to what extent. Fourth, if the abdominal defect involves fetal bowel, sonographic differentiation of stricture or dilation needs to be noted. Finally, with the presence of any sonographic fetal abdominal wall defect, thorough investigation, imaging, and description of all other areas of fetal, uterine and placenta anatomy need to be noted.

CAM IN THE FETAL LUNG

Cystic adenomatoid malformations (CAM) in the fetal lung are unilateral and broken into three subtypes: cystic, cystic and solid, and solid. CAM develops when an abnormal cystic tissue of the lung develops and occupies a large portion of where the normal lung should be. It can occur in either lung equally and over all prevalence is unclear but estimated at 1 in every 30,000 pregnancies with a slight male over female predominance. CAM is responsible for about 25% of all congenital pulmonary lesions. Sonographically, CAM may be diagnosed by a highly echogenic mass in the fetal thorax with cardiac displacement and a flat or everted diaphragm.

PENTALOGY OF CANTRELL

As its name suggests, the pentalogy of Cantrell is a rare disorder characterized by five fetal defects. The five defects are: abdominal wall defect, lower sternum defect, diaphragmatic hernia, pericardium defect, and intracardiac defects. This pentad of defects develops around the 6th – 7th gestational week, with abnormal abdominal mesoderm folding. In half of the cases, and atrial septal defect will be present. A number of noncardiac fetal defects are also associated with this condition. Sonographically, the heart will appear exposed or outside of the thorax and omphalocele will be present.

PULMONARY SEQUESTRATION

Pulmonary sequestration is further termed extralobar sequestration to describe a condition that develops in the fetus or neonate. Extralobar pulmonary sequestration is marked by the development of abnormal cystic lung tissue that does not have any connection to the tracheobronchial tree. Furthermore, this anomalous area receives its blood supply from the abdominal aorta rather than the pulmonary artery. Extralobar pulmonary sequestration can be seen in as many as 6% of all congenital thoracic anomalies. Prognosis is good in most cases. Diagnosis may be prenatal with Doppler studies or more often postnatal with a variety of work-ups leading to the diagnosis and extent.

MECONIUM ILEUS AND MECONIUM PERITONITIS

Meconium ileus is a condition in which the ileus portion of the small intestine fills with meconium causing an obstruction and/or dilation of the ileum at this point. With this finding, the colon will be smaller than expected for gestational age or may not be visualized at all. The presence of meconium ileus is highly correlated with cystic fibrosis. Meconium peritonitis is the result of perforated intestine/colon in utero. The intestinal contents (bowel and meconium) then leak into the abdominal/peritoneal cavity. Sonographic appearance of meconium peritonitis reveals hyperechogenic areas and punctate and linear calcifications throughout the fetal abdomen.

CAUSES OF FAILURE TO VISUALIZE THE FETAL STOMACH

The fetal stomach should be easily viewed via sonography after 14 gestational weeks. In the event of sonographic absence of the stomach, interval reevaluation should be scheduled and fetal anomalies considered. Anomalies that may be responsible for nonvisualization of the fetal stomach are largely centered on any condition that would impair fetal swallowing, central nervous system anomalies, and musculoskeletal defects. Other conditions that may not allow for sonographic visualization of the fetal stomach are: stomach displacement into chest or base of umbilical cord, an abnormally small stomach, reduced esophageal patency, decreased amniotic fluid production or failure to reach the amniotic cavity, and the presence of a normal stomach that has just emptied.

CLOACAL EXSTROPHY

Cloacal exstrophy is a rare set of birth anomalies occurring about once in every 250,000 live births. It is also known as OEIS complex, which better describes the set of anomalies that are present: Omphalocele, Exstrophy of the cloaca (open bladder with rectal communication), Imperforate anus, and Spinal defects (especially spina bifida). Diagnosis of cloacal exstrophy is with elevated AFP tests and sonograph. Sonographically, the OEIS complex will reveal a tissue mass inferior to the fetal umbilicus attachment site, a fluid-filled mass in the pelvis (cloaca), and often times the absence of the anterior pelvic bones. Due to prenatal diagnostic techniques, survival rate is improved but will likely result in a number of postnatal surgical procedures. Probable postnatal surgeries include: repair of omphalocele; repair of bladder and rectum/anus (creating bowel and bladder elimination routes), and often times surgical sexual determination and repair (males will be surgically made female, and females will have surgical vagina created).

GASTROSCHISIS

Gastroschisis is a condition in which fetal abdominal contents herniate through an opening in the abdominal wall, usually to the right of the fetal umbilical cord. Gastroschisis occurs in up to 2.5 per 1000 births and in slightly more males than females. In most cases of gastroschisis, the nonrotated small intestine is the only structure that herniates through the abdominal wall. Rarely will the liver, stomach or colon protrude through the opening. The exact mechanisms and risks for development of gastroschisis are unknown, but many theories involve obstruction of the omphalomesenteric vessels. Prenatal diagnosis with sonography and AFP testing is common. Associated fetal anomalies are rare, and usually are related to the defect itself. With increased technology and surgical repair methods, survival is up to 90%.

LBWC

Limb-body wall complex, also known as body stalk anomaly, is a rare birth defect occurring approximately once for every 10,000 pregnancies. Limb-body wall complex is primarily characterized by a severe abdominal wall defect, prominent kyphoscoliosis, and a poorly developed umbilical cord. A number of other defects may be present including, but not limited to, cranial and facial defects and limb anomalies. Forty percent of body stalk anomalies also have the presence of amniotic bands. The exact etiology of limb-body wall complex is unknown. Sonographically, the liver may appear attached to the placenta. Sonographic imaging of the umbilical cord may reveal its absence or a poorly developed and abnormally short umbilical cord. Significant spinal distortion will be present and, if identified, the limbs will be grossly abnormal. Body stalk anomalies are always fatal.

COLON ATRESIA

Colon atresia accounts for up to 10% of intestinal bowel atresias. Most colon atresias are secondary to vascular or nerve injury to the affected colonic portion. Colon atresia is not associated with increased amniotic fluid findings and may first be suspected or diagnosed in the third trimester when the colonic diameter exceeds 18 mm. The most common colon atresia is anorectal atresia, which is associated with cardiac, kidney, limb, vertebral, and upper GI tract anomalies. Colon atresia often coexists with a more proximal small bowel atresia. If not diagnosed before birth, the first signs of colonic atresia will be the absence of infant bowel movements, abdominal distention and vomiting.

DUODENAL ATRESIA

Duodenal atresia refers to a condition in which the duodenum is closed and does not allow for passage of stomach contents into the small intestines. The incidence of duodenal atresia is 1 in 10,000 births. Rarely is duodenal atresia an independent finding. Thirty percent are also associated with Down syndrome. Sonographically, duodenal atresia may be suspected and diagnosed with increased amniotic fluid and swollen stomach and proximal duodenum (double bubble sign), often seen after 24 gestational weeks. With early diagnosis and surgical repair, prognosis is good. Undetected and untreated duodenal atresia is fatal.

ESOPHAGEAL ATRESIA

Esophageal atresia is a congenital disorder in which the esophagus does not develop normally. There are several types of esophageal atresia, but two common conditions are: the failure of the upper esophagus to connect to its inferior portion and thus the stomach, and a fistula that develops between the esophagus and trachea. It is difficult to detect this directly with prenatal sonography, but in the presence of increased amniotic fluid and other congenital anomalies (cardiac, renal, limb, vertebral, and anal), esophageal atresia should be highly suspected. Prognosis is based on early detection and the extent of other anomalies.

TRACHEAL ATRESIA AND BRONCHOGENIC CYSTS

Fetal tracheal atresia is the absence of a normal or patent tracheal opening and is a very rare finding. Sonographically, the fetal lungs appear enlarged and hyperechogenic as a result of dilated alveoli. The heart will appear relatively small in the midline. Tracheal atresia is most common at the level of the larynx and is often associated with other fetal anomalies. Bronchogenic cysts are a rare condition that may result during fetal bronchi development later in pregnancy. The diagnosis is not usually made prenatally. The location rather than the size of the bronchogenic cysts determine outcome, with bronchogenic cysts at the carina being the most severe and life threatening.

HYDROCELE, CRYPTORCHIDISM, AND HYDROMETROCOLPOS

A hydrocele refers to a collection of serous fluid within the scrotum, surrounding the testes. In the developing fetus it may be a sign of a developmental anomaly or in a worst case scenario one developing fetal hydrops. Hydroceles are correlated with increase inguinal herniation. Cryptorchidism is the failure of one or both testes to descend from the pelvis/abdomen after 30 weeks gestation. This is commonly termed undescended testes. This may be an independent finding or associated with other anomalies. Hydrometrocolpos is a condition found in females in which excessive mucous secretions collect in the genitourinary tract, especially the uterus and vagina. Hydrometrocolpos and imperforate hymen are often used interchangeably.

NEUROBLASTOMA AND CONGENITAL MESOBLASTIC NEPHROMA

A neuroblastoma is a malignant tumor of embryonic nerve cells. A neuroblastoma can occur anywhere but about 30% of them are associated with the adrenal gland. Prenatal diagnosis may be difficult, but may appear sonographically as a mass invading the fetal kidney. Congenital mesoblastic nephroma is usually diagnosed postnatally as an abdominal or renal mass finding. It is the most common renal tumor of infancy, with greater than 60% being diagnosed in the first 3 months of life and 90% diagnosed by 1 year of age. They generally do not metastasize but can become large enough to invade surrounding tissue and compromise other organ function. Removal is curative.

BILATERAL RENAL AGENESIS

Bilateral renal agenesis is a genetic disorder in which the fetal kidneys fail to develop. This occurs in up to 1 in every 4000 births. In the absence of fetal kidneys, there is most definitely oligohydramnios. With insufficient amniotic cushioning, several other defects follow: limb contractures, flattening nose, low-set ears, bell-shaped thorax, and even sirenomelia. Further sonographic evaluation will reveal an elongated, flattened, and echogenic adrenal gland in the absence of no pelvic kidney or urinary bladder. Bilateral renal agenesis is always fatal ultimately secondary to hypoplastic formation of the pulmonary system.

HYDRONEPHROSIS

Hydronephrosis refers to enlargement of the fetal kidney secondary to urine back up from an outlet anomaly. This condition may be unilateral or bilateral. Sonographically, a dilated ureter may be seen in addition to the swollen kidney. Sonographically, the fetal kidney and bladder can be seen as early as 15 weeks gestation. By about 18 weeks, the renal sinus can be seen as a central echo. If the anterior to posterior kidney measurement of the renal pelvis is greater than 8 mm by the 20th gestational week or 10 mm after 20 weeks gestation, the diagnosis of hydronephrosis can be made. Hydronephrosis is the most common fetal anomaly detected, and account for about half of all genitourinary anomalies. Rarely is hydronephrosis and independent diagnosis, rather a symptom of another disorder. Prognosis is dependent upon pregnancy stage, unilateral or bilateral kidney involvement, and degree of kidney swelling/ureter dilation.

CLASSIFICATION OF RENAL CYSTIC DISEASE

Renal cystic diseases, also known as Potter's syndromes, are classified into four disease types using six criteria. The renal cystic disease type classification uses the Roman numeral system and labels the four types as: Potter's Type I, Potter's Type II, and etc. However, it is the first criteria of nomenclature type that probably best describes each of the four renal cystic disease classifications. The second and third classification criteria are based on location and sonographic appearance. The fourth criterion evaluates the volume of amniotic fluid associated with each type of renal cystic disease. The fifth classification criterion is based on outcome or prognosis. And finally, the sixth classification criteria labels risk of a fetus having renal cystic disease in future pregnancies.

DERMOID CYSTS AND PELVIC KIDNEY

The sonographic finding of a dermoid cyst during pregnancy presents as an echogenic and complex mass with posterior shadowing. Within the mass are the appearance of ectodermal structures such as hair, skin and teeth. Definitive and recommended treatment is removal. A pelvic maternal kidney may be an incidental sonographic finding during pregnancy. Sonographically it is viewed as either a complex or sold mass and may contain cysts located centrally within the mass. The presence of hydronephrosis is the greatest concern during pregnancy.

UNILATERAL RENAL AGENESIS AND RENAL ECTOPIA

Unilateral renal agenesis is a condition in which the fetus only develops one functional kidney. This condition is compatible with life. Sonographically, a normal appearing fetal kidney will be present as well as a normal urinary bladder and adequate amniotic fluid. In the space of the absent kidney will be the elongated and flattened adrenal gland. Renal ectopia describes a condition in which one or both kidneys are positioned outside of the normal renal fossa. The kidney(s) may be positioned anywhere from the chest to the pelvis and are often malrotated. Occurrence is 1 in 1,000 births but only 1 in 10 are diagnosed, usually as an incidental finding. If discovered, evaluate for other congenital abnormalities.

URETHRAL OBSTRUCTION AND PRUNE BELLY SYNDROME

Urethral obstruction appears sonographically as an enlarged renal pelvis, a dilated and/or twisted ureter, and a thickened bladder wall. In the male fetus, the most likely site of ureter obstruction is in the posterior urethral valves. In the female fetus, urethral obstruction is usually secondary to a cloacal anomaly. In cases of complete and severe urethral obstruction, the renal tissue will develop abnormally giving the kidneys a cystic or echogenic appearance. Prune belly syndrome, also known as Eagle-Barrett syndrome is a rare set of birth defects seen in the male fetus. Prune belly syndrome is characterized by absence of abdominal wall musculature, hydronephrosis, hydroureters, enlarged urinary bladder and undescended testes.

FETAL GENITAL MALFORMATIONS

Fetal genital malformation possibilities are numerous. They may be secondary to a chromosomal disorder or originate from improper embryonic development, closure and fusion. Defective genital formation affects both male and female fetuses and can result in ambiguous male/female. Adrenal hyperplasia can also result in fetal genital malformation. Many genital defects occur between the 12th and 16th gestational weeks, as this is the normal time in which differentiation occurs. Examples of male genital malformations are: penile agenesis and duplication, penile torsion, microphallus, scrotal agenesis, and penoscrotal transposition. Examples of female genital defects are: ectopic labium, labial adhesions, clitoral duplication, clitoral hypertrophy, and interlabial masses.

HETEROZYGOUS ACHONDROPLASIA

Heterozygous achondroplasia is a skeletal condition in which cartilaginous development of the long bones was disrupted. It is an autosomal dominant trait that is not fatal. However, up to 90% of cases are sporadic, which suggests the possibility of a mutation cause of transmission. It is characterized by rhizomelic shortened limbs and a normal thorax. Frontal bossing, trident hands, thoracolumbar kyphosis, and midfacial hypoplasia are common findings and characteristics of heterozygous achondroplasia. Prenatal, sonographic diagnosis is difficult and rare unless one of the parents has achondroplasia.

OPEN SPINA BIFIDA

Open spina bifida refers to a defect that results from failure of the fetal vertebrae to fuse and create a protective column for the spinal cord. Instead, the spinal cord is left exposed and sometimes can protrude. In spina bifida operta, the skin in this area does not come together either, and often the only barrier for the spinal cord to the environment is a thin meningeal membrane. This defect occurs within the first 5 gestational weeks. However, sonography may not detect spina bifida operta until later in pregnancy. Open spina bifida usually occurs in the lumbosacral region.

SPINA BIFIDA OCCULTA AND RACHISCHISIS

Spina bifida occulta is the mildest form of spina bifida. It affects up to 10% of the population. It occurs when the neural arch of the vertebra fails to close, but all overlying soft tissue is intact. Therefore, in spina bifida occulta the spinal cord is not exposed or protruding. Obstetrical sonography may not detect spina bifida occulta. X-ray films are usually diagnostic, after delivery. Examination of the newborn may reveal a skin dimple or a tuft of hair growing from the location in the spinal column where the defect exists, usually lumbosacral. Spinal rachischisis is the rarest and most severe form of spina bifida. Spinal rachischisis describes an open spina bifida involving the entire spinal column.

Radial Ray Abnormalities, Clubfoot Deformity, and Focal Femoral Hypoplasia

A radial ray anomaly refers to one in which there is a congenital absence of the radius and thumb. This congenital anomaly may be an independent finding or associated with a number of other conditions. A radial ray anomaly may be bilateral or unilateral. In the absence of the radius and thumb, the four fingers project perpendicular to the ulna. Clubfoot is a relatively common (up to 7 in 1000 births) anomaly found independently or in association with other disorders. Clubfoot is an anomaly in which the foot/feet are plantarflexed, adducted and inverted. Focal femoral hypoplasia refers to a usually independent birth anomaly of unilateral or bilateral femoral shortening. This is more common in females and correlated with maternal diabetes.

Thalidomide

Thalidomide is a pharmacological agent that was initially prescribed for hyperemesis associated with 'morning sickness' during pregnancy. Use of thalidomide as an antiemetic was primarily in the 1950 –1960 time period. Fetuses of mothers that took thalidomide suffered severe deformities including phocomelia. Phocomelia is the lack of development of arms and legs, but often with poorly formed hands and feet attached to the trunk (flipper appearance). Current indication for prescription of thalidomide is only for the treatment of a severe skin condition – erythema nodosum, when it occurs in an individual with leprosy. It is a pregnancy category X pharmaceutical agent now.

Finger Hypoplasia, Brachycephaly, and Cardiac Defects in Relation to Down Syndrome

Underdeveloped digits, specifically the 5th finger, may be a sonographic finding in the diagnosis of Down syndrome. When sonographically evaluating this, measurements of the middle 4th phalanx and the middle 5th phalanx should be taken. If the measurement of the 5th middle phalanx is only about 60% of that of the 4th middle phalanx, suspect Down syndrome. Brachycephaly is a common finding in Down syndrome; however, clear-cut definitions and measurements of the cephalic index have not been determined. The most common sonographic cardiac findings in Down syndrome are: atrioventricular canal defects and an echogenic portion in the left ventricle in the area of the papillary muscle.

Teratoma

Teratomas are masses that are made up of various tissues such as bone, teeth, thyroid tissue, and hair. Because of the multitude of tissues this mass is comprised of, the ultrasound appearance may include solid and cystic components, with many being completely solid. A commonality that may help with a diagnosis of a teratoma is the visualization of calcifications within the mass. Most teratomas are visualized in the lower portion of the spine, but those found in the neck may be located in the thyroid or anterolateral neck regions. The latter may have a similar appearance to a cystic hygroma, but it is important to document the size and origin whenever possible. Color Doppler will often display increased blood flow within the mass. The prognosis in this region, although benign, will often be determined by the patency of the fetal airway.

Fetal Intracranial Tumors, in Utero Intracranial Hemorrhage, and Intracranial Calcifications

The most common fetal intracranial tumor is a teratoma, although all fetal intracranial tumors are extremely rare. Fetal intracranial tumor should be suspected anytime sonography detects hydrocephalus or any mass-occupying lesion. Intracranial tumors may have low echogenicity on ultrasound. Prognosis is poor for all types of fetal intracranial tumors. In utero intracranial hemorrhage is also extremely rare and is usually the result of maternal problems. Fetal intracranial calcifications are a rare, late pregnancy sonographic finding. Intracranial calcifications are usually secondary to infectious agents. Associated sonographic findings may include lateral ventricular enlargement and a small-for-gestational-age head.

DERMOID CYSTS

Dermoid cysts (cystic teratomas) care a germ cell type tumor. Although they are rare in terms of all types of ovarian tumors, they are the most common ovarian tumor in patients 25 years of age and younger. Dermoid cysts are usually unilateral with a symmetrical shape. Average size is 15 cm but they may be as large as 40 cm. The sonographic appearance of a cystic teratoma is highly varied. Often times, the mass will contain material with hair, fat, teeth, bone, and cartilage-like material. Sonographically, the dermoid cyst can appear either solid or cystic with a great deal of shadowing. Approximately 70% of ovarian dermoid cysts are benign.

CONDITIONS CONFUSED WITH CYSTIC TERATOMA

Due to the highly variable appearance of cystic teratomas, they may be easily confused with other conditions on sonographic examination. Of equal concern is the misdiagnosis of dermoid cysts, when in fact another pelvic pathology is present. Other sonographically similar diagnostic possibilities to cystic teratoma include: ectopic pregnancy, distended bowel, fibroids (especially pedunculated), tubo-ovarian abscess, appendicitis, extraovarian lipomatosis, and any cystic mass with echogenic nodules. Furthermore, sonographic findings can appear "normal", thus the importance of the clinical history. Ovarian torsion or hemorrhage can be secondary to the cystic teratoma or independent of it.

NORMAL FETAL GROWTH IN TWIN GESTATION

Fetal growth in twin gestations should be similar to that of the single pregnancy growth parameters in the first and second trimesters. At about the third trimester is when we see the separation of growth parameters of singleton versus twin growth curves. In the third trimester the twins will still have steady growth but it will be much slower than that of a single pregnancy. Slight variation in crown-rump length (less than 5 days difference) is acceptable in the first trimester. Fetal weights should also be within 20% of each other; anything greater incurs greater risk for fetal complications. Theoretically, growth of monozygote twins should be similar and dizygotes may display slightly more variation.

INCREASED INCIDENCE OF COMPLICATIONS IN MULTIPLE GESTATION

Multiple gestation pregnancies carry greater risk of low birth weight babies and preterm delivery. Approximately 60% of twins are delivered preterm. This percentage increases with increasing number of multiples. Most preterm multiples are considered 'low-birth-weight' which is less than 5 ½ pounds. Again, the higher the number of multiples and the earlier the preterm delivery, the lower the birth weight measurements. Even before birth, multiple gestations are at increased risk of complications. Monozygote twins are at increased risk for twin-to-twin-transfusion syndrome and birth defects. Other defects that may be seen in multiple gestations include: embolization syndrome, umbilical cord entanglement, vessel anastomoses, and acardiac parabiotic syndrome. Maternal risks such as preeclampsia and gestational diabetes also increase when carrying multiples versus singletons.

FACTORS THAT INCREASE INCIDENCE OF MULTIPLE GESTATION

Several factors contribute to the increased likelihood of multiple gestation. Increased maternal age, increasing use of fertility treatment medications, and increased in vitro fertilization are responsible for the overall increased incidence of multiple births. The incidence is approximately 1 in every 80 births. Increased maternal parity is also responsible for the increased likelihood of multiple

175

gestation, especially if this number is greater than 6. There is a significantly increased incidence of dizygotic twins in certain African countries. A positive maternal family history of dizygotic twins increases the chance for multiple gestation. Paternal family history and race do not seem to contribute to increased incidence of multiple gestation. Monozygotic twinning also seems to be independent of any incidence variability.

ACARDIAC TWIN

The acardiac twin anomaly is also known as Twin-Reversed Arterial Profusion sequence or TRAP sequence. TRAP sequence is seen in only about 1 in 35,000 births. It is seen in monozygotic monochorionic gestations. The TRAP sequence occurs when there is a venous and arterial anastomoses that results in retrograde deoxygenated blood flow to the acardiac twin. This results in significantly compromised development that is seen essentially in all major organ systems from the waist and up in the acardiac twin. These structural abnormalities are diagnostic on ultrasound as well as retrograde umbilical flow of the acardiac twin on Doppler studies. The other twin often develops normally.

CLASSIC HYDATIDIFORM MOLE WITH NORMAL TWIN AND PSEUDO-PARTIAL HYDATIDIFORM MOLES

There are three situations that may sonographically appear similar to a partial hydatidiform molar pregnancy, and that must be differentiated from this condition. The first situation is a twin pregnancy in which there is one normal twin with a healthy placenta and the presence of a complete or classic hydatidiform mole. The second condition is that of fetal demise. The placental degeneration that takes place after a fetal demise can sonographically be similar to the "bunch of grapes" appearance seen in a molar pregnancy. Chromosomal testing may be necessary to differentiate this situation. Finally, a fetus with Beckwith-Wiedemann syndrome can mimic sonographic findings in partial mole pregnancies. With Beckwith-Wiedemann syndrome, fetal growth restriction will not be observed and fetal anomalies associated with the syndrome will be sonographically evident.

TWIN EMBOLIZATION SYNDROME

Twin embolization syndrome is a condition that is most commonly associated with monozygote monochorionic twins. It is a condition in which one fetus dies, often secondary to twin-twin transfusion syndrome. The demise of the one fetus results in embolization placental fragments, fetal thromboplastin, and any other number of necrosed fetal fragments. This embolized matter affects the surviving fetus or twin in a number of ways. The more vascular organs of the living twin are most notably affected including the brain and kidneys. Twin embolization syndrome can result in a number of central nervous system defects and anomalies in the surviving fetus. Furthermore, anomalies throughout the GI system and abdominal cavity (especially necrotic in nature) and even limb defects occur in the remaining fetus when TES is present.

CORD ENTANGLEMENT AND CONJOINED TWINS

Umbilical cord entanglement syndrome is a condition seen in approximately 50% of monoamniotic twins. The risk is high in this situation because of the shared amniotic sac and thus the lack of membranous separation of the umbilical cords of the two fetuses. This results in twisting, tangling and even knotting of the two umbilical cords and resulting fetal complications and even mortality that would be associated with a compromised blood flow to and from the fetus(es). Conjoined twins are rare but may develop from the partial division of a single fertilized ovum. This rare condition is readily diagnosed with sonography. Sonography is important in determining twin attachment site and shared organs. Their anatomical conjunction site further classifies conjoined twins. Common attachment sites are the abdomen and thorax (omphalopagus and thoracopagus).

DIAGNOSIS OF ACARDIAC TWINNING WITH ULTRASOUND IMAGING

Acardiac twinning is a complication that may only take place in a monozygotic twin pregnancy, and, of course, it will be of the same sex. Ultrasound indications of this malformation include the visualization of one twin that is extremely deformed, referred to as the acardiac twin. As the term acardiac suggests, this twin does not develop a heart, or the heart is severely malformed. Often, the superior body of this fetus has not been formed, and the head is either missing or microcephaly is present. The other twin is often fully developed and is referred to as the "pump" twin; this twin is at a higher risk for hydrops, polyhydramnios, or congestive heart failure. It is believed that this condition occurs as blood flows through an artery-to-artery anastomosis and a vein-to-vein anastomosis, and it is referred to as twin reversed arterial perfusion. The inferior portion of the acardiac twin tends to receive blood that is richer in oxygen, so these body parts are often well developed.

ULTRASOUND FINDINGS OF CONJOINED TWINS

Conjoined twins are an unlikely occurrence in a monozygotic pregnancy that will only take place in the presence of one amnion and a single chorion. If a sonographer identifies a twin pregnancy but cannot see an amniotic membrane separating the fetuses in the presence of one placenta, this should be a consideration. Conjoined twins can never occur when the amniotic membrane is present or in the presence of more than one placenta. Ultrasound clues of conjoined twins include fetal heads that are aligned at the same height, bodies and organs that cannot be identified as separate entities, fetuses that demonstrate extension of the neck while facing their twin, demonstration of more than three vessels in one umbilical cord, and polyhydramnios. Conjoined twins are most often characterized as thoracopagus (the most frequent anomaly when fetuses are joined at the chest), thoraco-omphalopagus (joined at the chest and abdomen), omphalopagus (joined at the abdomen), and craniopagus (joined at the head).

COMMON ABNORMALITIES ASSOCIATED WITH MULTIPLE GESTATIONS

Sonographers should understand that all multiple gestations are considered to be high-risk pregnancies not only for the fetuses, but also for the mother. Congenital abnormalities are found two to three times more often in pregnancies that are associated with twins than in a single gestation. Multiple gestations have escalated due to increasing maternal age and the use of infertility techniques. Like all obstetrical ultrasounds, it is important for the operator to determine the number of gestations as well as the presentation. It is also important to determine the number of amniotic sacs and placentas, which is more accurately identified in the first trimester. More anomalies are found in monozygotic pregnancies than those found in dizygotic pregnancies and include acardiac twinning, conjoined twins, twin-twin transfusion syndrome, vanishing twin, or a heterotopic multifetal pregnancy. It is important to correctly diagnose any anomaly as soon as possible so that the specialists can make the best decision for the patients.

ULTRASOUND FINDINGS OF TWIN-TO-TWIN TRANSFUSION SYNDROME

Twin-to-twin transfusion syndrome (TTTS) only takes place in monozygotic twins that share one placenta. This is a syndrome that actually affects the placenta instead of the twins, but because the blood flow is not dispersed evenly between the twins, it affects their growth differently. TTTS is believed to be caused when artery-to-vein anastomosis deflects blood flow away from one twin to the other. The connection tends to be from the umbilical arterial system of the twin that is displaying growth restriction, or the "donor" twin, to the larger "recipient's" umbilical vein. This shunting of blood creates a significant risk for both twins. Ultrasound findings will often reveal that a "donor" twin that is measuring smaller than expected is not moving and actually appears "stuck" in the presence of oligohydramnios. The larger "recipient" twin may have hydrops in the presence of polyhydramnios, with organomegaly and ascites.

HMG, GnRHa, AND CLOMID

Human menopausal gonadotropin (hMG) is a fertility treatment option that consists of injectable medication that stimulates follicular production. These medications are comprised of a variety of FSH and LH combinations. Gonadotropin-releasing hormone agonists (GnRHa) are used in a number of disorders, but their use in infertility stimulates release of FSH and LH, followed by a down regulation response and placing the body in a hypoestrogenic and hypogonadal state. Both of these states are reversible. This infertility treatment is often used in combination with others. Treatment of infertility with the medication Clomid is common as monotherapy and combination therapy. This medication down regulates estrogen, thus increasing FSH production and ovulation.

SELECTIVE REDUCTION OF MULTIFETAL PREGNANCY

Multifetal reduction is a procedure that may be carried out between 9 –24 weeks gestation. It may be considered in any multi gestation of 2 or more, but is more likely to be performed with higher order multiples of 4 or more. It is widely known that multiple gestation incur higher risks and complications to both the mother and fetuses than a singleton pregnancy. These risks increase significantly with increasing number of fetuses. Selective reduction of multifetal pregnancy is a term used when the number of fetuses is reduced to increase the likelihood that the pregnancy can continue. Furthermore, selective reduction of multifetal pregnancy is carried out in an effort to decrease morbidity and mortality risks to the mother and the remaining fetus(es). This procedure should only be considered if potential benefits outweigh risks and if the fetus(es) being terminated have a separate placenta. The procedure is performed by ultrasound-guided injection of potassium chloride into the heart of the fetus to be terminated.

PERGONAL, CLOMID, AND DANAZOL

Pergonal and Clomid are used in the treatment of female infertility. Pergonal is a gonadotropin stimulant and stimulates the production of FSH and LH. Possible side effects are multiple gestation and ovarian hyperstimulation syndrome. Clomid is also a gonadotropin stimulant fertility drug. This is a commonly used drug that competes with estrogen release in the hypothalamus, creating a negative feedback cycle. As with all fertility drugs, there is increased risk of multiple gestation. Danazol is a modified testosterone, primarily used for the treatment of endometriosis. Side effects are those associated with an amenorrheic state and female masculinization. This drug is contraindicated in pregnancy.

SONOGRAPHIC FOLLICULAR MONITORING FOR ASSISTED REPRODUCTIVE TECHNOLOGY TREATMENTS

Sonographic follicular monitoring is used in a number of assisted reproductive technology treatments. It is used to monitor women that are being treated for infertility clomiphene, insemination, and HCG. Sonographic follicular monitoring is useful for monitoring the above treatments to determine timing of inseminations, timing of cycles that cannot be monitored by the LH kit, and timing of cycles that are difficult to monitor by basal body temperatures. Furthermore, sonographic follicular monitoring is used to monitor complications of the above treatments, most notably ovarian hyperstimulation syndrome. If the ovaries are being hyperstimulated, sonography will reveal progressive ovarian enlargement and ascites in the pelvic and abdominal cavity.

IVF, GIFT, AND ZIFT

In-vitro fertilization (IVF) is an infertility treatment option that may be used when there is a defect in spermatogenesis. It attempts to use the infertile partner's sperm to fertilize an egg outside of the body. This technique is often used in combination with ET (embryo transfer). Gamete intrafallopian transfer (GIFT) attempts to treat infertility by removing an egg from the female ovary (after harvesting and injection with hCG) and mixing it with sperm outside of the body, and then laparoscopically placing it into the intact and functioning fallopian tube. Zygote intrafallopian transfer (ZIFT) is similar to the GIFT procedure, except that the egg and sperm are not returned to the intact fallopian tube until they are in their fertilized, zygote form. Therefore, ZIFT requires in vitro fertilization.

AMNIOCENTESIS

An amniocentesis is offered in cases that have an increased risk of chromosomal defects such as mothers who are ages 35 or older or in cases of positive prenatal screenings. They may also be performed if either parent has a known genetic disorder, if there is a history of malformations in earlier pregnancies (such as neural tube defects or Down syndrome), or if an ultrasound suggested possible deformities or could not find the cause of any abnormal labs. Although this exam is typically performed to diagnose chromosomal defects, it can also determine the blood type of the fetus or evaluate the maturity of the lungs. An amniocentesis examines the amniotic fluid, which contains chemicals released by the baby as well as fetal cells to assess for any birth defects. This study should be performed after 15 weeks to avoid the risk of dry taps.

PERFORMANCE UNDER ULTRASOUND GUIDANCE

The sonographer should always make sure that written consent is obtained and questions that the patient may have about an amniocentesis are answered prior to the procedure. Associated risks should also be communicated prior to the start of the exam. Prior ultrasound exams and reports should be obtained, if any were completed. An ultrasound survey should be performed prior to the start of an amniocentesis to determine fetal position, movement, presence of cardiac activity, placental location, and largest vertical pocket of amniotic fluid (this is found with a transverse position of the probe). The operator must be sure that the transducer is perpendicular to the mother's abdomen. Sterile technique must be performed during this procedure to decrease any risk of infection. The needle must always be visualized and especially before it is inserted into the amniotic cavity. It is ideal to withdraw 20 cc of fluid that does not contain cells from the mother for proper evaluation. The amniotic fluid should be labeled and sent to the lab for analysis.

ACETYLCHOLINESTERASE AND TRIPLE SCREEN TESTING

Acetylcholinesterase (ACHE) is a protein that can be evaluated during pregnancy to determine increased risks for the development of neural tube defects in a fetus. The test is usually only used after a positive AFP test. ACHE testing is done via amniocentesis. Although ACHE testing offers greater specificity for fetal neurological defect determination, it may also be positive in a number of other fetal abnormalities. It should be used in conjunction with other maternal screening tests and not independently. The triple maternal screen incorporates testing of AFP, unconjugated estriol, and human chorionic gonadotropin to determine risk for fetal chromosomal anomalies. Maternal triple screening specifically evaluates the risk of delivering a baby with Down syndrome and trisomy 18. False positive rates for the triple screen are as high as 6%.

BIOPHYSICAL PROFILE

The biophysical profile is one of several methods used to assess fetal well-being. The biophysical profile grades five areas of well-being, giving each category a score of "0" for abnormal or a score of "2" for normal. The five areas evaluated are: fetal breathing movements, fetal body movement, fetal tone, reactive fetal heart rate (nonstress test), and amniotic fluid volume. The scores are added together and a score of 8-10 indicates normal fetal well-being. A score of 6 is equivocal and a score of less than or equal to 4 is abnormal.

ACUTE FETAL DISTRESS

In terms of biophysical profile markers, acute fetal distress can be diagnosed with a score of "0" in any of the categories. Fetal distress is present if there are no fetal breath movements for 30 consecutive seconds in a 30-minute monitoring period. Acute fetal distress may be present if there are less than 3 fetal body/limb movements in 30 minutes. Fetal tone assessment that reveals a flaccid posture indicates fetal distress. A nonreactive nonstress test is consistent with acute fetal distress. Finally, inadequate amniotic fluid or no amniotic fluid indicates acute fetal distress. The biophysical profile defines inadequate amniotic fluid as the absence of amniotic fluid pockets greater than 1 cm after evaluation in two perpendicular planes.

PLACENTA PREVIA

Placenta previa is a condition in which the placenta is abnormally located in relation to the cervical os. Complete placenta previa is defined as a complete coverage of the cervical os by the placenta. Partial placenta previa is described when the border of the placenta covers only a portion of the cervical os. Marginal placenta previa is diagnosed if the placental margin is directly adjacent to the cervical os, but not covering the os. A low-lying placenta previa is described if any portion of the placenta is located near, but not directly adjacent to, the cervical os.

The dangers of placenta previa lie in the fact that the placenta is blocking the baby's exit during delivery. As the cervical os dilates and the cervix thins, during labor, the vessels of the placenta may stretch and tear. This causes life-threatening blood loss for both the mother and baby. Reported incidence with which placenta previa occurs varies greatly, from approximately one in every 200 pregnancies to one in every 500 pregnancies. Exact causes of developing placenta previa are unknown, but several risk factors exist. Multiparous women, multiple pregnancy, adhesions, smoking, maternal age greater than 35 years, drug use, and placenta previa in previous pregnancy increase the risk of placenta previa.

SIGNS, SYMPTOMS, AND DIAGNOSIS

Vaginal bleeding is the main sign of placenta previa. This can occur as spotting in the first or second trimester and as profuse and sudden bleeding in the third trimester. Once bleeding is present, cramping may develop but is rare. Blood loss is usually maternal in origin; therefore, signs of fetal distress are usually not apparent initially, but be weary of signs of maternal shock with large amounts of blood loss. Diagnosis of placenta previa is via ultrasound. Ultrasound allows for a precise description of the placental location, especially its relative location to the cervical os. The diagnosis should not be made before 20 weeks of gestation because of normal placental migration and localization. If placenta previa is suspected, digital pelvic exam should be avoided.

CHORIOCARCINOMA

Choriocarcinoma is the most severe of the gestational trophoblastic diseases. Choriocarcinoma is essentially a placental cancer. It can be localized to the uterus, but more likely it metastasizes to the brain and pulmonary and hepatic systems. Half of all cases of choriocarcinoma are preceded by a partial or classic hydatidiform molar pregnancy. The other half of choriocarcinomas occurs after spontaneous abortion, ectopic pregnancy termination, and normal pregnancies. Sonographically, choriocarcinoma must be differentiated from complete mole. Prognosis is dependent on metastasis, with brain and liver metastasis holding the poorest prognosis and response to chemotherapy.

PLACENTAL ABRUPTION

Placental abruption is the premature separation of the placenta from the uterine wall. This deprives the fetus of nutrients and oxygen and can cause maternal bleeding. The condition can be partial or complete and may be life-threatening to mother and baby. Signs and symptoms are similar to that of placenta previa but usually with greater pain and cramping symptoms. Ultrasound has little value in the diagnosis of placental abruption, and is primarily used to exclude placenta previa. Diagnosis is primarily clinical and with fetal monitoring. Hypertension is the most common cause of abruptio placentae.

PLACENTA ACCRETA

Placenta accreta should be suspected in any gravid female with placenta previa and an elevated serum alpha-fetoprotein. These findings should be further evaluated with sonography and sometimes MRI. Although definitive prelabor diagnosis is rare, there are characteristic sonographic findings that make the diagnosis more likely. If the muscular area behind the placenta is thinned to less than 2 mm on sonographic measurements, placenta accreta is likely. Irregular, "punched-out" areas of the placenta appearing alternatingly hypoechoic and anechoic are consistent sonographic findings of placenta accreta. Doppler studies can further accentuate these hypoechoic areas secondary to the rapid blood flow within them.

PLACENTAL INFARCTION

It is unusual to identify a placental infarction with ultrasound because they are often isoechoic to the placenta, and this can create difficulty in identifying them sonographically. Typically, most placental infarctions involve a minuscule portion of the placenta (less than 5%) and they do not affect the pregnancy. However, if a third or more of the placenta is affected, there is an increased chance of pregnancy complications including premature labor, intrauterine growth restriction, or possibly fetal demise. Placental infarctions are not generally visualized during a sonogram except when a hemorrhage is present, which tends to display a hypoechoic region surrounded by a hyperechoic rim. It has been determined that most infarctions are due to thrombosis of an artery connecting the placenta to the uterus, but some cases are due to hypertension and a pregnancy that has extended beyond the expected due date.

BENEFIT OF SMI DURING EVALUATION OF PLACENTA IF INFARCTION IS SUSPECTED

Superb microvascular imaging (SMI) is a new ultrasound technology that can detect blood flow that is moving at an extremely slow rate, which includes blood flow within tiny vessels. Often, these small vessels cannot be detected by conventional color or power Doppler imaging. SMI shows promise during OB exams in which a placental infarction is suspected. An infarction cannot typically be visualized sonographically because it appears isoechoic to the surrounding tissue of the placenta (unless it has a hemorrhagic component that appears hypoechoic). SMI is effective at detecting lower velocities because it removes the artifacts created by tissue motion. In a normal placenta, SMI can accurately portray the vessels that branch out to the peripheral villous components in the maternal surface. In cases of placental infarction, this demonstration of branching vessels cannot be visualized with SMI. SMI is also helpful because operators can increase the frame rate to help compensate for a fetus that is moving.

PLACENTA CIRCUMMARGINATE AND PLACENTA CIRCUMVALLATE

Both conditions affect the normal placental shape. The normal placenta is a discoid shape with membranous edges extending smoothly to the placental edges. Furthermore, the placenta attaches to the uterine wall. Conditions affecting the placental margin result in abnormal placental shape. A circummarginate placenta is a condition in which the fetal chorionic membrane does not reach to the edges of the placenta, from the center. In this situation, the edges of the placenta are covered with a smooth layer of chorion. Similarly, circumvallate placenta is an abnormality in which the fetal chorionic membrane is larger than the placenta and forms folds and prevents a smooth placental edge. Circumvallate placenta can be partial or complete; therefore, it is important to image the entire margin of the placenta. Complete circumvallate placenta is associated with fetal and labor problems. Partial circumvallate placenta and circummarginate placenta are generally not associated with fetal abnormality.

PLACENTA MEMBRANACEA AND PLACENTA SUCCENTURIATE

Both placenta membranacea and placenta succenturiate are conditions that affect normal placental shape. Placenta membranacea is a condition in which the villus of the gestational sac does not regress as through pregnancy. This results in the surface of the gestational sac being entirely covered by placenta. In this condition, the placental membrane will appear abnormally thin. A succenturiate placenta, also known as an accessory lobe, may form in the case of partial placenta membranacea. This accessory placental lobe forms with spotty regression of the villi. The succenturiate is attached to the primary placenta via uterine wall vessels. A succenturiate placental lobe may result in delivery complications.

ACCESSORY LOBE OF THE PLACENTA

It is important for ultrasound operators to assess the size and shape of the placenta because it is the lifeline for the fetus. An accessory lobe (succenturiate) is a mass of placental tissue that is connected to the main portion of the placenta by blood vessels. It is important to diagnose an accessory lobe because this area of the placenta may not be delivered with the main lobe of the placenta, and it could cause maternal bleeding after childbirth. Vasa previa is one of the main concerns for the correct identification of an accessory lobe because the vessels may be positioned between the cervix and the presenting fetal anatomy. This may lead to constriction of the blood vessels or rupture of the tissues. If vasa previa is diagnosed, a cesarean section is planned for the patient. An accessory lobe of the placenta is found about 5% of the time.

ULTRASOUND APPEARANCE

The placenta is a curved organ that attaches to the uterine wall during pregnancy. This organ supplies the fetus with oxygen and nutrients, and it clears wastes from the fetal circulation. The placenta is disk shaped, extremely vascular, and separated into maternal and fetal divisions. When a patient has an accessory lobe of the placenta, it can be classified as one of three types including succenturiate, bipartite, and annular placentas. A succenturiate lobe will be identified by ultrasound as an additional (yet smaller) component of the placenta that is connected to the main portion by blood vessels. A bipartite placenta (also referred to as a bilobed placenta) appears as two placental lobes also connected by blood vessels. As opposed to the succenturiate lobe, these divisions of the placenta are the same size and are connected by chorionic tissue that provides a thin connection of the two lobes. An annular placenta is one that forms a ring around the internal uterus. All of these are important to document so that placental retention does not create bleeding or infection after the child is born.

CHORIOANGIOMA

A chorioangioma is a benign vascular tumor of the placenta. As its name would suggest, it arises from chorionic tissue. Determining whether a chorioangioma is at high-risk for causing fetal or maternal difficulties is dependent on two variables: size and vascularity. Any chorioangioma greater than 5 cm increases the risk for complications. The greater blood flow (determined with Doppler studies), the more likely fetal complications will develop. Sonographically, a chorioangioma is usually visualized at the insertion site of the placental cord. It will appear as a clearly demarcated and round lesion. Careful evaluation of the fetus for conditions of volume overload and hydrops is necessary in the event of visualizing a chorioangioma. Regular sonographic monitoring is indicated.

PLACENTAL CALCIFICATIONS AND CYSTIC LESIONS

Placental calcifications are found in over half of pregnancies in the third trimester. Although this can be a normal finding, mothers that use tobacco products, heparin or aspirin therapy secondary to coagulation disorders, and mothers that have delivered fewer babies are more likely to have greater degrees of calcification. Common areas to image placental calcifications are at the septa, base, and around the chorionic and villous spaces. Cystic lesions may also be viewed on sonographic evaluation as a hypoechoic area almost anywhere on the placenta. They are common and usually insignificant.

OLIGOHYDRAMNIOS AND POLYHYDRAMNIOS

Oligohydramnios indicates insufficient amounts of amniotic fluid, usually less than 300 mL. Oligohydramnios may be defined in a number of ways. If using the AFI, oligohydramnios is present if < 5 cm. If sonographic measurement of vertical pockets in the uterine quadrants are < 2 cm, consider oligohydramnios. Oligohydramnios may occur with abnormalities in fetal urinary tract and kidney development as well as intrauterine growth restriction. Polyhydramnios is the presence of excessive amounts of amniotic fluid, usually > 2000 mL. Using the AFI, polyhydramnios is defined as a measurement of > 20 cm. Polyhydramnios may occur in any situation in which the fetal ability to swallow and absorb amniotic fluid is compromised.

AMNIOTIC BAND SYNDROME

Amniotic band syndrome is a condition in which many congenital malformations are present ranging from mild to complex. An example of a mild malformation is lymphedema of the digits due to constriction bands. An example of complex defects from amniotic band syndrome is fetal limb amputation. The constricting bands of tissue seen in this syndrome can affect almost any part of the fetal anatomy. Ambiguous genitalia, facial clefts and severe abdominal wall deformities are also seen in amniotic band syndrome. The prevalence of amniotic band syndrome is approximately 7 in every 10,000 live births. Amniotic band syndrome should be differentiated from body stalk anomalies and the presence of an amniotic sheet, versus constricting amniotic bands, when performing the sonogram.

TREATMENT OF RH INCOMPATIBILITY IN PREGNANCY

The best treatment of Rh Incompatibility in pregnancy is prevention. Maternal isoimmunization can be prevented with the RhoGam injection. This injection is an immunoglobulin that prevents the mother from making antibodies against the fetal Rh antigens. It can be given mid-pregnancy if the father is Rh positive. A second injection will then be given before delivery. If the infant has already been affected, treatment of jaundice includes hydration and phototherapy with bilirubin lights/blanket. In the event of hydrops fetalis, amniocentesis can be performed to determine severity and guide treatment. Intrauterine fetal transfusion, neonatal transfusion, labor induction, and treatment of fetal/newborn congestive heart failure may be performed in the presence of hydrops fetalis. If kernicterus is present, multiple exchange transfusions and phototherapy are necessary.

TURNER SYNDROME

Turner syndrome is a genetic disorder seen in females only. It may also be termed XO syndrome, Monosomy X, and gonadal dysgenesis. The incidence is 1 in 2,000 live births. There is a high rate of miscarriage in fetuses with Turner syndrome, miscarriage and prognosis is highly dependent on the presence and degree of fetal hydrops and pleural effusion. A potential sonographic finding associated with XO syndrome is cystic hygroma, which refers to multiple serous fluid collections, particularly around the shoulders and neck. Heart and kidney defects are probable sonographic findings in Turner syndrome.

IUGR

Intrauterine growth restriction (IUGR) is a condition or term used to define a fetal weight that is below the 10th percentile for gestational age. This is determined by fetal weight and gestational age tables. Further definition of IUGR includes a fetal abdominal circumference measurement less than the 2.5 percentile. Intrauterine growth restriction should be differentiated from 'small-for-gestational-age'. If a fetus is small-for-gestational-age, they are otherwise healthy and have reached their appropriate growth potential. Usually a diagnosis of small-for-gestational-age is made retrospectively and after delivery and evaluation. IUGR carries a high risk for perinatal mortality and morbidity. Accurate and early diagnosis, however, can reduce mortality rates.

RISK FACTORS AND CAUSES

There are several risk factors for the development of intrauterine growth restriction. Anatomical/physiologic risk factors include a small maternal uterus and placental abnormalities. High altitude is considered an environmental risk. Poor maternal nutrition and/or maternal use of drugs, alcohol, tobacco products, and certain prescription medications increase the risk for development of IUGR. Furthermore, maternal vascular and heart disease, diabetes, kidney disease, asthma, GI disorders, and bleeding/clotting disorders can contribute to the development of IUGR. Previous miscarriage, multiple pregnancy, and maternal infections (viral, parasitic, and bacterial) are causative for IUGR. Complications during pregnancy such as preeclampsia, eclampsia and HELP syndrome are correlated with IUGR. Fetal chromosomal abnormalities also increase the risk of comorbid IUGR.

TYPES

The two types of intrauterine growth restriction can be distinguished by sonography; they are asymmetric IUGR and symmetric IUGR. Asymmetric IUGR describes an unequal decrease in the size of fetal anatomical structures. In asymmetric IUGR, normal sonographic biparietal diameter measurements may exist, but abdominal circumference measurements may be well below the expected ranges. This is often times due to fetal malnutrition secondary to placental insufficiency. The fetus with asymmetric IUGR will direct its energy to maintaining the heart and brain (thus normal development) at the expensive of the liver and other structures. Symmetrical IUGR is the second type. Symmetrical IUGR reveals proportionate decreased measurements and size in all major fetal structures.

CORDOCENTESIS

Cordocentesis is also known as percutaneous umbilical blood sampling, which is more descriptive of the technique. Cordocentesis requires an ultrasound to locate the insertion point of the umbilical cord into the placenta. With ultrasound guiding, a needle is inserted through the maternal abdomen, through the maternal uterine wall, and into the umbilical cord to collect a small sampling of cord blood. The sample is collected from the umbilical vein. Note: cordocentesis cannot be undertaken unless the fetus is immobilized by use of intramuscular fetal injection of muscle relaxant. The blood sample is then sent for laboratory analysis. Cordocentesis may be performed when other testing methods such as amniocentesis and ultrasound are inconclusive. It is performed after 17 weeks of gestation.

Battledore Placenta, Velamentous Insertion, and Vasa Previa

All three terms describe abnormal umbilical cord insertion upon the placenta:

- Battledore placenta – a condition in which the umbilical cord inserts on the edge of the placenta rather than its normal central insertion site. This is usually clinically insignificant.
- Velamentous insertion – a condition in which the vessels of the umbilical cord separate and then insert into the edge of the placenta. The separation of the vessels leaves them without the protective gelatinous material. A velamentous insertion increases fetal abnormalities and complications, growth restriction, and preterm labor.
- Vasa previa – a condition in which the vessels of the umbilical cord separate, cross the cervical os and then attach to the edge of the placenta. Vasa previa occurs approximately once every 3,000 births and has a fetal mortality rate of at least 75%.

Short Cord Umbilicus Abnormalities

Abnormal embryologic development and folding of cord material usually starts at about the 4th to 5th week of development. The same conditions that result in complete lack of umbilical cord formation can also result in short cord syndrome. Sometimes an umbilical cord can form from fetal abdominal wall material (body stalk anomaly). A short umbilical cord restricts fetal movement resulting in a number of fetal abnormalities including: cord compression, placental abruption, limb abnormalities, body wall defects, fetal heart rate abnormalities and compromised fetal descent during labor. Insufficient amniotic fluid, multiple pregnancy, maternal use of cocaine, amniotic bands, and other fetal abnormalities correlate with the finding of short umbilical cord.

Vascular Umbilical Cord Abnormalities

The most common (1% of pregnancies) vascular abnormality of the umbilical cord is the presence of only one umbilical artery instead of two. This should be evaluated at the fetal end of the umbilical cord, not the placental end, to avoid arterial fusion, which is a normal variant. The absence of the second umbilical artery is likely from clotting in the artery, resulting in infarction. If a single umbilical cord artery is confirmed, about a 40% chance of other fetal abnormalities and malformation exists. Rarely, an increased number of umbilical cord vessels may be noted. This condition is known as a multivessel cord and is associated with conjoined twins and fetal malformation.

Abnormal Umbilical Cord Structural Formation

The presence of a structurally abnormal or absent umbilical cord usually has a fatal prognosis for the fetus. Structural cord abnormalities are secondary to an abnormal embryonic folding that results in fetal abdominal wall malformation. Without an umbilical cord, the fetus is directly attached to the placenta. On sonographic evaluation the umbilical cord will not be visualized and the fetal abdominal organs will appear herniated or outside of the fetal body. Limb abnormalities may also be visualized. This condition is also termed: congenital absence/aplasia of the umbilical cord, body stalk anomaly, or limb-body wall complex.

Long Cord Umbilicus Abnormalities

The term long cord is often synonymous with nuchal cord or nuchal loops. Nuchal loops may be found in up to 25% of pregnancies. Nuchal cords are a condition in which the umbilical cord is looped (at least twice) around the fetal neck. An abnormally long umbilical cord is more likely to be associated with cord knots and cord prolapse. Umbilical cord prolapse is seen in up to 1 in 300 pregnancies. A prolapse occurs when a portion or loop of umbilical cord slips into the vaginal canal after membranes rupture but before the baby descends into the birth canal. All of the above aforementioned conditions can still result in a healthy baby, but there may be a higher incidence of fetal heart rate patterns, amniotic meconium, and cesarean delivery. Nuchal cord and long cord abnormalities present complications because of the stretching and/or compression they place on umbilical cord vessels.

UMBILICAL CORD CYSTS

Three main types of umbilical cord cysts exist. If cysts are visualized in the first trimester, they may resolve or turn out to be a normal variant. Second and third trimester cysts may be associated with increased concern for fetal anomalies. The first type is omphalomesenteric duct cyst. This cyst arises from yolk stalk tissue and is viewed with ultrasound near the fetal end of the umbilical cord insertion. The second type of umbilical cord cyst is the allantois or urachus duct cyst. Embryologically, this structure extends from the fetal bladder to the umbilical cord. This type of cyst is often seen near the fetal end, separates the umbilical vessels, and is associated with fetal abnormalities. Thirdly, a pseudocyst is from inflammation of the Wharton's jelly. The umbilical vessels can travel through these cysts and the cysts are usually insignificant and sometimes resolve on their own.

UMBILICAL CORD MASSES

Umbilical cord hemangiomas are often seen near the placental end of the cord as an echogenic area. Edema may be visualized beyond the actual area of hemangioma. This may involve bleeding, fetal anemia and hydrops. A cord hemangioma can be differentiated by an umbilical cord teratoma by the presence of sonographic calcifications within the echogenic cord mass. An aneurysm is another cord mass that may be sonographically visualized as a local dilation of any of the umbilical vessels. These can clot and cause fetal death. An umbilical cord hematoma occurs in approximately 1 in every 500 births. Increasing incidence is secondary to increased amniocentesis and cord blood sampling. This can usually be seen near the fetal end of the umbilical cord and is usually the result of the fetal umbilical vein being ruptured. Fetal mortality is variable but as high as 50%.

SHIRODKAR PROCEDURE, MCDONALD'S PROCEDURE, AND CONE PROCEDURE

Shirodkar procedure is the placement of a permanent 'purse-string' type suture around the lower cervix. This is used in conditions in which the gravid female has an incompetent cervix, to prevent premature delivery. Cesarean delivery is then necessary. McDonald's procedure is also used to prevent premature delivery in incompetent cervix; however, the suture in this procedure is placed as a band around the superior portion of the cervix and is removable. This procedure is often used if cervical effacement of the inferior portion of the cervix has begun. A cone procedure is biopsy-like procedure used obtain a larger sample of cervical cells when evaluating an abnormal pap smear and/or colposcopy. This may be diagnostic as well as a treatment for removal of abnormal cells.

CERVICAL INCOMPETENCE AND CERVICAL CERCLAGE

Causes of premature cervical widening and thinning are a history of previous cervical incompetence, previous cervical surgery (cone biopsy) or injury, and previous dilation and curettage. Risk for cervical incompetence also increases with DES exposure and anatomical anomalies. The incidence of cervical incompetence is approximately 1% of all pregnancies, but it can cause up to 25% of all second trimester miscarriages.

Cervical cerclage is the treatment of choice for an incompetent cervix. It is performed after the 12th week gestation. It is a procedure in which the cervical os is sutured shut, to prevent preterm dilation, thinning, and bulging membranes.

HYDROSALPINX AND CYSTADENOMA

Hydrosalpinx is a fluid collection in one or both fallopian tubes that may become obstructing. It may occur as the result of a pelvic infection. The history of this in a pregravid female may raise fertility concerns. Found during obstetrical ultrasound, it may be visualized as a rounded cyst with multiple septations. Hydrosalpinx must be differentiated from a cystadenoma. A cystadenoma is the most common *cystic* ovarian tumor. The sonographic appearance varies greatly, from a cystic mass without septations to a cystic mass with multiple thin or thick septations. The sonographic appearance of nodules in a cystadenoma increases the concern for malignancy.

COEXISTING MATERNAL DISORDERS RELATED TO PELVIC MASSES

Many gynecological conditions may exist prior to a woman becoming gravid. These conditions may or may not have been symptomatic in the pregravid state. Pregnancy may result in these preexisting conditions becoming noticeable or identified if they were previously asymptomatic. On the other hand, if symptoms did exist prior to conception, they may intensify during pregnancy. Sonographically speaking, gynecological conditions can be broken down into 2 categories: the presence of a palpable and sonographically identifiable pelvic mass, and areas of referred pain that can be evaluated sonographically (flank, abdomen, and extremities). Sonographic masses less than 5 cm of non-obstetrical origin may be monitored with the watch and wait approach. Surgical consideration must be given to all other masses. The primary limiting factor in detecting pelvic masses is maternal obesity.

MATERNAL ALLOIMMUNIZATION

Maternal alloimmunization or isoimmunization is also known as Rh incompatibility. This occurs when a mother has rhesus or Rh-negative blood and her fetus has Rh-positive blood. When the mother's Rh-negative blood comes into contact with the fetus Rh-positive blood cells, through placental nourishment, the mother makes antibodies against the Rh-positive blood cells. These antibodies against the Rh-positive blood may cross the placenta and start to destroy fetal red blood cells. The first pregnancy is usually not affected, but successive pregnancies may be affected and Rh incompatibility can cause a range of problems for the fetus, from mild to fatal. Hemolysis can occur, resulting in a jaundiced baby. Severe and even fatal fetal complications of Rh incompatibility are hydrops fetalis and kernicterus.

POSTPARTUM HEMORRHAGE

Postpartum hemorrhage is defined as a maternal blood loss of at least 500 mL after vaginal delivery or at least 1000 mL after cesarean section. Postpartum hemorrhage is further defined by the timing at which it occurs. Primary postpartum hemorrhage develops within the first 24 hours after delivery. Maternal hemorrhage that develops after 24 hours of delivery is termed secondary postpartum hemorrhage. Postpartum hemorrhage is the leading maternal cause of death. The risks for primary or secondary postpartum hemorrhage include: lack of uterine constriction, trauma during delivery, maternal bleeding or clotting disorders, abnormal implantation of placenta, and retained products of conception.

PRETERM LABOR

Preterm labor is defined as regular contractions, cervical dilation, and ruptured membranes prior to gestational week 37. Approximately 12% of births are premature and of these, 25% are intentional or induced preterm labor for medical reasons. About 75% of preterm labors are spontaneous. Risk factors for preterm labor include maternal infection, smoking, drug/alcohol use, poor nutrition, and stress. Maternal infections, chronic maternal disease states and maternal socioeconomic status have also been implicated. Preterm labor is more likely with multiple gestation, placental abnormalities, maternal anatomical anomalies, and fetal abnormalities. Assessment of preterm labor includes evaluation of the maternal cervix and cervical secretions looking for the presence of a protein fibronectin. Monitoring of force and frequency of uterine contractions with a tocodynamometer may be used (less frequently) to assess risk of preterm labor. Sonographic assessment of preterm labor by measurement of cervical length measurement is a commonly used diagnostic tool as well.

NON-GYNECOLOGIC MATERNAL DISORDERS THAT PRESENT WITH PAIN

Several non-gynecological maternal disorders causing pain may coexist with a normal pregnancy. We will limit this discussion to disorders that have an increased propensity to develop during pregnancy and those that can be successfully evaluated and diagnosed with sonography. Acute cholecystitis may occur as the result of preexisting gallstones, or the development of stones during pregnancy. Appendicitis may occur during pregnancy. Sonographically, look for the appendix to be more superior and laterally located (in the gravid patient) to its normal anatomical position. Pyelonephritis may be sonographically evaluated in the presence of localized flank pain and a positive urine culture. Deep vein thrombosis can best be diagnosed with venous duplex ultrasound. Ureteral calculus may occur and may be diagnosed with sonography and/or intravenous urogram to assess obstruction.

COMPLICATIONS OF MATERNAL HYPERTENSION

The two most common pregnancy-induced hypertensive disorders are preeclampsia and eclampsia. Preeclampsia is defined as the development of the triad of hypertension, proteinuria, and edema during pregnancy. This is further subdivided into mild and severe depending on the degrees of the three conditions. Preeclampsia usually develops around the second half of pregnancy. Eclampsia is defined when all of the criteria for preeclampsia are met plus the presence of convulsions. Eclampsia is more commonly seen in the first 72 postpartum hours. Sonographic findings of intrauterine growth restriction, decreased placental volume or rapid placental maturation, insufficient amniotic fluid amounts, and fetal demise are correlated with a preeclamptic pregnancy. Doppler studies may show vascular resistance in the placenta.

PELVIC MASSES INVOLVING NON-GYNECOLOGICAL STRUCTURES

There are several other situations and pelvic structures that may be confused as a gynecological mass or pathology. It is important for the sonographer to find the origin of these other non-gynecological structures. If this is not possible, then documentation of normal appearing gynecological and non-gynecological structure is helpful as a 'process of elimination'. Diverticuli in the colon, abscessed colon, colonic mass, inflammatory bowel disease, and stool may be confused with a gynecologic mass. Appendicitis, urinary bladder distention, urinary diverticuli, and ureter stone or dilation also needs to be differentiated from gynecologic pelvic structures.

FETAL ANOMALIES THAT MAY BE ASSOCIATED WITH MATERNAL DIABETES MELLITUS

Gestational diabetes develops during pregnancy and usually after embryo development and primary organogenesis; therefore, the fetus does not suffer any major defects. However, pre-existing maternal diabetes can result in a number of structural fetal defects ranging from minor to severe. Greater-than-normal birth weight (macrosomia) is a common complication. Fetal absence of the bony sacrum and neural tube defects such as spina bifida are also highly associated with pre-existing maternal diabetes. Cerebellar encephalocele in the fetus is specific to maternal diabetes and a number of other central nervous system anomalies affecting the brain and cranium. Increased risk of cardiac abnormalities such as aortic coarctation and ventricular septal defect may also be present. Abdominal organ disorders, including many kidney anomalies, are potential complications. Even lower fetal limb fusion (sirenomelia) is possible with pre-existing maternal diabetes.

ANOVULATION AS A CAUSE OF INFERTILITY

Anovulation is responsible for about 30% of infertility. Signs of anovulation may be changes in menstrual flow (excessive, light, or absent), irregular basal temperatures, or change in premenstrual symptoms (presence or absence of PMS). Common causes of anovulation are: excess weight gain or loss, excess exercise, frequent travel, breast feeding, stress, thyroid disorders and polycystic ovary syndrome. Conception is dependent on the release of an egg from the ovary (ovulation), which then travels through the fallopian tube to unite with a sperm. If there is lack of cyclical egg release (anovulation), it follows that there is no chance of pregnancy. So identifying and attempting to correct the disorders that would prevent this are important. Restoration of regular ovulation may be done with lifestyle changes and medication.

PELVIC ULTRASOUND OF NONPREGNANT FEMALE PATIENT

The ultrasound of a nonpregnant female patient can be done in a longitudinal or transverse plane as well as the oblique plane. The uterus, including the fundus, cervix, and corpus, should be seen. The endometrium, both ovaries and fallopian tubes, and the vaginal canal should be imaged. Either transvaginal examination or transabdominal transducers can be used and an acoustic medium gel offers the best imaging medium. Measure any mass, cyst, or node imaged. Measure any uterine myomas in three dimensions and show it as intramural, submucosal, subserosal, or pedunculated. Investigate the cul-de-sac for fluid or mass. Document important laboratory tests and past medical history that may influence or support the images obtained with the ultrasound.

SAGITTAL SCAN SONOGRAM

The sagittal (or longitudinal) scanning plane is that which runs from the head to the foot and divides the patient into right and left halves. Some examples of structures that are seen in the sagittal plane are the uterus and cervix. The correct orientation of a saggital scan sonogram is as follows:

- Posterior is at the bottom of the sonogram
- For a sagittal scan through the pancreas and aorta, the direction of the patient's feet is on the right side of the sonogram
- For a sagittal scan in the right breast, the direction of the patient's head is on the left side of the sonogram.

TRANSABDOMINAL SONOGRAPHY, ENDOVAGINAL SONOGRAPHY, AND SONOHYSTEROGRAPHY

Transabdominal sonographs are commonly used to evaluate pelvic structures and organs. This technique is especially useful in evaluation of upper uterine and pelvic masses, ovaries and ectopic pregnancies. It is also widely used in the gravid female, for fetal monitoring and assessment. Transabdominal sonography may be synonymous with pelvic sonography. It may be done with a full urinary bladder to enhance the appearance of some structures. An endovaginal or transvaginal sonography allows for view of pelvic structures, especially those that are more inferiorly and posteriorly located. These sonographs are usually of greater quality. It is important for the technician to thoroughly describe this procedure to the patient prior to introducing the vaginal probe. Sonohysterography is used primarily to evaluate the endometrial structures, as a catheter is introduced into the endometrium, filling it with sterile saline solution.

ASSESSING PREMENARCHAL PATIENTS WITH ULTRASOUND

Menarche refers to a female's first menstrual period, often occurring between the ages of 11 and 14. Premenarchal refers to the time prior to the start of menstruation. Because most girls are virginal in this stage, transvaginal ultrasound (TVUS) is contraindicated, and, therefore, the transabdominal ultrasound (TAUS) technique should be used. This is performed while the patient has a full bladder to provide an optimal acoustic window. Anatomical structures that are identified during a pelvic ultrasound are the vagina, cervix, uterus, endometrium, ovaries, and bilateral adnexal regions. The anterior and posterior cul de sacs are also evaluated for the presence of free fluid. A quick survey of the patient's urinary bladder may also be performed. The advantage of a TAUS study over a TVUS study in this patient population is that it will allow for a wide field of view to provide a sufficient survey of the false pelvis during the postvoid portion of the exam. Any pathology that may have been shifted into the false pelvis by the distended bladder may be seen with this method.

PURPOSE

Premenarchal patients have not yet started their menstrual periods. Physicians may find it necessary to evaluate the pelvic organs in young patients for many reasons that include ambiguous genitalia (which is often noticed at birth), pelvic pain, palpable mass, or amenorrhea. Ultrasound findings in these situations may include an ovarian cyst or tumor, ovarian torsion, or an absent uterus. It is important to realize that neonatal females that are scanned may demonstrate a uterus or ovaries that are enlarged due to the effect of hormones from their mother. Around the ages of seven or eight, the uterus and ovaries tend to increase in size. The pediatric uterus will range from about 2.5 to 4 cm in length and about 1 cm wide. The endometrium will appear as a thin echogenic line when visualized — until puberty, when the patient begins her menstrual cycle. Ultrasound users may visualize ovarian follicles at any age, but the volume of pediatric ovaries when calculated tends to be less than 1 cm^3.

UPPER ABDOMINAL FINDINGS WITH PELVIC DISEASE

In addition to referred pain, the upper abdomen may contain clues to pelvic pathology on sonographic examination. Ovarian cancer should be considered if widespread serous fluid is imaged in the peritoneum or if a mass is imaged in the omental tissue. If liver metastases are sonographed, consider a primary cancer in the distal colon. Pelvic mass, inflammation, or pathology may affect the ureters, thus the demonstration of dilated kidney(s) on ultrasound. Incidental findings of widespread endometriosis and adhesions are often noted with laparoscopic appendectomy and cholecystectomy. Flexible sigmoidoscopy and colonoscopy findings obstructing or narrowing the patency of the colon may make one suspect pathology in surrounding structures.

ADULT FEMALE MENSTRUAL CYCLE

There are four main phases of the menstrual cycle. First is menstruation, counted from the first day of vaginal bleeding and lasting up to 4 days. During menstruation, the endometrium is shed which produces bleeding. Second is the follicular or proliferative phase lasting approximately from day 5 to 13? This phase is marked by maturation of follicles in the ovary by initially releasing FSH from the pituitary, then LH and estradiol. Estrogen then initiates formation of a proliferative layer of endometrium. Third is ovulation, approximately day 14, marked by a surge of LH and FSH. A mature ovarian follicle ruptures, releasing an egg. Fourth, the luteal or secretory phase is approximately day 15-28. The luteal phase is marked by a surge of progesterone, which converts the endometrial lining from a proliferative lining to a secretory lining.

IN UTERO DES EXPOSURE

The population that deserves the most consideration for complications and malformations associated with diethylstilbestrol (DES) exposure are those born between 1940 and 1970. At that time, DES was being given to pregnant women of high-risk pregnancies. It has been determined that fetal exposure to DES not only increases the risk of female organ cancer, but also increases uterine malformation as well. The inferior portion of the uterus, including the cervix, is the area most affected by the DES exposure. The endometrial canal and cervical os are severely narrowed by DES exposure. With this and the less affected fundus of the uterus, sonographic imaging with radiopaque material, often produces a "T" appearance of the endometrial cavity.

NORMAL ADULT UTERUS

From puberty through the teenage years, the uterine growth (along its longest axis) is up to about 3 more centimeters. The adult uterus weighs about 15 grams. At this stage the body of the uterus measures about 8 cm by 4 cm, while the cervix measures about 3 cm. The ratio of uterine body to cervix height is approximately 3:1 at this stage. The adult uterus is positioned centrally in the pelvic region with the urinary bladder anterior to it and rectum posterior to it. The broad ligaments attach to either side of the uterus laterally. There are several other smaller ligamentous networks that keep the uterus in its anatomical position.

AIUM GUIDELINES FOR PERFORMANCE OF ULTRASOUND EXAMINATION OF THE UTERUS

Sonographic evaluation of the uterus is not only important to diagnose uterine-related disorders, but often equally important as a reference point to evaluating other structures within the pelvic cavity. Thorough documentation of this structure is imperative. Document uterine size (in all planes), uterine shape and position, endometrial lining (thickness and both layers and all planes), myometrial lining (thickness and description), and cervical appearance (size, orientation, mass). If there is fluid present within any of these structures, do not include it in the measurement itself; rather, fluid gets its own description and measurement.

UTERINE DEVELOPMENT IN UTERO, INFANCY, AND CHILDHOOD

The uterus develops from Mullerian ducts that form the fallopian tubes. In normal cases, the fused ducts form the fallopian tubes and then the body of the uterus. Abnormal fusion of ducts leads to a variety of uterine malformations. From birth to about two years of age, the uterus slightly decreases in size. From the age of two to ten, the uterus takes on the size and shape of a pear. It remains a similar overall length measurement (3 cm) during this time, but the distribution changes. The uterus of a child has an equal ratio of uterine body length to cervix length. The ratio of uterine body length to cervix length doubles to triples at puberty. From about age 10 to 13 years of age, the total length of the uterus increases about 2 – 2.5 cm from its childhood length.

LEIOMYOMAS

Leiomyomas, more commonly termed uterine fibroids, are the most common benign pelvic mass in females. They usually develop after 30 years of age. The growths arise from the cells that make up the wall layers of the uterus. Patient complaints (increased menstrual flow and pain) and/or a mass palpated on pelvic exam prompts further evaluation. Ultrasound is diagnostic. Fibroids arising from the outer uterine layer may grow to a size larger than the uterus itself. Growth and development of leiomyomas appear to be the result of increased estrogen levels. Treatment options include: watchful waiting, medications, hysteroscopy, myomectomy, or hysterectomy.

DIDELPHYS UTERUS, DUPLEX BICOLLIS UTERUS, BICORNATE UTERUS, UNICORNUATE UTERUS, AND SEPTATED UTERUS

All are uterine malformations that develop when the Mullerian ducts do not fuse together correctly:

- Didelphys uterus – occurs when the Mullerian ducts don't fuse and develop into 2 separate cavities, forming 2 uteruses. They may have an individual or shared cervix and a single or divided vagina.
- Duplex bicollis uterus – two separate uteruses, two cervix and one vagina.
- Bicornate uterus – two fused uteruses (two uterine horns), one cervix and one vagina (upside down heart).

- Unicornuate uterus – occurs when only one of the Mullerian ducts forms. Often called a "one-sided uterus" or "half-uterus" (banana shape).
- Septated uterus – occurs when the Mullerian ducts fuse, but a partition remains. This septum usually just involves the body of the uterus, but may be seen as a complete partition from the uterus to the cervix and vagina.

ANATOMICAL STRUCTURES DOCUMENTED WITH SONOGRAPHIC EXAMINATION OF NONPAROUS UTERUS

In the nonparous female, a pelvic and transvaginal ultrasound may be performed. The pelvic portion gives an "overview" of pelvic structure, while the transvaginal approach allows for more detailed documentation of measurement and texture of structures. The size (in all major planes), angle, ratio, patency and positioning of associated structures of the uterus are documented. Major uterine anatomy includes the cervix, corpus (uterine body), cornu (where fallopian tubes enter uterus), and the fundus (above the cornu). Description of the thickness of the layers of the uterine wall should be included with emphasis on the innermost layer (endometrium) and the myometrium. The endometrium thickness can be dependent on the menstrual cycle, so LMP (last menstrual period) should be documented. Description of vasculature and of structures and spaces immediately outside the uterus are often documented (cul-de-sac of Douglas and vesicouterine pouch), especially if they contain fluid or are surrounded by adhesions.

CHANGES IN THE POSTMENOPAUSAL UTERUS

In the postmenopausal woman that is not on hormone replacement therapy, the sonographic appearance of her uterus will be much smaller than that of a premenopausal woman. The first thing to decrease in size is the muscular portion of the body of the uterus. By about five years, postmenopause, the ratio of length of uterine body to cervix is 1:1. In addition to uterine muscular shrinkage, the endometrium thins to less than 8 mm. The postmenopausal woman on hormone replacement therapy will maintain the sonographic uterine dimensions and appearance of an adult, premenopausal female.

LEIOMYOSARCOMA AND ADENOMYOSIS

Leiomyosarcoma of the uterus is an extremely rare cancer that arises from the smooth muscle cells of the myometrium of the uterine wall. Its prognosis is poor. The presence of uterine fibroids, even if severe, does not predispose a woman to the development of leiomyosarcoma. Adenomyosis is more commonly termed endometriosis. It is a noncancerous condition in which the cells that make up the layer of the inner uterus, endometrium, grow outside of the uterus. This can cause pain, menstrual irregularities and decreased fertility. The condition is diagnosed by patient history, physical exam, and usually confirmed with transvaginal ultrasound or laparoscopy.

MOST PRECISE MEASUREMENT OF THE ENDOMETRIAL THICKNESS

During routine grayscale imaging, axial resolution is superior to lateral and elevational resolution. Axial resolution is the ability to correctly portray two objects (front to back) that are located parallel to the main portion of the ultrasound wave. Axial resolution is not affected by the depth of the reflector, and it relies heavily on the spatial pulse length because shorter pulses create images with better detail. Lateral resolution is how two objects are portrayed when lying next to each other or perpendicular to the ultrasound beam. Elevational resolution tries to resolve the question of if the reflectors are within the beam or located above or below it. In this example, when measuring the thickness of the endometrium, the sonographer would want to take the measurement at an angle that is parallel to the beam so that the axial resolution is the most accurate.

SONOHYSTEROGRAPHY

Sonohysterography involves injecting sterile saline into the uterus by using a transcervical approach to evaluate the endometrium. This method provides clinicians with even more detail than a transvaginal ultrasound. This exam may be performed to better discern abnormal findings on a pelvic ultrasound; to better evaluate the endometrium when it appears thicker than normal; or in suspected cases of endometrial polyps, submucosal fibroids, cancer, or hyperplasia; to evaluate abnormal uterine bleeding; to investigate repeated pregnancy loss; or to determine if the patient's fallopian tubes are patent. If there is a greater amount of free fluid present after the saline is injected, there is patency of at least one of the fallopian tubes. It is important to note that sonohysterography should not be performed on patients who have extreme pelvic pain, are pregnant, or who may have a pelvic infection.

APPEARANCE OF ENDOMETRIUM ON SONOGRAM DURING THE MENSTRUAL CYCLE

The endometrium progressively thickens throughout the phases of the menstrual cycle. The endometrial lining can be as thin as 1 mm at the beginning of menstruation to as thick as 28 mm at the luteal phase. The most sonographic change is seen within the follicular phase. At its thinnest, the endometrium is echogenic. Later in the follicular phase the endometrial stripe becomes hypoechoic. At the latest follicular phase and during ovulation, the endometrium actually appears to have three layers. These layers are echogenic on either end, with the middle layer being hypoechoic. During the luteal or secretory phase, when the endometrium is at its thickest, the appearance is strictly echogenic.

ENDOMETRIAL ADHESIONS

Endometrial adhesions, synonymous with Asherman syndrome, are secondary to scar tissue formation within the uterus. This is most commonly secondary to aggressive or multiple dilation and curettage procedures, but may also be seen as a result of any pelvic surgery or infection. Asherman syndrome often results in infertility or recurrent miscarriage. Plain sonographic evaluation has limited value in the diagnosis of endometrial adhesions. Sonohysterography and hysteroscopy are more definitive tests, as these will demonstrate a characteristic webbed pattern. Testing is best done during the secretory phase of the menstrual cycle.

ENDOMETRIAL CARCINOMA

Endometrial carcinoma is considered an estrogen-dependent cancer. It is most common in the postmenopausal population and accounts for the leading type of female organ cancer in the United States. Endometrial carcinoma should be excluded first in any vaginal bleeding that occurs in a postmenopausal patient. There is a relationship between endometrial hyperplasia and the development of endometrial carcinoma, but it is not clear at what point or for what reason the hyperplastic state turns cancerous. A thickened and irregular end endometrium is present on sonographic evaluation, but this is true with many gynecological conditions. Echogenic tumors and myometrial involvement and irregularity may also be present. These findings may be further evaluated with sonohysterography or hysterosalpingography, but ultimately biopsy is definitive.

ENDOMETRIAL HYPERPLASIA

Endometrial hyperplasia is the result of thickening of the endometrial lining, without its cyclical sloughing. The increasing thickness is the result of prolonged and abnormal estrogen stimulation. This can occur when the body produces too much estrogen, when the body doesn't produce enough progesterone to balance estrogen production, conditions such as PCOS with anovulation but continued estrogen production, and certain medications such as estrogen-only hormone therapy and Tamoxifen. Sonograph is helpful in the diagnosis of endometrial hyperplasia, but may not differentiate it from endometrial cancer or polyps. Endometrial hyperplasia is most common in the perimenopausal female.

ENDOMETROID TUMORS, CLEAR CELL TUMORS, AND TRANSITIONAL CELL TUMORS

Endometroid tumors, clear cell tumors and transitional cell or Brenner tumors are all a type of surface epithelial-stromal tumor. They are far less prevalent than the others in the class (serous and mucinous cystadenomas). Sonographically, they are difficult to differentiate from each other. Endometroid ovarian tumors are unilateral or bilateral arising from endometrial cells, often making it difficult to determine if this is a primary endometroid ovarian tumor or from secondary endometrium cancer. Clear cell ovarian tumors have a very poor prognosis. They are unilateral or bilateral and arise from mesonephric tissue. Often endometriosis is in coexistence when a clear cell tumor is diagnosed. Brenner or transitional cell tumors are benign, small and usually unilateral. Sonographically, they are often solid with well-defined borders.

ENDOMETRIOSIS

Endometriosis is the growth and development of endometrial cells and tissue outside of the uterus. Endometriosis is seen in women in their 20s and 30s. The exact incidence is unknown, because there may be asymptomatic endometriosis. Often times diagnosis is incidental, through other abdominal/pelvic procedures. Although endometriosis can occur almost anywhere, common sites are the ovaries, uterosacral and rectovaginal areas as well as the colon itself. If there is a focal area of endometriosis, it is often termed endometrioma. Endometriomas may be detected on sonography, as they may appear as echoic cysts with debris, fine strands or they may present as a hemorrhagic cyst. Definitive diagnosis is with a combination of laparoscopic and histologic evaluation.

ENDOMETRITIS

Endometritis is an infection of the endometrial lining. Arguably, the terminology is incorrect, as infection can extend beyond the boundaries of the endometrium. In this case, the term metritis is more descriptive, and includes endometrial, myometrial and parametrial infection. Endometritis may arise after cesarean section, PID or dilation and curettage procedures. On sonography, the endometrial layer is irregular and thickened. Furthermore, metritis may be observed on sonography with uterine air bubbles and debris within the endometrium. However, sonographic finding may also be normal and debris may be mistaken for retained products of conception or an intrauterine hematoma.

HYSTEROSONOGRAPHY

A hysterosonogram should be scheduled after the patient's menstrual period, but prior to ovulation because this test should not be performed on pregnant women. Written consent should be obtained prior to the procedure with the sonographer obtaining images and measurements before the catheter is inserted. The physician performing this exam will place a speculum to access the cervix. The catheter should be flushed with sterile saline before it is inserted, and aseptic methods should be used to properly clean the cervix. Ultrasound should be used when saline is injected to demonstrate the filling of the endometrium with the appropriate images taken after the saline is injected to complete this exam. Color Doppler or 3D images may also be taken of any abnormal structures identified. The patient should be informed to contact her physician if any heavy bleeding or symptoms of infection occur afterwards.

POSSIBLE ULTRASOUND FINDINGS WHEN ASSESSING THE CERVIX

Blood or other fluids may be visualized within the cervix (endocervical canal) during an ultrasound evaluation. In addition to fluid, structures such as polyps may also be identified. A cervical polyp is a benign (noncancerous) mass, but it may create symptoms such as abnormal or heavy bleeding. The size and location of these polyps can be determined on ultrasound. Pap smears are the gold standard to determine abnormal cells of the cervix, but ultrasound will often demonstrate masses of the cervix. Cervical cancer is typically a hypoechoic or isoechoic lesion when visualized sonographically, but sometimes the only sign is an enlarged cervix. Ultrasound can also be used to determine if other adjacent structures are involved in the presence of a mass. Color Doppler evaluation may provide useful data pertaining to the vascularity of the tumor.

ULTRASOUND APPEARANCE OF NABOTHIAN CYSTS

Nabothian cysts are commonly visualized sonographically within the cervix in women of childbearing ages, after childbirth, or with any disorder that causes inflammation of the cervix. The cervix contains mucus that is produced by the glands located within, and nabothian cysts are produced when these glands become obstructed by the skin that covers them. Ultrasound demonstrates anechoic cysts that are typically very small (often less than 1 cm), and often more than one will be displayed in the cervical region. Color Doppler will not display blood flow within these structures. They do not typically cause symptoms, so surgical intervention is not required unless they become symptomatic and cause pain. Ablation or cryotherapy may be the primary treatment choices when these cysts need to be removed. These cysts can be diagnosed with transvaginal and transabdominal approaches.

ASSESSMENT OF CERVIX DURING PELVIC ULTRASOUND

The cervix is the lower portion of the uterus and is located just above the vagina. To visualize the cervix during a transabdominal pelvic ultrasound, the patient must have a full bladder. This typically provides a good acoustic window, but care must be taken if the length of the cervix is to be measured. A completely full bladder may improve visualization of the cervix while increasing the cervical length. This is especially important during the obstetrical (OB) ultrasound that is ordered to determine cervical incompetence. Cervical incompetence is demonstrated by a short cervix, so this must be considered during a transabdominal ultrasound (TAUS) approach. A transvaginal ultrasound (TVUS) or endovaginal ultrasound (EVUS) approach will require the patient to empty her bladder, and the measurement is taken between the internal and external cervical os. Yet another approach that can be used to visualize the cervix is a translabial technique, which is used if a patient is having any discomfort from the EVUS or TVUS method.

PID

PID is an infection that originates at the cervix and endocervix, often spreading superiorly to involve other pelvic structures. There are many causative organisms, but Chlamydia trachomatis and Neisseria gonorrhea are the most common. Oral contraceptive pills make the mucosa less favorable for PID to develop. Early in the disease, sonographic diagnosis may not be possible but is important to exclude other disorders such as ectopic pregnancy and appendicitis. Later, several characteristic sonographic findings may be present. If the fallopian tubes are affected, the "cogwheel" sign may be present with increased tubal thickening. The tube may also contain fluid and nodular, "beads on a string". Laparoscopy with or without culture is definitive, but not always necessary.

TORSION OF ADNEXAL MASSES OR CYSTS

Torsion refers to the twisting along the long axis of an adnexal mass or cyst, thus compromising blood supply. Torsion is always accompanied by a maternal complaint of pain, usually pelvic. Torsion can be very difficult to diagnose; therefore, whenever there is a maternal complaint of pain, one must maintain an increased index of suspicion for torsion. Furthermore, the diagnosis is broken into partial and complete torsion. Doppler evaluation is ideal but not always absolutely diagnostic due to varied blood flow to ovaries under normal circumstances. Sonography is most accurate when there is a small mass, torsion is then more obvious as the affected ovary becomes edematous, enlarged, and with multiple cysts.

PERITONEAL INCLUSION CYSTS

Peritoneal inclusion cysts are more likely to be seen in females with a history of pelvic inflammatory disease, multiple pelvic adhesions, and endometriosis. These develop from fluid produced by the ovaries, which does not absorb normally due to the thickened peritoneum. This fluid becomes entrapped within the fibrotic network, causing the cyst. This is not an ovarian cyst. Clinically and sonographically it is difficult, if not impossible, to differentiate from a paraovarian cyst. A thick layer of mesothelial cells lines peritoneal inclusion cysts. Inclusion cysts can be as large as 20 cm in size. Peritoneal inclusion cysts are synonymous with: benign encysted fluid and benign cystic mesothelioma.

CORPUS LUTEUM CYSTS

Corpus luteum cysts are benign cysts, but before diagnosing them, ectopic pregnancy should be ruled-out. The sonographic appearances of corpus luteum cysts are difficult to differentiate from that of the sonographic appearance of an ectopic pregnancy. A corpus luteum cyst forms from hemorrhage into the luteum after ovulation. Average size of a corpus luteum cyst is 4 cm but can be as great as 10 cm. These cysts are commonly seen early in pregnancy, reaching maximal size by 10 weeks of pregnancy. Rupture and spontaneous resolution occur by the end of the first trimester. Sonographic characteristics include: complex to cystic mass, central blood clot, and septations (lacy pattern) within the clot. Corpus luteum cyst and hemorrhagic cyst are often synonymous.

AIUM GUIDELINES FOR PERFORMANCE OF ULTRASOUND EXAMINATION OF THE ADNEXA

The American Institute of Ultrasound in Medicine (AIUM) has established examination and documentation protocols for evaluation of the adnexa. The ovaries are the primary structure that should be identified and thoroughly described in sonography of the adnexa. The ovaries should serve as the primary landmark in sonographic examination of the adnexa. In the case of an enlarged uterus or a postmenopausal patient, the ovaries may not be readily imaged; in every other instance, every attempt should be made to document visualization of the ovaries. Document size and thickness in all planes, location, and the presence of any masses and their description and measurements. Compare all findings to the opposite ovary. The fallopian tubes need to be part of the adnexal sonography and description. However, in the absence of pathology, fallopian tubes are generally not identified on sonography. Any fallopian tube visualization should contain all appropriate descriptors, measurements and notes on symmetry.

SONOGRAPHIC APPEARANCE OF UTERUS AND POSITION OF UTERINE ARTERIAL NETWORK

The sonographic appearance of the uterus should be uniform in composition and structure. Although the uterus itself is hypoechoic, the actual endometrium is echogenic. The amount of echogenicity is dependent on stage of menstrual cycle. Sonographic shadow are common on the edges of the uterus due to the network of muscular and ligamentous attachment surrounding the uterus. The broad ligament, of the uterus, contains the primary vasculature network. Sonographically, these are best visualized near the cervix and inferior most portion of the uterus. Sonographically, the fallopian tubes are difficult to visualize unless they contain pathologic findings.

APPLICATIONS OF COLOR DOPPLER WHEN EVALUATING NORMAL OVARIES

Sonographers should use color, power, and spectral Doppler during a pelvic ultrasound to better demonstrate any ovarian or adnexal pathology. Transvaginal ultrasound (TVUS) has provided a relatively low cost, noninvasive imaging technique. When TVUS is combined with color and/or power Doppler, improved sensitivity to the vascularity and flow within the ovary can be determined in normal and abnormal tissues. Color Doppler ultrasound can be used to demonstrate a normal flow pattern within the ovary or aid in the diagnosis of ovarian torsion. Vascularity within the ovary will change with the maturation of follicles, and arterial flow can be different in the dominant ovary when compared to the nondominant ovary. A corpus luteum will demonstrate a "ring of fire" upon color or power Doppler interrogation that reveals the physiology of this structure.

OVARIAN COLOR AND SPECTRAL DOPPLER VALUES WHEN BENIGN OVARIAN MASS IS PRESENT

The ovaries are supplied with oxygen-rich blood from the ovarian arteries. These arteries arise from the abdominal aorta just inferior to the renal arteries. However, the ovaries are considered to have a dual blood supply because the ovarian arteries join with the uterine arteries in the cornual part of the uterus. These branches can provide a collateral network of blood supply for the ovary in case either aforementioned artery becomes blocked. The ovarian veins carry blood away from the ovaries. The right ovarian vein drains blood directly into the inferior vena cava (IVC), whereas the left ovarian vein empties into the left renal vein and then continues to the IVC. Benign masses of the ovary tend to display blood flow around the peripheral margin of the mass. Spectral analysis of blood flow within a normal ovary offers data pertaining to the pulsatility index (PI) and resistivity index (RI). If the impedance is moderately high, a benign lesion is often assumed. The RI in a benign lesion is typically greater than 0.4. The PI for a benign mass tends to be greater than 1.0.

NORMAL POSITION OF OVARIES IN NULLIPAROUS ADULTS

Ovarian position changes after pregnancy and is not thought to return to its pregravid state. One ovary is found on either side of the uterus, each near the lateral wall of the pelvic cavity. The ovaries are situated inferior to the fallopian tubes and attach to the posterior side of the uterine broad ligament. Each ovary is contained within the ovarian fossa, a space created at the lateral pelvic wall. The external iliac vessels support the fossa superiorly, posteriorly by the ureter, and anteriorly by the umbilical artery. It is thought that the oval ovary is positioned in a vertical manner. The suspensory ligament of the ovary is on the superior end and contains the ovarian vessels. The ligament of the ovary, within the broad uterine ligament, attaches the inferior end of the ovary to the angle of the uterus.

NORMAL SONOGRAPHIC APPEARANCE OF OVARIES IN MENSTRUATING FEMALES

Usually pelvic and transvaginal ultrasound are both used to evaluate the ovaries; however, the transvaginal image often assesses the ovaries more completely. It is possible that neither ultrasound will visualize the ovary. The ovaries are generally visualized posteriorly and laterally to the broad ligament; however, several anatomical variations exist. The ovary itself is shaped like an oval or ellipse and is echogenic. The multiple follicles within the ovary are hypoechoic and should be less than 3 cm. Normal sonographic appearance of the ovary depends heavily on where the patient is in relation to her menstrual cycle. Prior to ovulation, it is not unusual for a single follicle to be greater in size than surrounding follicles, up to 2.5 cm.

SONOGRAPHIC APPEARANCE OF POSSIBLE OVARIAN CANCER

A high-degree of suspicion is important for detection of ovarian cancer in the patient who has abnormal or postmenopausal bleeding, pelvic mass, family history of ovarian cancer, personal history of cancer (especially female organ), and nulliparous women. Both pelvic and transvaginal sonography are recommended. Any adnexal or ovarian mass should be described thoroughly in terms of size and consistency. Cystic ovarian structures, fairly common and normal in a menstruating female, should increase concern in the postmenopausal ovary, especially if they are greater than 10 mm in size. Septations and nodules within an ovarian cyst are also a concerning finding for an ovarian cancer. Low resistive index with Doppler evaluation, of an ovarian mass, also increases concern for ovarian cancer.

SURFACE EPITHELIAL-STROMAL TUMORS

A mucinous cystadenoma is a benign ovarian tumor, usually unilateral, large (at least 15 cm), and it is not unheard of to have one of these weigh greater than 100 pounds. Ultrasound reveals a simple cyst with thin walls and multilocular septations. The cyst contains a thick, gelatin-like material. Mucinous cystadenocarcinoma is a malignant ovarian tumor that can be unilateral or bilateral, usually found in the menopausal patient. They are large tumors, much like that of the mucinous cystadenoma, but are more likely to rupture. On sonograph these have thick and irregular walls and septations. Mucinous cystadenocarcinomas also contain hypoechoic fluid, often with debris present. If a mucinous cystadenocarcinoma ruptures, it is called pseudomyxoma peritonei. Sonographically, pseudomyxoma peritonei reveals loculated ascites and mass effect. Pseudomyxoma peritonei can also be present from rupture of other mucinous tumors of other organs such as the appendix and bowel.

FIBROMAS AND THECOMAS

An ovarian fibroma is a type of gonadal stromal cell tumor; however, unlike other tumors in this category, it does not secrete hormones. Ovarian fibromas are often benign. They can vary greatly in size. Sonographically, the ovarian fibroma has smooth and regular borders, solid in appearance and often associated with ascites. An ovarian thecoma is also a gonadal stromal cell tumor that does produce hormone. Ovarian thecomas are benign and mostly unilateral with varying size. Differentiating ovarian thecomas from ovarian fibromas via sonograph is difficult.

FOLLICULAR OVARIAN CYSTS

Follicular cysts are normal sonographic findings in the menstruating female. Follicles are formed every time the ovary produces an egg. Follicles increase to maximal size at ovulation, and then burst to release the egg. It is when the follicles don't release the egg and continue to grow that we call them follicular cysts. Follicular cysts are greater than 2.5 cm, average about 6-8 cm and can be as big as 20 cm. They usually spontaneously regress over the course of a few menstrual cycles; this can be monitored by ultrasound. If follicular cysts do not shrink to less than 8 cm over the course of monitoring (3-5 cycles), consider further work-up and alternate diagnosis.

GRANULOSA CELL TUMORS AND SERTOLI-LEYDIG TUMORS

Granulosa cell tumors arise from the gonadal stromal cells. They are functional, meaning they produce hormones. These can affect all age groups but are more likely to be benign in older patients, but can lead to endometrial carcinoma in the menopausal patient. Granulosa cell tumors are primarily unilateral. Sertoli-Leydig tumors are more appropriately termed arrhenoblastomas (Sertoli-Leydig tumor of the ovary), as this differentiates them from Sertoli-Leydig tumors of the testes. They arise from gonadal stromal cells. These tumors are an average size of 10 cm and produce male hormone, thus patients with arrhenoblastomas will often demonstrate masculine characteristics.

KRUKENBERG TUMORS

Krukenberg tumor is a term used to describe a secondary ovarian tumor, or a tumor that has metastasized from another organ or site. Metastatic ovarian tumors are largely (80%) from a gastrointestinal (stomach and colon) site. Krukenberg tumors are often bilateral and contain signet-ring cells. They are a mucinous carcinoma and often infiltrative. Although the term Krukenberg tumor initially was used to describe metastatic tumors of the ovary from a gastrointestinal source, it is now commonplace to use it to describe ovarian metastatic tumors from all sources including the breast. Krukenberg tumors represent up to 10% of all ovarian tumors.

OVARIAN TORSION

Ovarian torsion is a condition in which the ovarian pedicle rotates on its axis. There may be complete or partial rotation. This is statistically more common in children and adolescence, with the right ovary, and in the presence of another benign adnexal mass. Clinically, ovarian torsion can act a lot like appendicitis. Fifty percent of the time there is a palpable mass. Sonographically ovarian torsion can vary. Imaged appearance is that of an edematous and enlarged ovary, usually greater than 4 cm. 'Classic' sonographic appearance of ovarian torsion is that of a hypoechoic mass surrounded by multiple small follicles. 'Common' sonographic appearance of ovarian torsion is of a completely solid adnexal mass. Doppler studies may reveal complete absence of blood flow to the ovary is torsion is complete or reduced blood flow to the ovary in partial torsion.

OVARIAN CARCINOMA

SCREENING

Pelvic examination, Pap smear, ultrasound, and tumor marker tests such as CA125 have all been evaluated for ovarian cancer screening. However, none of these individual options or combinations has stepped to the forefront for a variety of reasons: specificity, cost versus benefit ratio, and impact on overall survival rate, and the presence/absence of definitive treatment. Important to all of these is a thorough patient history, as there are several known risk factors for the development of ovarian carcinoma: family history, age >50, nulliparous, history of breast cancer, race, Jewish descent, HRT in postmenopause, and fertility drugs. The CA125 test is erroneous in the fact that it is nonspecific and often positive in premenopausal patient in a number of benign conditions. Furthermore, it does not detect all types of ovarian carcinomas at any age. Currently, if a patient possesses ≥ 2 risk factors, performing a CA125 and sonography is reasonable.

PREVALENCE, MORBIDITY AND MORTALITY

The prevalence of ovarian carcinoma, in the United States, annually is approximately 22,000 diagnosed cases. Of these, over half are fatal. Ovarian carcinoma represents about one-quarter of all female organ cancers and is the fourth leading cause of cancer death among women in the United States. Incidence of malignancy increases proportionately with age. Mortality is highly dependent upon the stage of cancer at the time of diagnosis. In general, for a variety of reasons, those with ovarian carcinoma usually present and are diagnosed later in the disease. The average 5-year survival rate, after diagnosis of ovarian carcinoma, is approximately 42%. Morbidity ranges from chronic pain, abdominal distension, bowel obstruction and multiple gastrointestinal symptoms, as well as numerous self-image and emotional difficulties.

PCOS

Polycystic ovary syndrome (PCOS) is the most common female hormonal disorder. It is a disorder marked by anovulatory cycles, partially due to the body producing excess androgens. This can be apparent by heavy or irregular menses, increased facial hair growth, insulin resistance, and fertility difficulties. Diagnosis is made with history, physical exam, lab tests, and ultrasound. The sonographic findings of enlarged ovaries and multiple cysts is not independently diagnostic of PCOS. Complications of PCOS are the development of diabetes, hypertension, lipid disorders, infertility, and endometrial cancer. Treatment options include dietary changes, weight-loss and exercise, hormones, fertility drugs, diabetic drugs (to help with insulin resistance), medications to decrease androgen production, and surgery.

SURFACE EPITHELIAL-STROMAL TUMORS

Serous cystadenoma is the most common benign ovarian tumor. Cystadenoma's are usually unilateral, smaller than mucinous cysts, more likely unilocular with thin but well-defined walls and thin septa. Serous cystadenocarcinoma are the most common ovarian cancer, often involving bilateral ovaries. Sonographically, serous cystadenocarcinoma are also smaller than mucinous cysts. The borders of serous cystadenocarcinoma are irregular and the walls are thick. This carcinoma is highly septated, multilocular and often has internal papillary projections. Cystadenofibroma are similar to the above two adenomas plus fibroids, as they display greater areas of solid tissue on ultrasound.

STRUMA OVARII, MATURE SOLID TERATOMAS, AND IMMATURE TERATOMAS

Struma ovarii are germ cell tumors that are usually benign, composed of mature thyroid-like tissue. As a result, struma ovarii produce thyroid hormone. They are hard to differentiate, sonographically, from a cystic teratoma. Mature solid teratomas are germ cell tumors that sonographically appear solid. They are slow growing and more common between the ages of 10 and 20 years. Immature teratomas are malignant germ cell tumors primarily affecting adolescents. Sonographically, immature teratomas appear solid but contain many tiny cysts and highly echogenic. Immature teratomas grow rapidly are usually unilateral.

THECA LUTEIN OVARIAN CYSTS

Theca lutein ovarian cysts are often the result of increased serum human chorionic gonadotropin circulation in the female. They are often comorbid to other conditions such as polycystic ovarian syndrome, gestational trophoblastic disease (hydatidiform mole and choriocarcinomas), multiple gestation, gestational diabetes, and sometimes as a result of some infertility medications. Theca lutein cysts usually spontaneously resolve or rupture by four months; however, they are at increased risk for torsion and hemorrhage. The patient with theca lutein cysts may complain of pelvic pain, dyspareunia, nausea and vomiting. Sonographically, bilateral ovarian enlargement will be present. Ovarian cysts will be multilocular and will also be found in both ovaries.

OVARIES OF POSTMENOPAUSAL WOMEN

Postmenopause finds the ovaries no longer ovulating and no longer the primary source of estrogen and progesterone production, as this tapers significantly during menopause and eventually ceases. The primary estrogen production then shifts to the fat cells of the body, but the rate of production is less than half of that of what the ovaries had produced. As a result of decreased hormonal production, the ovary shrinks. Typically, a postmenopausal ovary should not be larger than 2 cm along its long axis. Due to decreasing function and size, postmenopausal ovaries may be hard to detect with ultrasound. As a result of their decreasing function, they are also without many surrounding cysts that are often found around even a "normal" premenopause ovary. Hormone replacement therapy does not affect the sonographic appearance of postmenopausal ovaries.

CONDITIONS OF FALLOPIAN TUBES THAT CONTRIBUTE TO INFERTILITY

The fallopian tubes can contribute, directly or indirectly, to many unsuccessful fertilizations. Infections such as pelvic inflammatory disease (PID) and appendicitis can cause significant inflammation in the area. PID places a woman at high risk for developing an ectopic pregnancy, which in itself is a contributor to infertility. Ectopic pregnancy is a result of a fertilized egg and sperm implanting themselves within the fallopian tube rather than the uterus, this most commonly happens at the ampulla. Furthermore, endometriosis and adhesions can contribute to decreased patency and function of the fallopian tubes, leading to infertility. Elective infertility involving the fallopian tubes is a common occurrence. In a tubal ligation, or female sterilization procedure, the tubes are either "tied", a section removed, a section removed and tied, or severed.

DEVELOPMENT AND CHARACTERISTICS OF FALLOPIAN TUBES

Fallopian tubes, also called uterine tubes or salpinges, arise from the Mullerian ducts. The fallopian tubes are comprised of three main sections. The first section is the portion that connects the fallopian tubes to the lateral fundus of the uterus bilaterally. This section is the proximal-most portion defined by and narrow (near the uterus) and a straight isthmus (wider section as it moves distal to the uterus). The second section is the middle portion called the ampulla. The ampulla is the usual site of fertilization. The third section of the fallopian tubes is called the infundibulum. The infundibulum is the most distal portion of the fallopian tubes and is defined by its fimbriae at the end. The fimbriae are classically described as finger like projections. The fimbriae do not directly attach to the ovaries, but they aid in collecting the egg released by the ovary, for transport down the fallopian tubes.

PARAOVARIAN CYSTS IN OBSTETRICAL SONOGRAPHY

A paraovarian cyst is sonographically differentiated from an ovarian cyst by its location outside of the ovary. It is located within the broad ligament and arises as a result of the embryonic remnants of the Wolffian ducts. It is rarely symptomatic and therefore is usually an incidental sonographic finding. Its sonographic appearance is a rounded cyst with septae located adjacent to the ovary. Although usually asymptomatic, paraovarian cysts are noteworthy because of their risk of torsion. Risk of torsion is greater in the pregnant versus the nonpregnant patient.

PARAOVARIAN CYSTS AND PERITONEAL INCLUSION CYSTS

Paraovarian cysts often form as the result of a Wolffian duct remnant. Paraovarian cysts are benign and fairly common (10% of all pelvic masses. They are found in the broad ligament and do not arise within the ovary. This can often be differentiated with the transvaginal ultrasound and they are often visualized above the fundus. They have the sonographic appearance of a normal cysts but may be hemorrhagic and torse. Paraovarian cysts are generally less than 5 cm and their size will not fluctuate with the menstrual cycle. However, paraovarian cysts can increase in size and extend into the abdominal cavity, making determination of origin difficult.

COLOR AND SPECTRAL DOPPLER CHARACTERISTICS OF MALIGNANT OVARIAN MASSES

Malignant ovarian masses tend to have certain characteristics when compared to those that are benign. Gray-scale may show cystic components with thick walls, internal septa, and mural nodules. The borders of the mass may not be discerned well. Internal solid components may also be present, and masses that are solid are more likely to be cancerous. Color and power Doppler may demonstrate a disorganized pattern of vascularity that includes a spokelike pattern extending into the middle of the mass. A malignant lesion will typically show blood flow that has high velocity, but low impedance. If the pulsatility index is less than 1.0 and the resistivity index is less than 0.4, this suggests malignancy. Some machines enable the use of 3D power Doppler, which combines the two technologies and provides power Doppler in a 3D image. This has been useful to detect ovarian cancer earlier than the two technologies used separately, which is crucial in order for treatment to be effective.

CUL-DE-SAC

There is an anterior cul-de-sac and a posterior cul-de-sac, which themselves are really just a "space" or cavity versus an organ or structure. The anterior cul-de-sac is space between the pubic bone and uterus, with the bladder making up the bottom of this area. The posterior cul-de-sac is also called the pouch of Douglas. The pouch of Douglas is located posterior to the uterus. Making up the other borders of the posterior cul-de-sac are: superior portion of vagina, cervix, rectum and the uterosacral ligaments. The cul-de-sacs are frequent sites of infection and endometriosis, especially the pouch of Douglas. Although this area may be difficult to view with sonography techniques, it should always be evaluated and noted for the presence of mass or fluid. If either of these findings is present, they should be clearly defined and masses should be differentiated from bowel if possible.

SONOGRAPHIC PATHOLOGIES FOUND AT THE VAGINA AND CERVIX

An imperforate hymen is the most common vaginal-outflow obstruction anomaly in females. It may be diagnosed from the neonatal period through adolescence. It usually presents as a bulging vaginal mass, which is due to retained vaginal secretions. Ultrasound or MRI is the preferred definitive diagnosis when this is present versus aspiration. A transverse vaginal septum may also be present independently or with a imperforate hymen. Gartner's duct cysts are remnants, in the vaginal wall, of fetal development. If they remain after birth, they can retain fluid and develop mass-effect and infection. Nabothian cysts are common benign cystic masses of the cervix. They can be visualized clinically when performing a speculum examination, or sonographically. Cervical cancer is a pathology that may be seen at the cervix; however, it is rarely detected by sonography. Pap smear is the screening/diagnosis method of choice for cervical carcinoma.

INTRAVASCULAR FETAL TRANSFUSION

Intravascular fetal transfusion is performed to treat fetal anemia, whatever its cause. To perform an intravascular fetal transfusion, a cordocentesis is performed concurrently. The ultrasound-guided cordocentesis allows for baseline and post-transfusion blood levels, especially fetal hematocrit, Rh factor determination, blood-typing and a complete blood count. This is all performed with the fetus temporarily paralyzed, as needle placement and maintenance is crucial. It is standard to use a 20 gauge, 5-inch needle to insert into the umbilical vein near the placental insertion. After a baseline blood sample is taken, an IV bolus of pancuronium bromide is given and transfusion started. Transfusion is with Rh negative, type O blood, washed and irradiated packed cells that are CMV negative, and cross-matched with maternal blood. The rate of transfusion is about 3-5 mL/min. Sonographically, transfusion appears as bright speckles. A post-transfusion hematocrit should be determined. Ultrasound monitoring should continue several minutes after the needle is withdrawn to assess blood leakage.

C-SECTION AND POSTPARTUM INFECTION

A cesarean section (C-section) is the surgical delivery of the baby or babies through an abdominal and uterine incision. The fetus(es) are then delivered through this incision directly versus through the cervix and vagina. This procedure may be chosen in a situation where it is thought to reduce fetal and/or maternal morbidity and mortality. Such indications may include: previous cesarean delivery, placental abnormalities, active maternal herpes infection, breech presentation, fetal heart decelerations, fetal macrosomia, preeclampsia, and multiple gestation. Cesarean deliveries increase the risk of postpartum maternal infection up to 4-fold of that of a vaginal delivery.

CVS

Chorionic villus sampling (CVS) is a procedure that may be performed relatively early in pregnancy, between the 10th and 12th weeks. It may be performed before amniocentesis and is used to determine the sex of the baby and identify genetic problems with the fetus. Chorionic villus sampling is not generally done as a routine screening test, due to slight increase in risk of miscarriage. It is a test that is primarily considered if a fetus is suspected to be at higher risk of a specific chromosomal disorder. Chorionic villus sampling may be considered if the mother is older than age 35, she has a previous child with a chromosomal disorder, or there is a known family history of a specific genetic disorder. This test does not assess the risk of neural tube defects.

IMPORTANT TERMS

Hypertrophic Cardiomyopathy—describes a condition in which the muscle of the left heart ventricle is thickened, particularly the septal wall. This condition is seen in many congenital defects and is thought to be responsible for sudden cardiac death in athletes.

Hyperplasia—this describes the presence of increased cellular number in any organ or tissue.

Hyperemesis Gravidarum—describes severe vomiting or 'morning sickness' of pregnancy.

Hypertelorism—describes an abnormally increased distance between two anatomical structures.

Supine Hypotensive Syndrome—describes a condition seen in the third trimester, in which the gravid uterus presses on the inferior vena cava. This may result in decreased venous return in the mother, and fetal hypoxia.

Asynclitism—is used to describe any condition in which there is an absence of parallelism or symmetry of anatomical structures.

Anasarca—used to describe any anatomical area of connective tissue that becomes infiltrated with edematous fluid.

Ascites—describes a collection of serous fluid localized within the peritoneal region.

Sirenomelia—describes a congenital defect in which the legs are fused together, usually with the feet remaining unfused. Also known as "mermaid legs or deformity".

Hygroma—used to describe any increase or swelling in cystic collection of serous fluid.

Dolichocephaly—describes a cephalic index of less than 75% and a "long-head" appearance.

Brachycephaly—describes a head that appears disproportionately small and has a cephalic index greater than 80%.

Anencephaly—a severe congenital defect in which there is complete absence of the fetal skull, brain, and brainstem.

Holoprosencephaly—a congenital defect in which the forebrain fails to cleave, and a single lobe is present. This is often accompanied by facial defects.

Ventriculomegaly—describes a condition in which the fetal lateral brain ventricles are dilated to greater than 10 mm.

Polydactyly—describes a congenital defect in which there are greater than five digits on a hand(s) or foot (feet). The extra digit(s) usually are comprised of soft tissue only, but may contain bone.

Talipes—is used to define any number of congenital anomalies involving the ankle/foot region. One of the more common uses of this term is talipes equinovarus, which is the medical term for 'clubfoot'.

Clinodactyly—describes radial or ulnar deviation of the finger digits. This is a congenital anomaly.

Hypospadias—a male congenital defect in which the urethral opening is located more proximal and ventral on the penis, then its normal position.

Macrosomia—also known as 'big baby syndrome', describes a fetus that is large for gestational age (>90th percentile).

Superficial Structures and Other Sonographic Procedures

CORRELATING ULTRASOUND FINDINGS WITH OTHER IMAGING MODALITIES

Ultrasound is often the first modality that is used to evaluate patients that present with pain, swelling, palpable masses, or abnormal lab values. Sonographers should always determine if the patient has had prior imaging exams pertaining to this issue before starting the exam so that a comparison can be made. Often, the patient may recall having an exam but may be confused as to which exam was performed. It is also important for other technologists (computed tomography [CT], magnetic resonance imaging, nuclear medicine) to do the same and compare any imaging studies to prior ultrasounds. Along with the actual exam, it is important for any technologist to carefully read any report, especially in cases where a follow-up has been indicated. For example, if a patient has three nodules that were previously visualized in the liver on a CT of the abdomen, the sonographer must make sure that all three lesions are properly documented. Some systems allow the ultrasound operator to upload a prior CT exam into their ultrasound system so that the CT image is next to the live ultrasound exam so the radiologist knows that the information obtained is on the correct lesion.

PENILE ULTRASOUND

The penis is a structure that can now be interrogated with the current advancements in ultrasound. Color Doppler has enabled clinicians to study the vascularity of this anatomical structure by minimally noninvasive means. A high-frequency transducer (longitudinal and transverse images) can demonstrate the corpus spongiosum, corpora cavernosa, and urethra, as well as the blood vessels they contain. Within the corpora cavernosa are the cavernosal arteries, which are branches of the internal pudendal artery that supply the penis with the majority of the necessary blood. Penile ultrasound is commonly performed for erectile dysfunction (ED), in which the physician will perform an injection to increase blood flow to the penis. ED may be caused when the blood vessels are unable to constrict or dilate properly to fill with blood. Blood flow velocities can be measured with ultrasound. The ultrasound technician can also check for any masses, calcifications, or fractures of the penis, or he or she can check if stones are suspected in the urethra.

STRUCTURES EVALUATED

The urethra is embedded within the corpus spongiosum (ventrally), which runs along the shaft of the penis and morphs into the head of the penis (glans penis). The corpus spongiosum is typically more echogenic when compared to the corpora cavernosa. The corpora cavernosa is paired and positioned on the dorsal and lateral surfaces of the penis and considered to be the dominant erectile tissue. They are hypoechoic on ultrasound and surrounded by a line that appears hyperechoic, which is the tunica albuginea. Together, the aforementioned structures make up the body of the penis. Ultrasound can also be used to identify the urethra and blood vessels that are present within the penis and associated measurements.

POSTSTENOTIC TURBULENCE

Recall that the word patent refers to a structure that is open or clear. For example, a patent trachea (windpipe) is necessary for air to reach the lungs. When performing a carotid duplex exam, a patent artery is what the operator hopes to find. If a sonographer visualizes a stenosis on routine grayscale imaging, a narrowing of the blood vessel lumen (opening) is present. If the user adds color Doppler, the direction of flow may vary because the blood is attempting to enter and exit the stenotic region

205

of the blood vessel. When pulsed-wave Doppler is used, the sonographer may expect to obtain higher flow velocities within the stenosis, but an even greater measurement distal to the stenosis. This is known as poststenotic turbulence, which is located after the blood vessel has been narrowed. Eddy currents will likely be visualized because the blood is no longer moving as smoothly as it was before the stenosis. If a clinician listens to the blood flow in this region, a bruit may be revealed.

TRANSDUCER USED FOR THYROID ULTRASOUND

A sonographer would choose a linear sequential-array transducer to perform a thyroid ultrasound. A linear sequential array may also be referred to as a linear switched array transducer. This transducer may be selected because it has a relatively thin but wide footprint, so it is ideal to image the thyroid gland, which sits at the base of the patient's neck. A user would choose a higher frequency because the thyroid gland is a superficial location. The image displayed on the screen is in the shape of a rectangle; the image is never wider than the transducer face. There are a number of active crystals that are arranged in a straight line across the transducer face (120–250 in number). Modern focusing and steering are done electronically. Early linear sequential arrays were fixed focus. When the beams are steered, they become the shape of a parallelogram instead of a rectangle. Linear switched array transducers enable blocks of crystals to send signals at the same time in order to form the sound beam. The signals are sent straight out of the face of the transducer and will form another beam when the next group fires.

REASON FOR USING A TRANSDUCER WITH A THIN CRYSTAL

The crystal in an ultrasound transducer is referred to as the active element or piezoelectric lead zirconate titanate (PZT) crystal. Companies that construct ultrasound probes use PZT material that is of assorted thickness in order to offer customers transducers with different frequencies. The thickness of the active element for clinical ultrasound purposes is in the 0.2 to 1 mm range. Transducers with thicker PZT crystals will offer lower frequencies, whereas those with a thin PZT crystal will offer a frequency that is higher. To illustrate this relationship, imagine the difference between tapping a crystal dish with a spoon versus tapping on a glass bowl with a spoon. The crystal dish will create a higher pitched sound than will the glass dish.

ABNORMALITIES WHEN IMAGING THE POSTSURGICAL NECK

Sonographers will often be asked to image the neck after a thyroidectomy. If prior scans are available, be sure to acquire them and the reports for comparison. A complete history is important to determine why the thyroid was removed and which lobes. It is important to document multiple images of the thyroid bed in the longitudinal and transverse planes. The sonographer should also scan the lateral neck region, and any enlarged lymph nodes, cysts, or masses should be captured with B-mode (with measurements) and color or power Doppler. If a patient is status postsurgical for cancer of the head or neck, it is important to scan all of the various neck regions. Again, if abnormal lymph nodes are visualized, they should be documented and measured. It is important for sonographers to look at the shape of the node (round is abnormal); loss of fatty hilum and cystic or calcified areas are also considered abnormal. The exam should consist of documentation of the vascularity of the node with color or power Doppler.

ANATOMIC VARIANTS OR CONGENITAL ANOMALIES OF THE NECK

During development, the thyroid forms in the pharynx and eventually gravitates down to the base of the neck. The passageway that allows the thyroid to move will typically disappear after the thyroid is in the correct place. However, in some individuals this connection does not disappear, and, instead, it creates a pathway for cysts to materialize within. These cysts are known as thyroglossal duct cysts, and they can be seen on ultrasound located in front of the trachea in the middle of the patient's neck. They are one of the most common neck masses diagnosed in children, but they can also affect adults. Another congenital, benign cyst that may be visualized during a neck ultrasound is a branchial cleft cyst, which is in a lateral location of the neck. On ultrasound, they tend to display an anechoic or hypoechoic, ovoid appearance with thin walls. These masses tend to be compressible, and the lack of vascularity can be confirmed with color Doppler.

EVALUATION OF THYROID FOR FUNCTION AND/OR PERFUSION

High-frequency ultrasound imaging of the thyroid is the best method available to evaluate the size and location of palpable masses, provide fine-needle aspiration, further assess abnormal lab values, or provide follow-up on nodules or cysts found previously. Measurements of the thyroid lobes (right and left) should be taken in the longitudinal and transverse planes to provide 3D measurements. The isthmus should also be imaged and measured. Color, power, and spectral Doppler may provide useful information pertaining to any nodules of the thyroid or any abnormalities of the neck (blood vessels or lymph nodes) and to demonstrate blood flow within the thyroid. The parathyroid may be imaged in cases of hyperparathyroidism, especially after the removal of the glands.

THYROID ABNORMALITIES THAT MAY BE DIAGNOSED WITH COLOR DOPPLER ULTRASOUND

The thyroid gland is vascular; it is supplied by four thyroid arteries (two supply the superior lobes, and two supply the inferior portion of the lobes). During a thyroid ultrasound, the sonographer may notice hyperemia (increased vascularity than normal) of the thyroid gland once color or power Doppler is applied. This is often seen in patients with Graves' disease, which, in the United States, is the most common form of hyperthyroidism (too many thyroid hormones are produced) and is considered to be an autoimmune disorder. When scanning the region of the neck lateral to the thyroid gland, the sonographer may incidentally observe a stenosis in the carotid artery or a blood clot (thrombus) in the jugular vein. Color Doppler is helpful to determine the extent of both of these findings.

BENEFITS AND PITFALLS OF USING ULTRASOUND TO DETECT PARATHYROID ABNORMALITIES

Ultrasound is a noninvasive, painless method that does not require radiation to produce images. The lower risk is also a reason why physicians will order an ultrasound first when neck masses are present or if the patient's laboratory results are abnormal. There are typically four parathyroid glands that sit on the posterior poles of the thyroid gland. Two are superior and the other two are attached to the inferior poles. Normal parathyroid glands are not often seen during an ultrasound study because of their size (3–5 mm). However, if a patient has a parathyroid adenoma, cancer, or hyperplasia (enlarged parathyroid glands), the ultrasound operator is often able to detect them. In patients that also have a multinodular goiter, it may be more difficult to penetrate the thyroid gland and parathyroid pathology may not be discerned as readily. Color or power Doppler can provide clues as to whether a mass separate from the thyroid is a lymph node or an adenoma. Parathyroid adenomas can be identified as the feeding vessels branch off of the thyroidal arteries, and they are often singular, hypoechoic, oval-shaped masses that measure less than 3 cm.

IMPORTANCE OF CAREFULLY EVALUATING LYMPH NODES IN THE NECK WITH ULTRASOUND

When a physician can palpate what is believed to be a lymph node, an ultrasound will be ordered, especially if the patient is not sick and the mass is nontender. Lymphadenopathy may be visualized incidentally when scanning other structures in the neck such as the thyroid gland. When evaluating lymph nodes, regardless of their location in the body, it is important to evaluate the shape, size, and fatty hilum of the node. Lesions in the neck that have borders that are well defined and display low-level echoes are likely lymph nodes. Ultrasound users should always apply color or power Doppler when imaging lymph nodes because a mix of peripheral and hilar (versus flow only in the hilum) flow may be an indication of a malignant node, as is a node that has lost its elliptical shape and has become more rounded.

SALIVARY GLANDS

The salivary glands are responsible for producing saliva and releasing it into the mouth. There are three pairs of major salivary glands, they are:

- The parotid glands. These glands are located in the upper part of each cheek (near the ears). The glands release saliva at the back of the mouth (near the molars of the upper jaw).
- The submandibular glands. These glands are located in the floor of the mouth and release saliva behind the lower front teeth.
- The sublingual glands. These glands are located under the tongue and release saliva onto the floor of the mouth.

BLOOD VESSELS OF THE NECK

Blood is supplied to the head (through the neck) via the aortic arch. The subclavian and the common carotid arteries arise from the aortic arch. The thyrocervical trunk arises from the subclavian artery. The common carotid artery splits into two branches called the internal carotid artery and the external carotid artery. Blood is drained from the head (through the neck) via the internal and external jugular veins (the internal jugular vein is much larger than the external jugular vein). The jugular veins connect to the right subclavian vein and the brachiocephalic vein respectively.

ANATOMY OF THE NECK

The neck is the site of many connections from the head to the rest of the body. It includes air and food passages (trachea and esophagus), major blood vessels (including the carotid arteries and jugular veins), nerves, and the spinal cord. The neck can be divided into two distinct anatomical triangles. They are:

- The anterior triangle is made up of the front border of the sternocleidomastoid muscle, the midline of the neck, and the mandible bone.
- The posterior triangle is bordered by the back border of the sternocleidomastoid muscle, the trapezius muscles, and the clavicle bone.

The neck also contains many lymph nodes that are located within the triangles.

COMMON SUPERFICIAL STRUCTURES EVALUATED FOR MASSES BY ULTRASOUND

The thyroid gland is one of the most common superficial structures that can be evaluated with ultrasound when it is assumed that there is a mass. Often, a physician will feel an enlarged thyroid during a physical exam or the patient may have difficulty swallowing or breathing. The thyroid gland is a butterfly-shaped gland located anterior to the trachea in the inferior portion of the neck. Ultrasound can offer clinicians information such as the presence of a mass, the number and location of masses, whether the masses are cystic or solid, as well as the vascularity or demonstration of calcifications within the mass. A goiter is an enlargement of the thyroid gland, and it is the most common reason that a thyroid gland is bigger than the normal size. Other common ultrasound findings of a goiter include a heterogeneous, nodular appearance that may be difficult to penetrate well due to inflammation.

GRAVE'S DISEASE

Grave's disease is an autoimmune disease that occurs when a person's immune system attacks the thyroid gland. When this happens, the thyroid gland becomes damaged and manufactures too much of the thyroid–specific hormone (thyroxine) that regulates the body's metabolism (called hyperthyroidism). Hyperthyroidism can increase the body's metabolism by sixty to one-hundred percent. It is more common in women than men, and is the most common cause of hyperthyroidism in the United States. Symptoms may include bulging eyeballs (Grave's ophthalmopathy), anxiety, irregular heartbeat, difficulty sleeping, weight loss, and the presence of a goiter (swelling of the thyroid gland).

The following ultrasound feature is present:

Increased vascularity of both lobes of the thyroid gland (using color Doppler)

PARATHYROID HYPERPLASIA

Parathyroid hyperplasia is a disease in which all four parathyroid glands show enlargement. This enlargement is due to an increase in the number of cells making up of the parathyroid gland itself. Similar to parathyroid adenomas, hyperparathyroidism (in which excess parathyroid hormone is produced) may result. Hyperparathyroidism causes the bones to release excess calcium into the blood (resulting in hypercalcemia). Symptoms may include bone weakness, lethargy, confusion, muscle pain, kidney stones, and nausea. Parathyroid hyperplasia is responsible for about fifteen percent of all cases of hyperparathyroidism. It is more common in patients with a family history of the disease.

HASHIMOTO'S THYROIDITIS

Hashimoto's thyroiditis is an autoimmune disease that occurs when a person's immune system attacks the thyroid gland. When this happens, the thyroid gland becomes damaged and cannot manufacture the proper amount of thyroid-specific hormone (thyroxine) that regulates the body's metabolism (called hypothyroidism). It is more common in women than men, and is the most common cause of hypothyroidism in the United States. Symptoms may include, fatigue, depression, muscle weakness, and the presence of a goiter (swelling of the thyroid gland).

The following ultrasound feature is present:

A diffuse enlargement of the thyroid with a heterogeneous echo texture.

CANCERS OF THE NECK

Neck cancers are typically squamous cell carcinomas (tumors that develop in the tissue lining the hollow organs of the body). Risk factors for cancers of the neck (and mouth) include cigarette smoking, chewing tobacco, heavy drinking, and pre-existing white patches in the mouth (called leukoplakia). The tumor types that may be seen include:

- Lymphoepithelioma
- Spindle cell carcinoma
- Verrucous cancer
- Cancers of the lymph nodes (called lymphoma)

Malignant lymph nodes show the following sonographic features:

- A rounded shape
- The echo-texture is heterogeneous

- Intranodal calcification
- Absence of an echogenic hilum

PARATHYROID ADENOMA

Parathyroid adenomas are benign tumors that appear on the parathyroid glands (four pea sized glands located at the front of the neck). Typically, only one of glands is affected and shows enlargement. The tumor may damage the parathyroid gland's ability to regulate the amount of calcium in the blood. This causes a condition called hyperparathyroidism (in which excess parathyroid hormone is produced). Hyperparathyroidism causes the bones to release excess calcium into the blood (resulting in hypercalcemia). The condition usually affects women over sixty years old, especially if there is a family history of the disease. Symptoms may include bone weakness, lethargy, confusion, muscle pain, kidney stones, and nausea.

The following ultrasound feature is present:

Homogeneous, hypoechoic, solid, oval-shaped nodules

THYROID CANCER

Thyroid cancer usually begins with a nodule on the thyroid gland. Simply having a nodule on the thyroid gland is a common occurrence (especially as one ages). In most cases the nodule is benign. Symptoms may include hoarseness, neck pain, and enlarged lymph nodes. The disease typically appears in patients over thirty years old and women are affected three times more than men. The most common type of thyroid cancer is papillary or mixed (papillary and follicular). This type accounts for more than two thirds of all cases. A ten-megahertz linear array transducer will provide the most optimum scan for nodules on the thyroid gland.

BEST TRANSDUCER FOR SMALL-PARTS SCANNING

Linear sequential (switched) transducers are the best choice for small-parts ultrasound exams. The design of the probe, which is long and narrow, allows for easier skin contact of the area being interrogated because these regions of the body are often smaller or more difficult to reach. The shape that results from this probe is rectangular, which is the most appropriate because sector images provide a wide field of view in the far field that is not necessary with these types of exams. The lateral resolution changes with scanning depth, but it is better in the far field because these probes have higher frequencies. Of course, the lateral resolution is the best at the focal point where the beam is the absolute narrowest, so the best way to optimize the lateral resolution is to use the highest number of focal zones.

POST-TRAUMATIC SONOGRAPHIC FINDINGS OF THE SCROTUM

B-mode and color Doppler ultrasound is the first imaging modality used for patients that present with scrotal injuries. Clinicians can quickly determine if surgery is necessary in order to preserve the testis. Testicular rupture can be diagnosed if the operator visualizes an interruption of the tunica albuginea. The normal ultrasound appearance should display two echogenic lines that are parallel to each other. When ruptures are present, often the underlying testicular tissue will demonstrate an irregular shape and heterogeneous appearance. Color Doppler should also be used to determine blood flow characteristics because a rupture typically results in interruption of blood flow to at least part of the testicle. A bilateral comparison of blood flow should be documented so that physicians can quickly determine if a rupture or torsion has occurred. A fracture of the testicle will appear as a straight, hypoechoic line that does not display blood flow. The epididymis may also be affected during trauma and will often appear enlarged and hyperemic.

VARICOCELE

A varicocele is a mass of enlarged veins that develops in the spermatic cord. The spermatic cord is made up of blood vessels, lymphatic vessels, nerves, and the duct that carries sperm from the body (vas deferens). If the valves that regulate blood flow from these veins become defective, blood does not circulate out of the testicles efficiently, which causes swelling in the veins above and behind the testicles. It usually occurs only in the left testicle since the left spermatic vein drains into the renal vein between the superior mesenteric artery and the aorta. These two arteries can compress the renal vein and thus impede blood flow from the spermatic vein. The condition is also associated with infertility.

The following ultrasound feature is present:

Varicoceles appear as a collection of tortuous tubular structures.

SONOGRAPHIC APPEARANCES OF TESTICULAR TORSION

Sonographers should be aware that a gray-scale ultrasound of a testicular torsion may be unremarkable in the first couple of hours after the torsion has occurred. This is the reason why it is important to also evaluate the testes with color, power, and spectral Doppler. If there is a partial torsion or if torsion is taking place during an exam, the ultrasound operator may still see blood flow, but the waveform may not show diastolic flow (or it will be reversed or will be less than normal). Color Doppler may show flow in the testis that is twisted, but it will have the color flashing, which demonstrates absent diastolic flow. In this case, it would be helpful to have the radiologist present or to take a cine clip of a side-by-side comparison with color flow Doppler turned on. The epididymis should also be evaluated with gray-scale and color Doppler because it will not demonstrate blood flow, but it may be enlarged. The scrotal wall may be thickened when torsion has taken place, and the testis may appear hypoechoic. The testes should be measured to determine enlargement. The head, body, and tail of the epididymis should also be examined with gray-scale and color Doppler.

TESTICULAR TORSION

Testicular torsion occurs when blood flow (to the testicle) is obstructed due to the twisting action of a mobile testicle. This condition affects patients that have a smaller than normal bare area where the blood vessels, lymphatics, nerves, and spermatic ducts are connected to the testicle. A small remnant stalk of the tunica vaginalis allows the testicle to become mobile and revolve around the stalk thereby cutting off the blood flow and causing severe pain. This is a severe condition and death of the testicle can occur within twenty-four hours without treatment.

The following ultrasound features are present:

- The testicle appears normal within the first four hours of torsion (however color and pulsed Doppler scans may show some abnormalities).
- After four hours the testicle appears enlarged and hypoechoic and may show an enlargement of the epididymus, a reactive hydrocele, and scrotal wall thickening.

ANATOMICAL STRUCTURES OF THE SCROTUM AND EVALUATION FOR PERFUSION

The scrotum can be evaluated sonographically to aid in the diagnosis of a multitude of symptoms the patient may experience due to trauma or infections. These include scrotal pain, swelling, mass, questionable hernia, possible torsion, varicoceles, or even to find a testis that is not palpable. The imaging technique includes documentation of the testes in the longitudinal and transverse planes with pertinent measurements. Color and spectral Doppler should also be applied, especially in cases in which torsion is a concern. The use of split-screen imaging in gray-scale and color Doppler is helpful in patients that are experiencing pain. Power Doppler may also be useful, but it should not be used without spectral interrogation. The color Doppler parameters may have to be adjusted to detect the slow flow of the testes. The spermatic cord should also be evaluated in suspected testicular torsion if possible. If a testis is not found within the scrotum, the inguinal canal must be imaged to provide further information for the clinician.

UNDESCENDED TESTICLE

The undescended testicle is a congenital anomaly that results when a testicle does not descend to the scrotum (from the retroperitoneum where it is formed) in the male shortly before birth (or early in the neonatal period). It is usually caused by a lack of hormonal stimulation (due to a lack of gonadotropin). It can also be caused by physical factors such as adhesions or barriers due to malformations of anatomical structures. If left untreated, the testicle will become atrophied and put the patient at higher risk of testicular cancer. The undescended testicle is typically oval-shaped, hypoechoic, and appears smaller than normal.

EPIDIDYMIS

The epididymis is located on the back side of the testicle. It is made up of a head (caput), body (corpus), and tail (cauda). The head is about one quarter to one half inch wide and is also known as the globus major. A small growth may be seen on the head which is called the appendix of the epididymis. The head is located over the upper pole of the testicle. The body and tail follow the back side of the testicle to the lower pole. The efferent ducts empty into the epididymis where the spermatozoa are stored, mature, and complete the migration from the testicle to the vas deferens.

SEMINIFEROUS TUBULES

The seminiferous tubules make up the testicular lobules (usually one to three tubules per lobule). This is the glandular part of testicles that contain the sperm producing cells. The epithelium of each tubule consists of sustentacular (or Sertoli) cells. These are tall, column-like cells that line the tubule. Located between the Sertoli cells are spermatogenic cells, which differentiate through meiosis (the cell division of reproductive or germ cells) to sperm cells. The seminiferous tubules converge to form a structure that resembles a network of tubules (called the rete testis). The rete testis then funnels the sperm cells into the efferent ducts (or vasa efferentia).

VAS DEFERENS

Beginning at the tail of the epididymis, the vas deferens is a narrow, muscular tube that connects the testicles to the urethra. The vas deferens is connected to the prostate and ultimately carries semen to the urethra.

SCROTUM
BLOOD SUPPLY

Blood is supplied to the testicles from the testicular artery which is connected to the aorta. The vas deferens and epididymis receive their blood supply from the deferential artery (a branch of the vesical artery). The pertesticular tissue receives blood from the cremasteric artery (a branch of the inferior epigastric artery). Both the deferential and cremasteric arteries are connected to the testicular artery. Blood is drained from the testicles through a network of veins originating in the mediastinum. This forms the pampiniform plexus located within the spermatic cord. The pampiniform plexus connects with three veins (the testicular, deferential, and cremateric). The right testicular vein drains into the vena cava and the left testicular vein drains into the left renal vein.

GENERAL ANATOMY

The scrotum is a part of the male anatomy that contains the testicles. It takes the form a two-sided pouch. The scrotum is separated into left and right sides by a septum (called the median raphe). Each side of the scrotum contains a testicle, an epididymus, a vas deferens, and a spermatic cord. The parietal layer of the tunica vaginalis provides an internal lining within the scrotum. The visceral layer of the tunica vaginalis surrounds the testicle except of a small bare area (located behind the testicle). The blood vessels, lymphatics, nerves, and spermatic ducts are connected to the testicle through this bare area. The scrotum has the ability to expand and contract (usually in reaction to temperature).

TESTES

The testes (or testicles) are part of the male reproductive organs. The testes are glands (made up of several hundred lobules) that produce and store sperm cells used for reproduction. In addition, they serve an endocrine function by producing testosterone. Testosterone is a hormone that stimulates the production of sperm and causes male traits such as a deeper voice, larger muscles, and thick facial hair growth. They are two oval-shaped glands measuring about one inch in diameter and about one and one-half inches in length. A thick fibrous capsule called the tunica albuginea protects the testicular parenchyma. The parietal layer of the tunica vaginalis surrounds the tunica albuginea.

SEMINAL VESICLES

The seminal vesicles are two sack-like glandular structures that produce part (about seventy percent) of the thick fluid (semen) that contains sperm. The thick secretions contain proteins, enzymes, fructose, mucus, vitamin C, flavins, phosphorylcholine and prostaglandins. These nutrients help the sperm cells stay alive and travel through the female reproductive system. Each vesicle is about two inches long. The vesicles are located at the base of the bladder just above and to the rear of the prostate gland.

The following ultrasound feature is present:

The seminal vesicles appear as hypoechoic, symmetrical, irregularly shaped structures.

SCROTAL HERNIA

A scrotal hernia occurs when a section of the bowel bulges into the scrotum. The affected patient usually presents with an enlarged scrotum.

The following ultrasound feature is present:

- Peristalsing loops of the bowel are observed in the scrotum.

HEMATOMA OF THE TESTICLE

Trauma to the testicle may cause injury and bleeding.

The following ultrasound features are present:

- The normal homogeneous appearance of the testicle may be altered.
- Hematomas of the epididymis or scrotal wall will have variable appearances.
- The age of the hemotoma affects the observed features.
- At first, the hematoma will appear hypoechoic.
- As the hematoma ages, the appearance becomes more echogenic.

SEMINOMA

Seminomas are cancerous tumors that develop from the germ cells of the testicle (the cells that produce sperm). There are two main types of tumors that are called classical (or typical) seminomas and spermatocytic seminomas. Over ninety five percent of seminomas are classical. They usually affect men in their late thirties to early fifties. The average age of men diagnosed with spermatocytic seminoma is about fifty-five. This is ten to fifteen years older than the average age of men with classical seminomas. Spermatocytic tumors are different from classical seminomas in that they grow very slowly and typically do not spread to other parts of the body. This usually results in a good prognosis for patients diagnosed with spermatocytic seminomas

SPERMATOCELES

Spermatoceles are painless, benign, cysts that usually grow in the head of the epididymis. They can be singular or multiple in number and are usually filled with a milky or clear colored fluid containing nonviable sperm. Over time, spermatoceles may remain constant in size or they may grow.

The following ultrasound features are present:

- Spermatoceles appear as cysts, are anechoic with posterior enhancement, and have rounded, well-defined walls.
- Spermatoceles cannot be differentiated from simple cysts of the epididymis (that are filled with clear fluid rather than sperm).
- Simple cysts of the epididymis are much less common than spermatoceles.

TESTICULAR MICROLITHIASIS

Testicular microlithiasis is a rare (it occurs in up one-half percent of men) benign condition that causes multiple minute calcifications throughout the testicles. It usually causes no symptoms. In up to eighty percent of cases both testicles are affected. Testicular microlithiasis has been associated with testicular cancer, cryptorchidism (the absence of one or more testicles from the scrotum), infertility and intraepithelial germ cell neoplasia (abnormal tissue growth).

The following ultrasound features are present:

- Multiple, echogenic, non-shadowing areas throughout the testicles.
- The calcifications may obscure other features of the testicle.
- An echo-poor (or complex abnormality) within the testicle may indicate the presence of an abscess, orchitis (infection), torsion, or tumor.

ULTRASOUND FEATURES OF MALIGNANT TESTICULAR TUMORS

The following ultrasound features are typically present for malignant testicular tumors:

- The tumors appear as well-defined masses.
- The masses are hypoechoic although they sometimes appear heterogeneous.
- Seminomas take on a hypoechoic appearance and are more homogeneous than nonseminomatous germ cell tumors.
- Choriocarcinoma tumors may have cystic features caused by necrosis and bleeding.
- Tumors of the sex cord stroma (Leydig and Certoli cell tumors) may appear as non-homogeneous testicles.
- Germ cell tumors larger than one half inch typically have many blood vessels and a disorganized blood flow.

PRIMARY TESTICULAR CANCER

Up to ninety five percent of primary testicular tumors originate in the germ cells (the cells that produce sperm). Primary testicular cancer typically occurs in men between the ages of fifteen and thirty-four. Usually there are no symptoms present, although in some cases (ten to fifty percent) there is acute pain in the scrotal area. Invasive testicular germ cell cancers begin as a noninvasive form of the disease (called carcinoma in situ or intratubular germ cell neoplasia). It takes about five years for carcinoma in situ to progress to the invasive form of germ cell cancer. When testicular cancer becomes invasive, its cells penetrate the surrounding tissues and spread (through blood circulation or lymph nodes) to other parts of the body.

SCROTUM AND PROSTATE ULTRASOUNDS

The ultrasound of the scrotum can detect carcinoma, cryptorchidism or undescended testis, and polyorchidism or the presence of more than two testes, torsion, and hernia. The ultrasound should find a small amount of fluid in the scrotal sac surrounding each testis and the vascular structures known to be present. Care should be taken to protect the privacy of the patient when performing the scrotal ultrasound. The testis should measure 4 cm in length and 2 cm in height and 3 cm in width in an adult male patient. If the measurements are far from the normal expected, suspicion of testicular carcinoma should be considered. Use the highest frequency linear transducer to obtain the best depth and clear image. Place the penis on the lower abdomen and cover with a towel for privacy. Evaluate the scrotum from the superior to the inferior walls and medial to lateral in both sagittal and transverse planes. Use a transabdominal or endorectal transducer for the prostate examination.

EPIDIDYMITIS

Epididymitis is an infection of the epididymis that eventually spreads to the testicle. The scrotum typically becomes swollen and tender. In most cases, the infection occurs on one side of the scrotum. Patients usually present with fever and painful urination.

The following ultrasound features are present:

- The head of the epididymis shows enlargement (with decreased echogenicity in the swollen area).
- A reactive hydrocele (an accumulation of anechoic fluid in the scrotum surrounding the testicle and epididymis) may be present.
- Color Doppler shows an increased amount of blood flow in the affected epididymis.
- In the event an abscess has formed, complex cystic structures may be observed.

ORCHITIS

Orchitis is the term for an infection that has spread to the testicle.

The following ultrasound features are present:

- The testicle may appear normal to enlarged in size.
- Echogenicity of the testicle may be decreased (or heterogeneous).
- Increased blood flow can be observed using color Doppler.
- In cases of chronic orchitis, layers of heterogeneous testicular parenchyma are present.
- Focal orchitis does not affect the epididymis and appears the same as a testicular tumor. The presence of a fever and an increased white blood count are indicative of orchitis.

ULTRASOUND APPEARANCE OF THE EPIDIDYMIS

A complete scrotal ultrasound should include an evaluation and measurements of the testes as well as the epididymis. The epididymis consists of a head, body, and tail. The head is located posterior to the superior portion of the testis and the tail courses posterior and lateral to the inferior pole, where it evolves into the vas deferens. The ultrasound appearance of a normal epididymis tends to be coarser than the adjacent testis, but it is isoechoic to it. Epididymitis (inflammation of the epididymis) is often caused by a sexually transmitted infection or urinary tract infection, and it is a common diagnosis that can be made with ultrasound. Ultrasound evaluation of the epididymis includes bilateral interrogation with longitudinal and transverse images. Measurements of the epididymal head should be included because it will often appear edematous and hyperemic on color or power Doppler. Instead of isoechoic, the epididymis may appear hypoechoic when compared to the testis.

ECTASIA OF THE RETE TESTIS

During a testicular ultrasound, a thin echogenic line may be visualized in the middle (hilum) of the testes. This line is the mediastinum testis, which is a continuation of the tunica albuginea (the fibrous capsule that encases the testes) and contains blood vessels, nerves, and seminiferous tubules. The rete testis is a region in which the various tubules join together to propel sperm out of the seminiferous tubules. When ultrasound detects ectasia of the rete testis, multiple anechoic cysts will be visualized in the testicular hilum due to obstruction of the efferent ductules. Color flow will not be present in this area of dilation, and this is often seen bilaterally, especially in older men. Sonographers must be able to discern ectasia of the rete testes from any neoplasm that may have internal cystic elements but will also contain solid components.

EVALUATING PARENCHYMAL DISEASES OF THE TESTES

When a patient presents with a palpable scrotal mass, swelling, or pain, he will be sent to the ultrasound laboratory for evaluation. Intratesticular neoplasms tend to be malignant, whereas extratesticular masses tend to be associated with a benign process. Intratesticular lesions can be easily identified with ultrasound, and these can include primary or metastatic tumors. Primary lesions will typically look like a hypoechoic, hyperemic mass with borders that are clearly defined. This mass may display cystic components as well. Microlithiasis is frequently diagnosed by ultrasound and appears as multiple echogenic foci within the testes. Orchitis will demonstrate as an enlarged testicle with a heterogeneous appearance. It is helpful for diagnosis to determine if a patient has elevated labs, fever, or chills because orchitis is an infection that has spread, but it may look similar to a malignant tumor.

BREAST ULTRASOUND

The breast region is a common anatomical structure that is evaluated by ultrasound. This can be performed on men or women, especially when a lump is felt to further investigate whether the mass is solid or cystic and its shape, vascularity, and borders. Breast lesions that are cystic are typically benign processes such as a cyst. Patients often present with a lump or lumps that can be palpated with or without tenderness, nipple inversion, dimpling of the skin, or infections of the breast. Ultrasound may be performed without or in conjunction with a mammogram, depending on the patient's age and medical history or to offer guidance during a cyst aspiration or breast biopsy. In patients who are positive for breast cancer, it is common to see a hypoechoic mass that is taller than it is wide, with irregular borders and possible microcalcifications. Color Doppler and more recently, elastography, are useful methods to use when breast cancer is suspected.

BREAST MASSES

Breast masses are typically cystic or solid lesions. Ultrasound can distinguish between ninety six to one hundred percent of these masses. Cystic masses have the following ultrasound features:

- The cyst will show smooth walls
- The front (anterior) and back (posterior) of the cyst will show sharply defined borders
- There will be no internal echoes
- The cyst will show posterior enhancement

Solid masses that show signs of malignancy have the following ultrasound features:

- A mass that is taller than it is wide
- Spiculation is present
- The mass shows angular margins
- The presence of a markedly hypoechoic solid lesion

Normal lymph nodes have the following ultrasound features:

A small, ovoid structure with a hypoechoic rim and echogenic hilum.

TDLU IN THE BREAST

The adult mammary gland forms a stalk and branches (originating at the nipple and continuing the structure to the lobules). The lobules are the functional units of the breast and are responsible for producing milk. The milk begins its passage through the breast by being expelled from the short intra-lobular terminal ducts and the longer extra-lobular terminal ducts. It then moves through the collecting ducts and finally to the nipple (through the lactiferous ducts). When the mammary gland is in the resting state, the terminal lobules (both the intra and extra) are referred to as the terminal-ductal-lobular-unit (TDLU).

SONOGRAPHIC EVALUATION OF THE BREAST

The proper transducer that will provide the most optimal imaging is the ten-megahertz linear array. Proper indications for breast ultrasound include:

- Differentiation of cysts from solid masses
- Evaluation of a palpable mass that is not visible in an x-ray.
- Assessment of a mass that is not viewable in a normal mammogram (possibly due to its location)
- Evaluation of a young patient with a palpable mass

The patient should be positioned properly to conduct the examination. For example, if the patient has a right lateral breast mass, the patient should be placed in the left posterior oblique position with their right arm abducted.

ABNORMALITIES RELATED TO TRAUMATIC EVENTS

Ultrasound can be a great tool to quickly evaluate the presence of free fluid in post-traumatic injuries. Clinicians can use the Focused Assessment with Sonography for Trauma method to help determine the best care for the patient without having to expose them to radiation. This is especially important in children, women that are pregnant, or when multiple victims are sent to the emergency department at once. Physicians and sonographers can evaluate the chest, abdominal, and pelvic cavities for evidence of a pericardial or pleural effusion, pneumothorax, or ascites.

Ultrasound may also aid in the diagnosis of an injury involving the liver, spleen, and/or kidneys. The inferior vena cava may also be imaged when the patient has lost a lot of blood. Sonographers should be aware that anechoic fluid visualized within the abdomen or pelvis when the patient is status post-trauma is likely due to a hemorrhage. However, blood may vary in appearance and may even be difficult to discern from the normal surrounding tissue of the solid organs.

IMPORTANCE OF DOPPLER ANGLE WHEN MEASURING VELOCITIES DURING CAROTID DUPLEX EXAM

In order for the sonographer to obtain the most accurate measurement during a carotid duplex exam, the moving red blood cells should be located parallel to the transducer. In this case, the measurement reflects the velocity located in all parts of the ultrasound wave. A positive Doppler frequency occurs when the velocity of the returning signals from blood cells moving toward the transducer is greater than the transmitted velocity. When the blood is not moving exactly parallel to the sound beam, the velocity measurement will not be as accurate. For example, if the angle cursor is larger than the actual Doppler angle, the velocity will be too high. If the angle cursor is lower than the angle that is parallel to the vessel wall, then the velocity will be underestimated.

OPTIMIZING COLOR FLOW OF PATENT CAROTID ARTERY IN WHICH COLOR IS NOT IMMEDIATELY SEEN

If a sonographer cannot visualize color during a carotid duplex exam, the first thing that can be done is to determine the angle of the color box with the direction of blood flow. It is important for sonographers to remember that if the color box is perpendicular (at a 90-degree angle) to a vessel, color will never be visualized. Modern systems allow color boxes to be steered with linear transducers, which will prevent the beam from being perpendicular to the vessel. Next, the user can increase the color gain. This demonstrates the amplification of signals within blood vessels, but it will not show blood flow if it is not actually present. The velocity scale is also important to adjust if blood flow is not well demonstrated or if aliasing occurs.

CAROTID BODY TUMOR

Carotid body tumors are the most common of all the paragangliomas. Paragangliomas are tumors that arise from the paraganglion. In this case, the paraganglion is located on the outer surface (adventitia) of the carotid artery at the point where it splits (bifurcates) into the internal and external carotid arteries. It affects more women than men, and becomes more likely in patients that are fifty-years old (or older). Patients usually present with a painless neck mass that is less than one inch in diameter. Only about five to ten percent of carotid body tumors turn out to be malignant.

HEPATOBLASTOMA

Hepatoblastoma is a rare form of liver cancer that usually occurs in infancy and early childhood (the median age is one year old with most cases being diagnosed by age two). It occurs in an otherwise healthy liver. Prior hepatitis infection is not associated with the occurrence of this cancer, and it may be of genetic origin. The cancer typically appears as an abdominal mass without any symptoms. In some cases, it may be accompanied by symptoms such as weight loss, abdominal pain, loss of appetite, anemia, fever, vomiting and jaundice. The cellular structure of the tumor is epithelial or mixed (containing structural elements such as osteoid tissue).

During an ultrasound examination of the tumor, the following feature is present:

Blood flow patterns are echogenic or cystic (with internal separations).

MESENCHYMA HAMARTOMA

Mesenchymal hamartoma is a rare cystic tumor that primarily affects children under two years of age. This is the second most common benign liver tumor of childhood. It is mostly found on the right lobe of the liver. It is usually discovered through observation of an abdominal distension (caused by a non-tender mass). The tumor can be large (up to five pounds). It is made up of cysts containing clear fluid and gelatin-like material. There is some evidence that this type of tumor regresses naturally, however surgical removal is the recommended course of action.

During an ultrasound examination of the tumor, the following features are present:

Well defined blood-flow patterns, mostly echo-free, with some web-like patterns at the border of attachment to the right lobe of the liver.

RISK FACTORS FOR DDH

Developmental dysplasia of the hip (DDH) is a term used to describe a number of malformations of the hip joint. The signs of this may not always be recognized once the child is born, so this term has replaced congenital hip dysplasia. The hip is a ball-and-socket joint, but often the femoral head (ball) is not completely covered by the acetabulum (socket). Many factors play a role in this process, and it is important for the sonographer to get a thorough history from the child's caregiver, but DDH is often due to a breech position, large gestational size, oligohydramnios, or it may tend to run in families. This tends to be more prevalent in girls, especially those that are firstborn, and the left hip is impacted more often from DDH than the right side. Other clinical findings that may warrant further investigation with ultrasound for DDH include legs that are different lengths or if the folds in the thigh appear asymmetrical.

ULTRASOUND APPLICATIONS IN HIP ANOMALIES

Ultrasound can be used in infants and children to assess when a dislocated hip is suspected or in symptoms of hip pain or when a child begins to limp. In order to diagnose a hip dislocation on ultrasound, the sonographer can perform the scan with the infant's hips flexed 90 degrees while in a transverse plane. An unstable hip is assumed when the ultrasound operator can see a difference in the relationship of the femoral head and the acetabulum when light pressure is applied from a more posterior and lateral approach. Synovitis can often be seen with ultrasound in children who are between the ages of three and eight. If the distance between the femoral neck and the external layer of the hip capsule measures more than 5 mm, then a joint effusion can be assumed. A measurement can also be taken of the contralateral side, and if the same measurements are more than 2 mm thicker on the side that is painful, a joint effusion is also diagnosed.

EVALUATING THE THYMUS GLAND

The thymus gland can be readily evaluated with ultrasound, especially in neonates and infants due to lesser degree of ossification of their sternum and ribs. The thymus gland is part of the endocrine and lymphatic systems and is located within the mediastinum between the lungs, superior to the heart, and posterior to the sternum. The ultrasound appearance is a homogeneous, somewhat hypoechoic (when compared to the thyroid, spleen, and liver) gland with internal echogenic strands that give it a "starry sky" appearance. A normal thymus demonstrates smooth borders. Upon color Doppler interrogation, a normal thymus gland is relatively avascular. An abnormal thymus gland will have a heterogeneous, lobular appearance, often with calcifications. The size of the thymus gland varies with age as it reaches maximum size during puberty, but it is then replaced by fat and shrinks.

MESOBLASTIC NEPHROMA

Mesoblastic nephroma is the most common benign renal tumor identified in newborn children (the peak age is three months). This tumor is sometimes confused with the congenital Wilms' tumor. It usually occurs in the first six months of life. These tumors can be quite large and take up the entire kidney area. The tumor itself has a homogeneous rubbery appearance, and (unlike Wilms' tumors) is not prone to bleeding. Symptoms may include hematuria, hypertension, vomiting, and hypercalcemia (these are usually seen in a minority of cases).

The following ultrasound features are present:

- A large, echogenic mass with a homogeneous echotexture.
- Any heterogeneity may suggest areas of necrosis (tissue death) or bleeding (hemorrhage).

NEONATAL HEAD ULTRASOUND

An ultrasound of the head in neonates and infants may be ordered to evaluate for congenital abnormalities, evaluate the brain when intrauterine growth restriction is present, if there are seizures or hemorrhage, or if the size of the head appears abnormal. Ultrasound can also be performed as part of a post-traumatic workup or prior to surgery. Color Doppler can also be used to evaluate the blood vessels of the brain for any issues. A thorough exam will include images obtained from the coronal and sagittal planes with additional views added when necessary. Anatomical structures examined during an ultrasound of the brain include the ventricles, carpus callosum, cavum septi pellucidi, lobes of the brain, and brain stem, among others. Ultrasound of the head should be performed with transducers that offer the best resolution while being able to penetrate as needed. Older infants may require the use of a lower frequency probe to penetrate the skull.

ULTRASOUND OF THE SPINE ON PEDIATRIC PATIENTS

OB ultrasounds include imaging of the fetal spine for any indication of spina bifida. After birth, the infant's spine may also be examined with ultrasound when a clinician suspects any spinal defect or an abnormal spinal cord, when a sacral mass is present, there is an abnormal sacral dimple or a cluster of hair or birthmark in the region of the spinal cord, or when the infant has other birth defects. Magnetic resonance imaging may be necessary (or it may be the exam of choice in cases in which infection is a concern) especially after three months of age because the spinal cord may not be visualized well due to the ossification of the vertebral column. Longitudinal and transverse imaging should be performed with a high-frequency transducer. The ultrasound operator may perform a limited exam of the lumbar and sacral portions depending on the reason for the exam, or the entire spine may be evaluated. The spinal cord is located within the central portion of the spinal canal, and it appears hypoechoic except for the central portion, which will be more echogenic; the conus medullaris should end at the L2-L3 disk space or higher. Extended field of view documentation may be beneficial when counting spinal segments.

SCANNING AN INFANT HIP FOR DEVELOPMENTAL DYSPLASIA OF THE HIP

Ultrasound is often the first imaging modality chosen to help diagnose developmental dysplasia of the hip. Ultrasound can be performed in infants because the hip joint is still rather cartilaginous. The examiner should scan both hips for comparison, and this exam should not take place prior to the baby being four weeks old because the hip tends to be rather flexible (unless there is a suspected dislocation of the hip). The sonographer should document the hip in a coronal plane with the patient relaxed and in a neutral position to take any measurements. The acetabulum is best evaluated with a coronal view, and the acetabular angle can be measured. If the angle is greater than or equal to 60 degrees, this indicates a normal depth of the acetabulum. A transverse plane should be used when the hip is flexed and while performing stress views. If the femoral head changes position within the joint after light pressure is applied from a posterior approach, instability can be assumed.

SONOGRAPHIC INDICATORS OF INTUSSUSCEPTION

Intussusception is often referred to as the "telescoping" of one part of the intestine within an adjacent portion, typically occurring in the region in which the small and large intestines join. This is often accompanied by inflammation and can create an obstruction. Patients often present with a right upper quadrant mass with intermittent abdominal pain, nausea, and vomiting, and often their stools will contain blood. An ultrasound of the abdomen should be performed with a high-frequency transducer, and graded compression should be used to displace any bowel gas that is present. It is important to scan the entire colon. Typical ultrasound appearances of intussusception in cross section are a target or bull's-eye appearance. A longitudinal image will often demonstrate a stacked pancake sign, and an oblique view will mimic a kidney.

PYLORIC STENOSIS IN INFANTS

Patients who have hypertrophic pyloric stenosis (HPS) will often be dehydrated, not gaining weight as expected, present with a palpable abdominal mass, and experience projectile vomiting (that does not contain bile) after being fed. HPS is the result of a thickened muscular layer of the lower third of the stomach called the pylorus. The pyloric canal allows for the passage of milk into the small intestine, but when this region is too thick, the contents are unable to continue past this point. HPS is the most common reason for surgical intervention in the first couple of months of life. Ultrasound should be performed after the baby has been fed in order to provide a dynamic study to determine if the contents are able to pass through the pyloric canal. A high-frequency transducer should be used, and the depth should be adjusted so the pylorus can be seen. With the patient supine, the pylorus can be found just posteromedial to the gallbladder and should be measured. The hypoechoic muscular layer should be less than 3 mm; an elongated pyloric canal may also be visualized, but it is a less reliable measurement (normal is less than 12 mm).

APPENDICITIS IN PEDIATRIC PATIENTS

When appendicitis is suspected in pediatric patients, ultrasound may be the modality of choice because it does not subject the patient to ionizing radiation. A high-frequency transducer should be used, and sonographers often ask the patient to place the probe over the region of maximum tenderness (when the patient is old enough to communicate this). Sonographic evaluation uses graded compression in order to move bowel gas out of the way and improve resolution to better visualize the appendix. The sonographer can move the transducer to the right lower quadrant to identify the ileum and cecum because the cecum is the proximal portion of the large intestine in which the appendix is located. The normal diameter of the appendix in children is 4.2 mm (6 mm in adults), and it should be compressible. Acute appendicitis will be greater than 6 mm in diameter and will not compress. Often, an inflamed appendix appears as a bull's-eye, is filled with fluid, and is hyperemic. However, an appendix that has perforated may not demonstrate blood flow. If an abscess is demonstrated, this also indicates a perforation. An appendicolith may suggest perforation, although these may be seen in patients with a normal appendix.

WILMS' TUMOR

A Wilms' tumor is the most common renal tumor detected in the pediatric population. These are often found in patients younger than the age of five, with most cases diagnosed when the child is three or four years old. This is the most common malignant cancer diagnosed in childhood. These masses are often noticed by the child's parents because a lump may be felt in the abdomen. The child may also have abdominal pain and/or hematuria (blood in the urine). A Wilms' tumor is also referred to as a nephroblastoma. The ultrasound appearance of a nephroblastoma is a predominantly solid mass found within the kidney that may be heterogeneous in the presence of necrosis or hemorrhage. The tumor may also contain fat or calcifications. It is important to note that a nephroblastoma is typically unilateral, but it may occur in the right and the left kidneys. When a solid mass is present, the sonographer must check the renal vein(s) and inferior vena cava to determine if there is vascular extension of the mass.

SCANNING THE ADRENAL GLANDS DURING PEDIATRIC EXAMS

The adrenal glands are part of the endocrine system and are found superior to the kidneys. The adrenal glands consist of an inner medulla and an outer cortex, and in newborns even normal adrenal glands are readily visible because higher frequency transducers can be used. The right adrenal gland can be seen more often than the left. Every pediatric abdominal ultrasound should include the adrenals to exclude any suprarenal masses such as a neuroblastoma. The adrenal glands can be difficult to visualize and require a skilled ultrasound operator, but newer ultrasound technology such as 3D, spatial compounding, and harmonic imaging have proved to be advantageous. Gray-scale is useful to determine if lesions are cystic or solid. Color and power Doppler can be used to determine if blood flow is present within any masses.

ULTRASOUND GUIDANCE FOR VASCULAR ACCESS PROCEDURES

Ultrasound can be a useful tool when vascular access procedures are required so that clinicians can be sure that the line is placed correctly. The use of ultrasound has proven beneficial because it does not expose the patient to ionizing radiation like fluoroscopy does. Physicians that are trained to perform these procedures with ultrasound guidance can also determine that there is patency of the vessel, the size and depth of the vessel, and tell when the needle is in the best location. It is also possible to visualize if the needle has passed through the posterior wall of a vessel. Surrounding anatomical structures can be visualized within vessels, for example, a valve in a vein or adjacent to the vessels. Ultrasound systems can also assist physicians because they can turn on color Doppler so that there is no doubt of whether the structure is a vein or artery.

ULTRASOUND-GUIDED FINE-NEEDLE ASPIRATION OR BIOPSY

Ultrasound-guided fine-needle aspirations and biopsies are common exams done in an ultrasound laboratory. These studies use ultrasound to improve diagnostic confidence because physicians can actually track the needle going into the target tissue or fluid in question. The material that is removed can then be sent to the laboratory for further evaluation. Ultrasound also serves as an aid to avoid anatomical structures such as blood vessel and nerves as the needle is being inserted. It is important that the region of interest is scanned and shown to the clinician performing the procedure. The sonographer should be sure that all consent forms and supplies are present and to maintain a sterile field. It is important that the physician has the correct supplies so that once the material is withdrawn, it can quickly be sent to the laboratory for further evaluation. Common fine-needle aspiration procedures include thyroid or parathyroid nodules, lymph nodes, breast cysts, or superficial abscesses. Biopsies may include tissue from the breast, prostate, and liver.

ROLE OF SONOGRAPHER

Sonographers are often required to assist during needle biopsy procedures. The sonographer must make sure to have the correct patient and explain the procedure to him or her before the clinician comes into the room. Any prior imaging exam and report should be provided for the physician. It is important that all consent forms are in the room so that the patient can sign them (either on paper or electronically) after they speak with the physician that will be performing the procedure. The sonographer will set up the sterile tray and gather any necessary supplies that the clinician may need. It is important to maintain a sterile field during the procedure to prevent an infection. The sonographer will often be scanning during the procedure, so communication with the physician is crucial in order to reach the target and save the necessary images so that the radiologist can generate a report. The patient should closely monitor the patient during the procedure, wipe off any gel, and provide follow-up information after the procedure including how the patient will receive their results. Sonographers should be sure that the collection containers are sent to the laboratory as soon as possible with the correct patient identifiers.

Assistance and Guidance of Sonographers During Procedures

Sonographers offer various types of assistance during ultrasound procedures. Regardless of the type of exam, the patient's safety is the most important concern of the sonographer. If a physician will be performing an ultrasound-guided procedure, the sonographer will have many roles. The sonographer must make sure that the correct patient, exam, and consent forms are gathered along with prior exams and reports. Sterile trays should be set up with other necessary supplies available. The sonographer should choose the correct equipment and ultrasound settings in order to obtain optimal resolution. It is important that enough space is available for the physician and that he or she can easily access the patient as well as see the ultrasound monitor. If the sonographer is to scan the patient, it is imperative to don sterile gloves and practice aseptic technique. If any specimens are collected, it is important that the sonographer correctly identifies them and sends them to the laboratory as soon as possible. Postprocedural steps include watching for signs of infection or bleeding and indicating how the patient will receive results.

Ultrasound Guidance for Injections

In the past, if physicians used guidance to inject a patient, it was often done by fluoroscopy; which is live X-ray. X-rays obviously use ionizing radiation, and the equipment is large and expensive. Ultrasound has become a more common method for physicians wanting a low-cost, nonionizing, portable technique for injections. Ultrasound-guided joint injections are performed to aid the physician when injecting corticosteroids that are used to help relieve pain and inflammation. Hyaluronic acid can be injected into the knee joint to provide a cushion and lubricate the knee joint to remove some of the pain from osteoarthritis. Ultrasound can be used to make sure the needle is in the correct location to provide the optimum amount of relief to the patient instead of having the physician inject blindly. Ultrasound also gives extra information to the physician so that other anatomical structures such as blood vessels and nerves can be avoided during an injection.

Measurement of the Achilles Tendon

Many methods are available to obtain an accurate measurement of the Achilles tendon. However, some of these processes tend to be quite invasive. Ultrasound can be used as a noninvasive technique while enabling users to obtain accurate measurements of the Achilles tendon. It is a painless, fast, and inexpensive method that can also be used for follow-up studies. The Achilles tendon in adults is longer than the face of an ultrasound transducer, and many ultrasound machines have extended field of view or panoramic imaging capabilities. Ultrasound is also sensitive to measure the thickness of the Achilles tendon, which does not require extended field of view images, but this information can be useful in cases of tendinopathy. Achilles tendons that have greater thickness measurements tend to be at a greater risk for tendinopathy.

MSK Imaging

Musculoskeletal (MSK) ultrasound applications offers patients and clinicians a more cost-effective and dynamic imaging modality without the use of ionizing radiation. Ultrasound can be used for patients that have contraindications for magnetic resonance imaging such as pacemakers, neurostimulators, aneurysm clips, cochlear implants, or even for those patients who are claustrophobic. This modality is still advancing because newer technology offers better resolution when evaluating soft tissue, muscles, tendons, ligaments, and nerves. MSK ultrasound may also be used to diagnose nerve entrapment and tears of muscles, tendons, or ligaments. Ultrasound can quickly give physicians comparisons of the contralateral structures for better diagnosis and treatment options and can be used to demonstrate real-time imaging of a dynamic movement. For example, the shoulder can be imaged while the patient is performing various motions and muscles can be imaged with the patient contracting and relaxing the muscle.

SONOGRAPHIC EVALUATION OF TENDONS

The proper transducer that will provide the most optimal imaging is the twelve-megahertz linear array. Tendons appear highly echogenic with a fibrillar echotexture. In comparison, normal muscles show oblique, parallel, echogenic fibers against a hypoechoic background. Proper technique is very important to avoid false hypoechogenicity due to the oblique incidence of the beam to the tendon axis.

The following ultrasound features are present in cases of tendonitis (inflammation of the tendon):

- There is a thickening of the tendon
- Echogenicity is decreased
- The margins of the tendon appear blurred
- In cases of chronic tendonitis, calcifications are present

IDENTIFYING INFECTIONS WITHIN SUPERFICIAL STRUCTURES

An abscess is one type of infection that may be diagnosed and evaluated with ultrasound. A physician may choose to drain an abscess under ultrasound guidance once it has been diagnosed. An abscess may have a wide array of appearances, but a collection of fluid that is either anechoic or hypoechoic, often displaying posterior enhancement is suggestive of an abscess. The borders of an abscess may be difficult to discern, and overlying soft tissues may appear edematous. Internal septa, gas, and floating particulates may be seen within the abscess, especially when light pressure is applied. Color or power Doppler will usually show peripheral blood flow or flow within adjacent tissues due to inflammation, but absent internal blood flow. When ultrasound guidance is used for aspiration of an abscess, the fluid should be sent to the lab for confirmation of an infection. A larger needle may be necessary in order to withdraw fluid in the presence of infection.

ULTRASOUND FINDINGS OF SUPERFICIAL FOREIGN BODIES

Foreign bodies that are not radiopaque can be difficult to diagnose and are common reasons for malpractice cases because retained objects can lead to complications from infections. The use of high-frequency transducers provides clinicians with better resolution when evaluating superficial structures in situations in which the use of X-ray was not successful in locating the object. Although locating a foreign body depends on the skill of the operator, size, and depth of the object, other clues can be helpful in the location attempt. Inflammation will be evident if the object has been in place for a while. The sonographic appearance of foreign bodies will be hyperechoic and will likely display some sort of artifact (reverberation, comet tail, or shadowing). Edematous tissue or an abscess will be represented by a ring around the object that is hypoechoic. Ultrasound can provide clinicians with important information such as the size of the object, depth, and how close the object is to blood vessels, muscles, tendons, and nerves.

LIPOMAS

Lipomas are common masses that sonographers may be required to scan, although physicians often diagnose these clinically without medical imaging. They are a benign, fatty, elliptical subcutaneous mass that are often compressible and contain echogenic strands running parallel to the skin line. Color Doppler may display a wide array of vascularity. Lipomas may be associated with weight gain, and patients may have more than one lipoma. Lipomas are usually fairly small with a diameter of less than 3 cm, but they can grow into larger masses. Ultrasound is useful to determine the size and location of these masses. Subcutaneous lipomas are the most common type of these masses, and they are often visualized in the proximal portions of the extremities, neck, and back. Lipomas that are deeper may have similar appearances to a sarcoma because these borders are more difficult to visualize and are less compressible. They can be located within, above, below, or between muscles and may need to be evaluated further by magnetic resonance imaging.

PLEURAL EFFUSION

Pleural effusions are common in individuals with cirrhosis, lung cancer, bacterial pneumonia, and heart failure or in those that have had open heart surgery. Ultrasound can be used not only to identify the pleural effusion, but to estimate the amount of fluid present and provide real-time imaging during a thoracentesis. Ultrasound operators should evaluate suspected pleural effusions while the patient is upright using a 2–5 MHz transducer in a longitudinal plane where the diaphragm can be visualized starting just posterior to the axillary line. The operator should see the lung, diaphragm, liver or spleen, and fluid. The fluid can be assessed as either a simple or complex collection. Ultrasound can also determine whether any septa are present. Ultrasound may also be used to evaluate masses within the wall of the chest cavity. These cases are best scanned using high-frequency transducers using B-mode, color, and spectral Doppler.

CHEST WALL LESIONS

Ultrasound can often be used as a follow-up method when a mass of the chest wall is visualized on X-rays. Radiographs may be unable to determine the various types of lesion because many of the findings are indistinguishable. Ultrasound of malignant chest masses can contribute information such as the location of the lesion, if adjacent structures are involved, if the lesion is completely solid or if it has a complex appearance, the vascularity of the lesion, and if there is a corresponding pleural effusion. Common malignant chest tumors are Ewing sarcomas and lymphomas. Benign (noncancerous) tumors that are found in the chest wall may include an abscess, lipomas, hemangiomas, and desmoid tumors. These benign processes are found more often than malignant tumors. Again, ultrasound can be used to determine the location, whether the mass is cystic or solid, the vascularity, and size.

HERNIAS

The abdominal wall can bulge and tear due to a natural weakness or an injury caused by strain (such as heavy lifting). This allows the lining of the abdomen to bulge through the tear and create a void. Sometimes a portion of the intestine (or other abdominal tissue) slips into this area causing pain and/or intestinal blockage. This condition is called a hernia. Most hernias occur near the groin (femoral). They sometimes occur at the navel (umbilical) or along a previous incision (ventral). Symptoms may include a physical bulge at the site of the hernia, pain during movement, or a dull ache.

Ultrasound is the modality of choice to help diagnose hernias that cannot be diagnosed clinically, especially those that tend to be small. Ultrasound is invaluable in the diagnosis of hernias because it offers a real-time visualization of the hernia contents as it protrudes through the neck. Ultrasound can be performed supine and upright, which is important because some hernias tend to reduce when the patient is lying down. The Valsalva maneuver can also be performed to increase the amount of pressure on the abdominal wall. Ultrasound can help determine if the hernia is fat containing or if the bowel is involved. Sonographers can also demonstrate reducibility of a hernia upon compression. Ultrasound machines today offers the ability to store cine clips to better demonstrate the hernia, especially during a Valsalva maneuver. Ultrasound can provide even more information such as the specific location (direct or indirect inguinal, femoral, incisional, or periumbilical hernia).

WHEN TO CONTACT A PHYSICIAN

A physician should be contacted when the ultrasound findings would indicate an immediate intervention. Urgent findings would include an ectopic pregnancy, abruptio placentae, or a leaking aneurysm. These are examples of the need for emergent surgical intervention. Fetal death, fetal anomalies, and abnormal fetal heart rate are examples of pathology that may need an intervention and should not wait for a dictated report to be sent to an office; calling the physician at the completion of the examination is the standard. Other serious conditions that should be phoned to the physician include: unexpected neoplastic masses; large hematomas; renal artery occlusion in kidney transplant patients; obstructed bile ducts; and placenta previa and bleeding.

ARRT Practice Test

1. Which term represents the degree of echo amplification or brightness of an ultrasound image?

    a. Zoom
    b. Gain
    c. Scatter
    d. Absorption

2. What type of image does the linear array offer in real-time imaging?

    a. Trapezoidal image
    b. Pie-shaped image
    c. Large-field image
    d. Rectangular image

3. Pulsed Doppler is used for what diagnostic purpose?

    a. To determine blood flow through arteries and veins
    b. To view large organs
    c. To determine solid masses
    d. There is no diagnostic purpose for pulsed Doppler.

4. The wave characteristic of frequency is measured by what unit of measurement?

    a. Gain
    b. Color
    c. Length
    d. Hertz

5. The comet tail image indicates which of the following to the ultrasound technician?

    a. The edge of the organ
    b. Artifact
    c. The sign of an abscess
    d. The right depth of the transducer

6. You are performing an ultrasound exam of the abdomen and pelvis of a patient with an unexplained fever. You understand the purpose of the exam is to look for which of the following?

    a. Abscess, inflammation, or mass
    b. Enlarged lymph nodes
    c. Both a and b
    d. Neither a nor b

7. What is an appropriate way to store color images of an ultrasound scan?

    a. Images can be scanned and stored in the memory of the equipment in gray scale, color, or real-time imaging.
    b. Images must be printed immediately because storage and memory are unreliable.
    c. Images can be stored as numbers or images.
    d. Images can only be stored in gray scale in the memory of the equipment.

8. Which term defines the first beam transmitting from the transducer?

   a. The reflected beam
   b. The incident beam
   c. The transmitted beam
   d. The harmonic beam

9. The purpose of a diagnostic ultrasound transducer is best described in which of the following descriptions?

   a. It is easy on the technician's hand and can be easily gripped.
   b. It is shaped with a round end for the best imaging.
   c. It is used to convert electrical energy into sound energy and sound energy to electrical energy.
   d. The transducer really has no definite purpose; the computer equipment actually does the scan.

10. What is the most significant side effect of sound waves on the patient who is undergoing an ultrasound?

   a. There is only a minimal possibility of adverse effects from the heat produced by the sound wave.
   b. There is no possibility of adverse effect from an ultrasound exam.
   c. Neonates have the only chance of any adverse side effects from an ultrasound.
   d. There are serious side effects from having an ultrasound, and the technician must explain those to the patient before every exam.

11. Which statement best defines the ALARA principle?

   a. The principle states that the lowest reasonable energy should be used to produce the clearest image.
   b. The principle states that the highest reasonable energy should be used to produce the clearest image.
   c. The principle states the level of energy is not included in when deciding what technique to use to get a clear image.
   d. The principle states that the lowest reasonable energy should be used with minimal exposure for obtaining the clearest image.

12. What is the lowest intensity value of ultrasound imaging?

   a. SATA
   b. SPPA
   c. SATP
   d. SPTP

13. What aspects of patient care and safety should be of concern to the ultrasound technologist?

   a. Identify the patient by name and offer privacy
   b. Address the patient by name, explain the procedure, and offer privacy
   c. Address the patient by name, explain the procedure clearly, offer privacy, select proper equipment, and follow the ALARA principles
   d. Explain the procedure, offer privacy, and minimize conversation

14. What physical abnormalities or illnesses may distort the results of an ultrasound of the gallbladder and may alter the interpretation of the images?

    a. The patient's history of chemotherapy, AIDS, a recent meal, or hepatitis
    b. Gallbladder stones
    c. An empty stomach
    d. Ascites

15. The ultrasound for an abscess can be difficult to image due to which of these pitfalls?

    a. A full stomach
    b. A full bladder
    c. An empty stomach
    d. Confusing the bowel with a possible abscess

16. Which statement explains the pitfalls of using ultrasound as a diagnostic tool for scanning the abdomen?

    a. There are no pitfalls. It is the best available test for abdominal pathology.
    b. The right kidney axis is unpredictable and often can shadow or imitate pathology when scanning the abdomen.
    c. Air, fluid, and tissue density will not affect the absorption and scatter in abdominal scans.
    d. The liver is too fatty to be noted on ultrasound.

17. Pertinent information that must be obtained prior to performing a fine needle aspiration of the thyroid includes all of the following except:

    a. reviewing prior imaging and reports.
    b. a signed and dated script for an FNA of the thyroid.
    c. a signed consent form.
    d. a prepared sterile tray.

18. The testicles are suspended within the scrotum by the:

    a. vas deferens.
    b. epididymis.
    c. seminiferous tubules.
    d. spermatic cord.

19. The least invasive type of thyroid biopsy that may be performed on a solitary thyroid nodule is a(n):

    a. fine needle aspiration.
    b. complete thyroidectomy.
    c. core biopsy.
    d. excisional biopsy.

20. A 16-year-old male presents to the emergency department with left-sided scrotal pain, nausea, and vomiting for the past several hours. He denies any recent trauma to his genitals. During sonographic evaluation, an enlarged left testicle with decreased echogenicity was documented. After further evaluation with color and spectral Doppler, intratesticular vasculature was noted to be absent. The patient most likely presents with:

    a. orchitis.
    b. torsion.
    c. an abscess.
    d. a hematocele.

21. Which arteries course along the renal pyramids within the kidney?

    a. Segmental arteries
    b. Arcuate arteries
    c. Interlobular arteries
    d. Interlobar arteries

22. A 27-year-old female presents to the ultrasound department for evaluation of the spleen. The patient complains of left upper quadrant pain. She was in a motor vehicle accident that occurred six months ago. All of the following sonographic findings may be present except:

    a. hypovolemic shock.
    b. left pleural effusion.
    c. splenomegaly.
    d. hematoma.

23. The portal triad includes the:

    a. common bile duct, common hepatic duct, and the main portal vein.
    b. common bile duct, hepatic vein, and the main portal vein.
    c. common hepatic duct, hepatic artery, and the main portal vein.
    d. common bile duct, hepatic artery, and the main portal vein.

24. Twinkling artifact may aid in the diagnosis of:

    a. cholelithiasis.
    b. hemangioma.
    c. portal hypertension.
    d. abdominal aortic aneurysm.

25. A 68-year-old male presents to the ultrasound department for evaluation of the liver. The patient complains of having anorexia, fatigue, and weakness for the past several months. His abdomen is enlarged. His labs indicate an increase in serum alpha-fetoprotein. Which is the most likely diagnosis?

    a. Focal nodular hyperplasia
    b. Hepatoma
    c. Cavernous hemangioma
    d. Liver cell adenoma

26. Which of the following is false regarding acute tubular necrosis?

a. It is the most common cause of renal failure
b. It causes an increase in arteriole resistance
c. It causes a decrease in arteriole resistance
d. It results in normal echogenicity of the renal cortex

27. The ureter inserts into the bladder at the trigone posteriorly and:

a. medially.
b. laterally.
c. superiorly.
d. inferiorly.

28. When acute pancreatitis is present, serum amylase and lipase levels both:

a. increase at the same rate, but lipase concentration stays elevated longer.
b. increase at the same rate, but amylase concentration stays elevated longer.
c. decrease at the same rate, but lipase concentration stays decreased longer.
d. decrease at the same rate, but amylase concentration stays decreased longer.

29. The main pancreatic duct is also known as the:

a. common bile duct.
b. duct of Santorini.
c. duct of Wirsung.
d. duct of Vater.

30. Clinical indications that may warrant a sonogram of the parathyroid gland to rule out a parathyroid adenoma include all of the following except:

a. hypophosphatemia.
b. hypercalcemia.
c. hypoparathyroidism.
d. hyperparathyroidism.

31. A patient presents to the ultrasound department for evaluation of the gallbladder. The patient complains of a recent onset of RUQ pain, nausea, and vomiting. The halo sign is visualized sonographically. What is the most likely diagnosis?

a. Acute cholecystitis
b. Chronic cholecystitis
c. Cholelithiasis
d. The patient has not been fasting

32. Which of the following indication may warrant a sonogram of the scrotum?

a. Trauma
b. Infertility
c. Scrotal enlargement
d. All of the above

33. Which of following vessels is NOT a branch of the celiac trunk?

a. Common hepatic artery
b. Right gastric artery
c. Left gastric artery
d. Splenic artery

34. A 17-year-old female presents for a viability sonogram. By her LMP, she should be 13 weeks and 4 days. The patient complains of hyperemesis, pelvic fullness, and bloating. The HCG levels are grossly elevated. Sonographically, a soft tissue-like mass fills the endometrial cavity. The mass appears heterogeneous, and is described as having a snowstorm appearance. What is the most likely diagnosis?

a. Choriocarcinoma
b. Invasive mole
c. Partial mole
d. Complete hydatidiform mole

35. Which of the following ligaments attaches the cornua of the uterus to the anterior pelvic wall?

a. Ovarian
b. Broad
c. Round
d. Cardinal

36. Which of the following best describes intrauterine insemination?

a. Embryos are developed outside of the body and are delivered into the uterus through a catheter
b. Embryos are developed outside of the body and are placed into the fallopian tube
c. Both parents' gametes are placed within the fallopian tube
d. The male gamete is inserted into the fundus of the uterus with a catheter

37. A didelphys and bicornuate uterus are congenital anomalies of the uterus that occur due to the:

a. failure of formation.
b. failure of fusion.
c. failure of dissolution.
d. failure of disappearance.

38. The normal evaluation of the genitourinary system includes evaluation of all of the following structures except the:

a. kidneys.
b. stomach.
c. bladder.
d. adrenal glands.

39. A patient is 18 weeks and 5 days pregnant. She presents to the ultrasound department for a fetal anomaly screening. The renal pelvis is seen and measured. What are the normal limits of the AP measurement of the renal pelvis at this age of pregnancy?

   a. Less than 2mm
   b. Less than or equal to 5 mm
   c. 5 to 10mm
   d. Greater than or equal to 10 mm

40. A fetus demonstrates frontal bossing of the cranium. The cerebellum is dislocated and there is obliteration of the cistern magna. What is a likely diagnosis?

   a. Spina bifida
   b. Anencephaly
   c. Iniencephaly
   d. Encephalocele

41. Sonographic evaluation of the fetal cranium demonstrates a large cystic space. The face is also evaluated and demonstrates proboscis and cyclopia. What is the most likely diagnosis?

   a. Hydranencephaly
   b. Porencephaly
   c. Hydrocephaly
   d. Holoprosencephaly

42. Which type of osteogenesis imperfecta is lethal?

   a. Type 1
   b. Type 2
   c. Type 3
   d. Type 4

43. All of the following are true regarding twin-to-twin transfusion syndrome except:

   a. it occurs with monozygotic/monochorionic twins.
   b. there is an artery-to-vein anastomosis that shunts blood away from the donor twin to the recipient twin.
   c. the donor twin measures large for dates.
   d. the recipient twin may demonstrate polyhydramnios.

44. All of the following may be typically visualized sonographically in a patient with gestational diabetes except:

   a. IUGR.
   b. macrosomia.
   c. a single umbilical artery.
   d. a thickened placenta.

45. Hematometra displays as which of the following?

   a. Pus in the uterus
   b. Water in the uterus
   c. Blood in the vagina
   d. Blood in the uterus

46. The umbilical cord is made up of:

    a.   one artery and two veins.

    b.   one artery and one vein.

    c.   two arteries and one vein.

    d.   two arteries and two veins.

47. Evaluation of the right ovary demonstrates sonographic evidence of a highly echogenic mass that displays shadowing and obscures the posterior wall of the mass. What is the most likely diagnosis?

    a.   Dermoid tumor

    b.   Dysgerminoma

    c.   Yolk sac tumor

    d.   Fibroma

48. A patient presents for a pelvic ultrasound. She complains of fever, lower abdominal pain, and vaginal discharge. Her labs indicate leukocytosis. What is a likely diagnosis?

    a.   Endometriosis

    b.   Pelvic congestion syndrome

    c.   Urinary tract infection

    d.   Pelvic inflammatory disease

49. All of the following are true regarding trisomy 21 except:

    a.   it is also known as Down syndrome.

    b.   it is also known as Edward's syndrome.

    c.   it may be present if the nuchal fold measures greater than 6mm between 15 to 21 weeks' gestation.

    d.   intellectual disability and abnormal physical characteristics may be present.

50. Fetal evaluation demonstrates macroglossia, gigantism, cardiac malformations, and placental enlargement. What is a likely diagnosis?

    a.   Pentalogy of Cantrell

    b.   Meckel-Gruber syndrome

    c.   Beckwith-Wiedemann syndrome

    d.   VATER association

Answer Key and Explanations

1. B: Gain is the term that identifies the degree of echo amplification or brightness of an image. Gain can be adjusted up or down to get the clearest image possible. Zoom allows magnification of an area, scatter refers to an unclear image of random sound waves, and absorption refers to the loss of the sound wave from the organ or area being scanned.

2. D: A linear array offers a rectangular image of an area. The vector format offers a trapezoidal image, a sector format offers a pie-shaped image, and the curved array provides a large-field image.

3. A: Pulsed Doppler is used to study the flow of blood through arteries and veins. It can also determine the pressure in those vessels. It is not used for solid organ diagnosis unrelated to blood flow or solid masses, unless the solid mass is obstructing the blood flow in a vessel. It is a valuable diagnostic tool in sonography.

4. D: Hertz is a unit of measurement used to measure a wave characteristic. Gain, color, and length are other characteristics or ways a sound wave is imaged.

5. B: The comet tail is an artifact, and the technician would know to redirect the transducer or change position or pressure to get a clear image.

6. C: In the presence of high fever with no source, an abdominal or pelvic ultrasound may be ordered to look for abscesses, enlarged lymph nodes, and inflammation, which can be a source of fever. The scan may also reveal tumors or masses that can be causing the body to react with fever.

7. A: Images can be stored, depending on the equipment, as gray scale images, colored images, or real-time imaging and video. Images can be displayed as numbers or images. The equipment type and capacity direct how a scan is archived.

8. B: The incident beam is the very first sound beam sent from the transducer. A transmitted beam is the beam that continues to travel. The reflected beam is the beam that returns to the transducer and helps to form the images.

9. C: The transducer is what contains the conductive material that converts electrical energy to sound energy and sound energy to electrical energy when received back to the transducer.

10. A: There is minimal adverse effect from an ultrasound exam, and that occurs from the heat generated by conducted energy. Neonates, more so than others, need to be protected from the possibility of heat injury, but heat injury should be considered when doing any exam.

11. D: The as low as reasonably achievable (ALARA) principle stresses the use of the lowest reasonable energy when obtaining the clearest image and minimal exposure to the patient. The principle also stresses that the FDA regulates the ultrasound instruments used because of the bioeffects of ultrasound and the effects on patient safety. Choices a, b, and c are not correct.

12. A: SATA is the spatial average-temporal average of a sound beam and is the lowest level of intensity. SPPA refers to spatial peak-pulse average and is measured during the time of the pulse. SATP refers to spatial average-temporal peak and is the average intensity of a beam at the highest point. SPTP is spatial peak-temporal peak and is the peak intensity of the beam in both space and time, being the highest intensity measurement for a sound beam.

13. C: It is important to identify the patient by name, explain the procedure clearly, protect privacy, select the proper equipment, and follow the ALARA principles for safety. The other choices are only partially correct.

14. A: A history of chemotherapy, ascites, hepatitis, AIDS, or a recent meal may alter the interpretation of the gallbladder ultrasound. The other choices are only partially correct or incorrect.

15. D: It is a common pitfall to confuse the bowel with a possible abscess. A full stomach or a completely empty stomach or a full bladder can assist in telling the difference between the bowel and an abscess, and often the patient is asked to drink water to fill the stomach after scanning with an empty stomach. The bladder is often also filled to help to determine the bowel from an abscess or other organs.

16. B: The right kidney axis is different in each person and can lead to misinterpretation of imaging of the abdomen. There are other tests that will be done to diagnose abdominal pathology along with the ultrasound, because the ultrasound alone can be inconclusive. Air, fluid, and tissue will affect the absorption and scatter of sound beams in the abdomen, making images false or unclear. The liver is not too fatty to be noted on an ultrasound exam.

17. D: Though a prepared sterile tray is necessary for a fine needle aspiration of the thyroid, it is not pertinent information. Reviewing prior images and reports, a script from the referring physician, and a signed consent form are all pertinent information that must be obtained prior to an invasive procedure such as an ultrasound-guided FNA of the thyroid.

18. D: The spermatic cord suspends the testicles in the scrotum. The vas deferens transports sperm to the urethra. The epididymis stores and excretes sperm. The seminiferous tubules produce sperm.

19. A: A fine needle aspiration (FNA) of the thyroid gland is a minimally-invasive procedure that involves the use of a very thin needle, usually an 18 to 25-gauge needle. The needle is guided directly into the nodule under ultrasound and is moved around within the nodule to shear off as many cells as possible. An FNA is the least invasive of the procedures listed, but warrants the poorest results. An excisional biopsy or a complete thyroidectomy are more invasive but allow the pathologist to examine the tissue makeup, which increases the chance of a definite diagnosis. A core biopsy also provides the pathologist with a larger sample of tissue. An FNA provides the pathologist with cells examined under cytology, whereas the other choices provide the pathologist with tissue samples examined under histology and increase the chance of diagnosis.

20. B: Torsion occurs when the spermatic cord becomes twisted, cutting off blood supply to the testicle. It occurs more commonly in adolescents than in adults and more often in the left testicle. The patient may present with scrotal pain, nausea, and vomiting. Sonographically, the testicle may appear enlarged with decreased echogenicity, a hydrocele may be present, and interrogation of the intratesticular vasculature may be absent with color and power Doppler evaluation. Torsion is considered a medical emergency and must be treated immediately to prevent complete infarction of the testicle. Orchitis is inflammation of the testes and presents as scrotal pain. Sonographically, orchitis may have a variable appearance ranging from hypoechoic with hyperemic vasculature under color and spectral Doppler evaluation to atrophic testes. Abscess may occur due to untreated orchitis. The patient may present with scrotal pain and swelling. An avascular, sonolucent, or complex mass may be seen on the sonogram. A hematocele most often occurs after trauma and causes blood to accumulate within the scrotum. It often mimics torsion and varies in sonographic appearances from sonolucent to complex with septations.

21. D: The main renal artery enters the renal hilum and branches into the segmental arteries. The segmental arteries then course through the renal pelvis region and branch into the interlobar arteries. These arteries course along the renal pyramids, pass over the base of the pyramids, and branch into the arcuate arteries. The arcuate arteries branch into the interlobular arteries.

22. A: Hypovolemic shock is caused by severe blood loss and may result in multiple organ failure. The patient may present with systemic symptoms of hypovolemic shock; therefore, it is not a sonographic appearance of the spleen. Left pleural effusion, splenomegaly, and a hematoma are pathologies that will be displayed sonographically.

23. D: The common bile duct, hepatic artery, and the main portal vein make up the portal triad. Sonographically, the "Mickey Mouse" sign may be visualized at the porta hepatis. The hepatic vein contains the right, left, and middle branches, which converge with the inferior vena cava. The common hepatic duct converges with the cystic duct to form the common bile duct. The hepatic duct and the hepatic vein are not part of the portal triad.

24. A: Twinkling artifact aids in the diagnosis of gallstones. When color Doppler is applied, a twinkle of color is visualized posterior to the stone where shadowing would be displayed. A hemangioma may show enhancement artifact. Portal hypertension and an abdominal aortic aneurysm will not display twinkling artifact.

25. B: Hepatoma (hepatocellular carcinoma) is the most common primary liver malignancy. Patients may present with hepatomegaly; and elevated levels of AST, ALT, and serum AFP. Focal nodular hyperplasia, cavernous hemangioma, and liver cell adenoma are all benign neoplasms of the liver. They may show similar signs and symptoms, or they may be asymptomatic.

26. C: Acute tubular necrosis is the most common cause of renal failure. Renal failure occurs due to ischemia, causing an increase in arteriole resistance. The echogenicity in the majority of cases does not change from its normal sonographic appearance.

27. D: The ureter inserts into the trigone posteriorly and inferiorly.

28. A: In the presence of acute pancreatitis, serum amylase and lipase increase at the same rate but lipase will stay elevated longer than amylase.

29. C: The duct of Wirsung is the main pancreatic duct that joins the common bile duct within the pancreatic head at the Ampulla of Vater where they dump into the second portion of the duodenum. The duct of Santorini is the accessory duct of the pancreas.

30. C: Hypophosphatemia, hypercalcemia, and hyperparathyroidism are all clinical indications that would warrant a sonogram to rule out a parathyroid adenoma.

31. A: Acute cholecystitis can be characterized by the halo sign sonographically. The halo sign describes a thick, edematous gallbladder wall. A non-fasting patient may also demonstrate a similar appearance, which is why it is important to take a good patient history. Chronic cholecystitis is visualized as a contracted gallbladder with thick, hyperechoic walls. Cholelithiasis is characterized as gallstones.

32. D: Ultrasound evaluation of the scrotum may be indicated for trauma, infertility, or scrotal enlargement.

33. B: The common hepatic artery branches off the celiac trunk and courses toward the porta hepatis. The left gastric artery branches off the celiac trunk and courses toward the stomach. It is not typically visualized sonographically. The splenic artery branches off the celiac trunk and courses toward the splenic hilum. This vessel tends to be tortuous. Only the right gastric artery is not part of the celiac trunk.

34. D: A complete hydatidiform mole is the most common type of gestational trophoblastic disease. A complete mole will demonstrate a heterogeneous mass filling the endometrium sonographically. Partial mole is associated with triploid. It transforms the placenta and causes severe IUGR. It is lethal to the pregnancy. Invasive mole will invade the myometrium. Choriocarcinoma is a highly metastatic tumor.

35. C: The round ligament attaches the cornua of the uterus to the anterior pelvic wall. It is located anterior and inferior to the broad ligaments and fallopian tubes. The ovarian ligament attaches the ovary to the uterine cornu. The broad ligament extends from the lateral aspect of the uterus to the lateral pelvic walls. The cardinal ligaments are the primary support of the uterus. They course superiorly and laterally from the uterus and arise inferiorly from the vagina.

36. D: IUI is best described as the male gamete being inserted into the fundus of the uterus with a catheter.

37. B: A didelphys and bicornuate uterus are congenital anomalies of the uterus that occur due to the failure of fusion.

38. B: The stomach is part of the gastrointestinal system. The kidneys, bladder, and adrenal glands are part of the genitourinary system. All structures should be evaluated sonographically.

39. B: The normal renal pelvis measurement for a fetus between 13- and 20-weeks gestational age is 5 mm.

40. A: Spina bifida occurs due to the lack of closure of the spinal vertebral column. Intracranial sonographic evaluation may demonstrate the lemon sign and the banana sign. Iniencephaly sonographically demonstrates as a hyperextended fetal head. Encephalocele appears sonographically where the brain tissue is herniated outside of the skull. Anencephaly sonographically demonstrates the absence of portions of the fetal cranium and intracranial structures.

41. D: Holoprosencephaly may demonstrate sonographically as a large midline cystic space. The face may display a proboscis and cyclopia. There are three types of holoprosencephaly which are alobar, semilobar, and lobar.

42. B: Osteogenesis imperfecta may result in fractured limbs, limb bowing, and bruising. Types 1 and 4 have the best prognosis. Type 2 is lethal.

43. C: When twin-to-twin transfusion syndrome is present, the donor twin will present as small for dates. Blood is shunted away from the donor twin to the recipient twin through an artery-to-vein anastomosis. The recipient twin may demonstrate polyhydramnios, but the donor twin may display severe oligohydramnios. This syndrome occurs with monozygotic/monochorionic twins.

44. A: IUGR may be seen sonographically in patients with gestational hypertension. Patients with gestational diabetes may demonstrate fetal macrosomia, a single umbilical artery, and a thickened placenta.

45. D: Hematometra is blood in the uterus. Pyometra is pus in the uterus. Hydrometra is water in the uterus. Hematocolpos is blood in the vagina.

46. C: The umbilical cord is made up of two arteries and one vein. The arteries carry deoxygenated blood away from the fetus and the vein carries oxygenated blood to the fetus.

47. A: Dermoids are the most common benign germ cell tumor. They may display the tip of the iceberg sign sonographically. They may cause ovarian torsion.

48. D: The patient with PID may complain of symptoms of infection. With the labs being positive for increased white blood cells, the most likely diagnosis is PID.

49. B: Edward's syndrome is known as trisomy 18. Down syndrome is trisomy 21. Patau's syndrome is trisomy 13.

50. C: Beckwith-Wiedemann syndrome is associated with macroglossia, gigantism, omphalocele, cardiac malformations, and placental enlargement. It may be known as an overgrowth syndrome. Children with this syndrome have a chance of developing a cancerous tumor known as Wilms' tumor. They are also at risk for the development of liver cancer known as hepatoblastoma. Pentalogy of Cantrell is associated with an omphalocele and ectopic cordis. Meckel-Gruber syndrome is associated with encephalocele, polycystic kidneys, cleft lip, and polydactyly. VATER association or VACTERL stands for vertebral anomalies, anal atresia, cardiac anomalies, tracheoesophageal atresia, renal anomalies, and limb anomalies.

How to Overcome Test Anxiety

Just the thought of taking a test is enough to make most people a little nervous. A test is an important event that can have a long-term impact on your future, so it's important to take it seriously and it's natural to feel anxious about performing well. But just because anxiety is normal, that doesn't mean that it's helpful in test taking, or that you should simply accept it as part of your life. Anxiety can have a variety of effects. These effects can be mild, like making you feel slightly nervous, or severe, like blocking your ability to focus or remember even a simple detail.

If you experience test anxiety—whether severe or mild—it's important to know how to beat it. To discover this, first you need to understand what causes test anxiety.

Causes of Test Anxiety

While we often think of anxiety as an uncontrollable emotional state, it can actually be caused by simple, practical things. One of the most common causes of test anxiety is that a person does not feel adequately prepared for their test. This feeling can be the result of many different issues such as poor study habits or lack of organization, but the most common culprit is time management. Starting to study too late, failing to organize your study time to cover all of the material, or being distracted while you study will mean that you're not well prepared for the test. This may lead to cramming the night before, which will cause you to be physically and mentally exhausted for the test. Poor time management also contributes to feelings of stress, fear, and hopelessness as you realize you are not well prepared but don't know what to do about it.

Other times, test anxiety is not related to your preparation for the test but comes from unresolved fear. This may be a past failure on a test, or poor performance on tests in general. It may come from comparing yourself to others who seem to be performing better or from the stress of living up to expectations. Anxiety may be driven by fears of the future—how failure on this test would affect your educational and career goals. These fears are often completely irrational, but they can still negatively impact your test performance.

Elements of Test Anxiety

As mentioned earlier, test anxiety is considered to be an emotional state, but it has physical and mental components as well. Sometimes you may not even realize that you are suffering from test anxiety until you notice the physical symptoms. These can include trembling hands, rapid heartbeat, sweating, nausea, and tense muscles. Extreme anxiety may lead to fainting or vomiting. Obviously, any of these symptoms can have a negative impact on testing. It is important to recognize them as soon as they begin to occur so that you can address the problem before it damages your performance.

The mental components of test anxiety include trouble focusing and inability to remember learned information. During a test, your mind is on high alert, which can help you recall information and stay focused for an extended period of time. However, anxiety interferes with your mind's natural processes, causing you to blank out, even on the questions you know well. The strain of testing during anxiety makes it difficult to stay focused, especially on a test that may take several hours. Extreme anxiety can take a huge mental toll, making it difficult not only to recall test information but even to understand the test questions or pull your thoughts together.

Effects of Test Anxiety

Test anxiety is like a disease—if left untreated, it will get progressively worse. Anxiety leads to poor performance, and this reinforces the feelings of fear and failure, which in turn lead to poor performances on subsequent tests. It can grow from a mild nervousness to a crippling condition. If allowed to progress, test anxiety can have a big impact on your schooling, and consequently on your future.

Test anxiety can spread to other parts of your life. Anxiety on tests can become anxiety in any stressful situation, and blanking on a test can turn into panicking in a job situation. But fortunately, you don't have to let anxiety rule your testing and determine your grades. There are a number of relatively simple steps you can take to move past anxiety and function normally on a test and in the rest of life.

Physical Steps for Beating Test Anxiety

While test anxiety is a serious problem, the good news is that it can be overcome. It doesn't have to control your ability to think and remember information. While it may take time, you can begin taking steps today to beat anxiety.

Just as your first hint that you may be struggling with anxiety comes from the physical symptoms, the first step to treating it is also physical. Rest is crucial for having a clear, strong mind. If you are tired, it is much easier to give in to anxiety. But if you establish good sleep habits, your body and mind will be ready to perform optimally, without the strain of exhaustion. Additionally, sleeping well helps you to retain information better, so you're more likely to recall the answers when you see the test questions.

Getting good sleep means more than going to bed on time. It's important to allow your brain time to relax. Take study breaks from time to time so it doesn't get overworked, and don't study right before bed. Take time to rest your mind before trying to rest your body, or you may find it difficult to fall asleep.

Along with sleep, other aspects of physical health are important in preparing for a test. Good nutrition is vital for good brain function. Sugary foods and drinks may give a burst of energy but this burst is followed by a crash, both physically and emotionally. Instead, fuel your body with protein and vitamin-rich foods.

Also, drink plenty of water. Dehydration can lead to headaches and exhaustion, especially if your brain is already under stress from the rigors of the test. Particularly if your test is a long one, drink water during the breaks. And if possible, take an energy-boosting snack to eat between sections.

Along with sleep and diet, a third important part of physical health is exercise. Maintaining a steady workout schedule is helpful, but even taking 5-minute study breaks to walk can help get your blood pumping faster and clear your head. Exercise also releases endorphins, which contribute to a positive feeling and can help combat test anxiety.

When you nurture your physical health, you are also contributing to your mental health. If your body is healthy, your mind is much more likely to be healthy as well. So take time to rest, nourish your body with healthy food and water, and get moving as much as possible. Taking these physical steps will make you stronger and more able to take the mental steps necessary to overcome test anxiety.

Mental Steps for Beating Test Anxiety

Working on the mental side of test anxiety can be more challenging, but as with the physical side, there are clear steps you can take to overcome it. As mentioned earlier, test anxiety often stems from lack of preparation, so the obvious solution is to prepare for the test. Effective studying may be the most important weapon you have for beating test anxiety, but you can and should employ several other mental tools to combat fear.

First, boost your confidence by reminding yourself of past success—tests or projects that you aced. If you're putting as much effort into preparing for this test as you did for those, there's no reason you should expect to fail here. Work hard to prepare; then trust your preparation.

Second, surround yourself with encouraging people. It can be helpful to find a study group, but be sure that the people you're around will encourage a positive attitude. If you spend time with others who are anxious or cynical, this will only contribute to your own anxiety. Look for others who are motivated to study hard from a desire to succeed, not from a fear of failure.

Third, reward yourself. A test is physically and mentally tiring, even without anxiety, and it can be helpful to have something to look forward to. Plan an activity following the test, regardless of the outcome, such as going to a movie or getting ice cream.

When you are taking the test, if you find yourself beginning to feel anxious, remind yourself that you know the material. Visualize successfully completing the test. Then take a few deep, relaxing breaths and return to it. Work through the questions carefully but with confidence, knowing that you are capable of succeeding.

Developing a healthy mental approach to test taking will also aid in other areas of life. Test anxiety affects more than just the actual test—it can be damaging to your mental health and even contribute to depression. It's important to beat test anxiety before it becomes a problem for more than testing.

Study Strategy

Being prepared for the test is necessary to combat anxiety, but what does being prepared look like? You may study for hours on end and still not feel prepared. What you need is a strategy for test prep. The next few pages outline our recommended steps to help you plan out and conquer the challenge of preparation.

STEP 1: SCOPE OUT THE TEST

Learn everything you can about the format (multiple choice, essay, etc.) and what will be on the test. Gather any study materials, course outlines, or sample exams that may be available. Not only will this help you to prepare, but knowing what to expect can help to alleviate test anxiety.

STEP 2: MAP OUT THE MATERIAL

Look through the textbook or study guide and make note of how many chapters or sections it has. Then divide these over the time you have. For example, if a book has 15 chapters and you have five days to study, you need to cover three chapters each day. Even better, if you have the time, leave an extra day at the end for overall review after you have gone through the material in depth.

If time is limited, you may need to prioritize the material. Look through it and make note of which sections you think you already have a good grasp on, and which need review. While you are studying, skim quickly through the familiar sections and take more time on the challenging parts.

242

Write out your plan so you don't get lost as you go. Having a written plan also helps you feel more in control of the study, so anxiety is less likely to arise from feeling overwhelmed at the amount to cover.

STEP 3: GATHER YOUR TOOLS

Decide what study method works best for you. Do you prefer to highlight in the book as you study and then go back over the highlighted portions? Or do you type out notes of the important information? Or is it helpful to make flashcards that you can carry with you? Assemble the pens, index cards, highlighters, post-it notes, and any other materials you may need so you won't be distracted by getting up to find things while you study.

If you're having a hard time retaining the information or organizing your notes, experiment with different methods. For example, try color-coding by subject with colored pens, highlighters, or post-it notes. If you learn better by hearing, try recording yourself reading your notes so you can listen while in the car, working out, or simply sitting at your desk. Ask a friend to quiz you from your flashcards, or try teaching someone the material to solidify it in your mind.

STEP 4: CREATE YOUR ENVIRONMENT

It's important to avoid distractions while you study. This includes both the obvious distractions like visitors and the subtle distractions like an uncomfortable chair (or a too-comfortable couch that makes you want to fall asleep). Set up the best study environment possible: good lighting and a comfortable work area. If background music helps you focus, you may want to turn it on, but otherwise keep the room quiet. If you are using a computer to take notes, be sure you don't have any other windows open, especially applications like social media, games, or anything else that could distract you. Silence your phone and turn off notifications. Be sure to keep water close by so you stay hydrated while you study (but avoid unhealthy drinks and snacks).

Also, take into account the best time of day to study. Are you freshest first thing in the morning? Try to set aside some time then to work through the material. Is your mind clearer in the afternoon or evening? Schedule your study session then. Another method is to study at the same time of day that you will take the test, so that your brain gets used to working on the material at that time and will be ready to focus at test time.

STEP 5: STUDY!

Once you have done all the study preparation, it's time to settle into the actual studying. Sit down, take a few moments to settle your mind so you can focus, and begin to follow your study plan. Don't give in to distractions or let yourself procrastinate. This is your time to prepare so you'll be ready to fearlessly approach the test. Make the most of the time and stay focused.

Of course, you don't want to burn out. If you study too long you may find that you're not retaining the information very well. Take regular study breaks. For example, taking five minutes out of every hour to walk briskly, breathing deeply and swinging your arms, can help your mind stay fresh.

As you get to the end of each chapter or section, it's a good idea to do a quick review. Remind yourself of what you learned and work on any difficult parts. When you feel that you've mastered the material, move on to the next part. At the end of your study session, briefly skim through your notes again.

But while review is helpful, cramming last minute is NOT. If at all possible, work ahead so that you won't need to fit all your study into the last day. Cramming overloads your brain with more information than it can process and retain, and your tired mind may struggle to recall even previously learned information when it is overwhelmed with last-minute study. Also, the urgent nature of cramming and the stress placed on your brain contribute to anxiety. You'll be more likely to go to the test feeling unprepared and having trouble thinking clearly.

So don't cram, and don't stay up late before the test, even just to review your notes at a leisurely pace. Your brain needs rest more than it needs to go over the information again. In fact, plan to finish your studies by noon or early afternoon the day before the test. Give your brain the rest of the day to relax or focus on other things, and get a good night's sleep. Then you will be fresh for the test and better able to recall what you've studied.

STEP 6: TAKE A PRACTICE TEST

Many courses offer sample tests, either online or in the study materials. This is an excellent resource to check whether you have mastered the material, as well as to prepare for the test format and environment.

Check the test format ahead of time: the number of questions, the type (multiple choice, free response, etc.), and the time limit. Then create a plan for working through them. For example, if you have 30 minutes to take a 60-question test, your limit is 30 seconds per question. Spend less time on the questions you know well so that you can take more time on the difficult ones.

If you have time to take several practice tests, take the first one open book, with no time limit. Work through the questions at your own pace and make sure you fully understand them. Gradually work up to taking a test under test conditions: sit at a desk with all study materials put away and set a timer. Pace yourself to make sure you finish the test with time to spare and go back to check your answers if you have time.

After each test, check your answers. On the questions you missed, be sure you understand why you missed them. Did you misread the question (tests can use tricky wording)? Did you forget the information? Or was it something you hadn't learned? Go back and study any shaky areas that the practice tests reveal.

Taking these tests not only helps with your grade, but also aids in combating test anxiety. If you're already used to the test conditions, you're less likely to worry about it, and working through tests until you're scoring well gives you a confidence boost. Go through the practice tests until you feel comfortable, and then you can go into the test knowing that you're ready for it.

Test Tips

On test day, you should be confident, knowing that you've prepared well and are ready to answer the questions. But aside from preparation, there are several test day strategies you can employ to maximize your performance.

First, as stated before, get a good night's sleep the night before the test (and for several nights before that, if possible). Go into the test with a fresh, alert mind rather than staying up late to study.

Try not to change too much about your normal routine on the day of the test. It's important to eat a nutritious breakfast, but if you normally don't eat breakfast at all, consider eating just a protein bar. If you're a coffee drinker, go ahead and have your normal coffee. Just make sure you time it so that the caffeine doesn't wear off right in the middle of your test. Avoid sugary beverages, and drink enough water to stay hydrated but not so much that you need a restroom break 10 minutes into the test. If your test isn't first thing in the morning, consider going for a walk or doing a light workout before the test to get your blood flowing.

Allow yourself enough time to get ready, and leave for the test with plenty of time to spare so you won't have the anxiety of scrambling to arrive in time. Another reason to be early is to select a good seat. It's helpful to sit away from doors and windows, which can be distracting. Find a good seat, get out your supplies, and settle your mind before the test begins.

When the test begins, start by going over the instructions carefully, even if you already know what to expect. Make sure you avoid any careless mistakes by following the directions.

Then begin working through the questions, pacing yourself as you've practiced. If you're not sure on an answer, don't spend too much time on it, and don't let it shake your confidence. Either skip it and come back later, or eliminate as many wrong answers as possible and guess among the remaining ones. Don't dwell on these questions as you continue—put them out of your mind and focus on what lies ahead.

Be sure to read all of the answer choices, even if you're sure the first one is the right answer. Sometimes you'll find a better one if you keep reading. But don't second-guess yourself if you do immediately know the answer. Your gut instinct is usually right. Don't let test anxiety rob you of the information you know.

If you have time at the end of the test (and if the test format allows), go back and review your answers. Be cautious about changing any, since your first instinct tends to be correct, but make sure you didn't misread any of the questions or accidentally mark the wrong answer choice. Look over any you skipped and make an educated guess.

At the end, leave the test feeling confident. You've done your best, so don't waste time worrying about your performance or wishing you could change anything. Instead, celebrate the successful completion of this test. And finally, use this test to learn how to deal with anxiety even better next time.

> **Review Video: Test Anxiety**
> Visit mometrix.com/academy and enter code: 100340

Important Qualification

Not all anxiety is created equal. If your test anxiety is causing major issues in your life beyond the classroom or testing center, or if you are experiencing troubling physical symptoms related to your anxiety, it may be a sign of a serious physiological or psychological condition. If this sounds like your situation, we strongly encourage you to seek professional help.

Online Resources

Due to our efforts to try to keep this book to a manageable length, we've created a link that will give you access to all of your online resources:

mometrix.com/resources719/sonography

It's Your Moment, Let's Celebrate It!

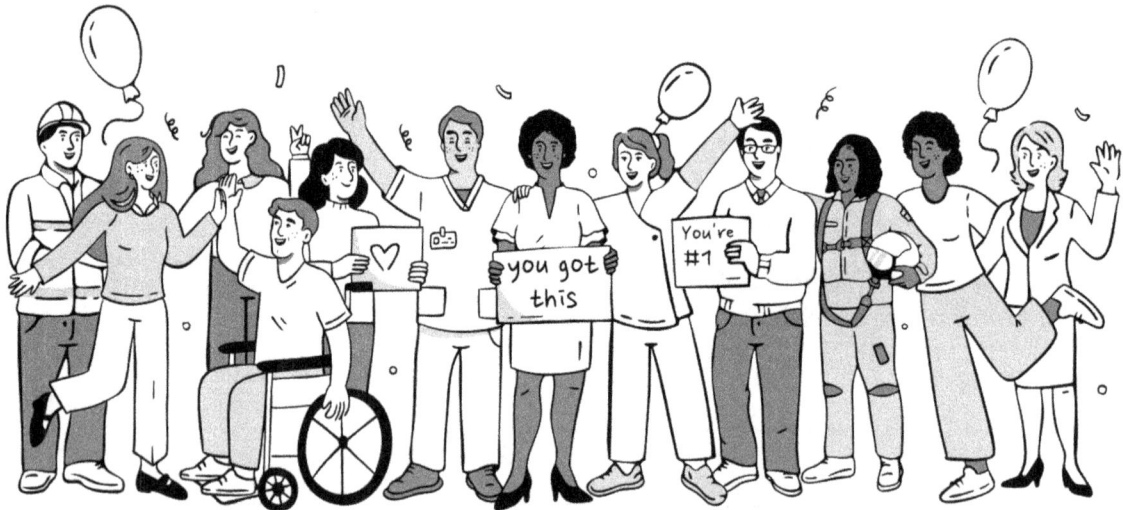

Share your story @mometrixtestpreparation